Diagnostic Parasitology for Veterinary Technicians

Fifth Edition

Diagnostic Parasitology for Veterinary Technicians

Fifth Edition

Charles M. Hendrix, DVM, PhD
Professor
Department of Pathobiology
College of Veterinary Medicine
Auburn University
Alabama

Ed Robinson, CVT
Shakespeare Veterinary Hospital
Veterinary Technology Program Instructor
Penn Foster Career Schools
Member of the American Heartworm Society
Fairfield, Connecticut

ELSEVIER

ELSEVIER

3251 Riverport Lane
St. Louis, Missouri 63043

Library of Congress Cataloging-in-Publication Data

ISBN: 978-0-323-38982-2

Content Strategist: Brandi Graham
Content Development Manager: Ellen Wurm-Cutter
Content Development Specialist: Katie Gutierrez
Publishing Services Manager: Hemamalini Rajendrababu
Project Manager: Radhika Sivalingam
Design Direction: Brian Salisbury

Printed in United States of America.

Last digit is the print number: 9 8 7 6 5

Working together
to grow libraries in
developing countries

www.elsevier.com • www.bookaid.org

In previous editions of this veterinary parasitology textbook, I sang the praises of my wife, Rebecca, my daughter, Charlotte, and my mentor in veterinary parasitology, Dr. John C. Schlotthauer. These loved ones provided a lot of love and support along my academic journey of over 40 years. I continue to be surrounded by their love.

For this present edition, I want to dedicate my textbook to the individuals who made my career so enjoyable over the last 35 years—the extremely dedicated and talented veterinary students at Auburn University's College of Veterinary Medicine. Their love for and dedication to the veterinary profession were a true inspiration to me. Without them, this endeavor would not have been possible. This current edition is dedicated to them.

CMH

To Thomas A. Milos, DVM, who taught me that the greatest thing about veterinary parasitology is helping others learn about the field.

ER

Veterinary clinical parasitology is one of the most important disciplines in any veterinary curriculum, be it a curriculum that trains veterinary students or one that trains veterinary technicians.

ORGANIZATION

This new edition was prepared to follow the educational structure used in parasitology classes in veterinary technology education. Our textbook is intended to inform the reader of the most commonly encountered internal and external parasites of both domesticated and laboratory animals. The text begins with a chapter detailing the language of parasitology, the many terms that describe the intricate host-parasite relationships of veterinary parasitology. These terms are the "framework" of the discipline, the means of communication among veterinarians, veterinary technicians, and their clients. Every veterinary practitioner, veterinarian, veterinary technician, and student must learn to effectively communicate in this language. Each succeeding chapter describes a different parasite group: protozoans (one-celled organisms), trematodes (flukes), cestodes (tapeworms), nematodes (roundworms), acanthocephalans (thorny-headed worms), arthropods (insects, mites, and ticks), hirudineans (leeches), and pentastomes (tongue worms). As with the last edition, each of these parasite groups is described in detail, with special emphasis placed on morphology, uniqueness of the life cycle, and important parasites within the group.

NEW TO THIS EDITION

Information on the parasites has been updated, and new information has been added to better prepare the technician for the parasites currently seen in veterinary practice. A brief synopsis of each parasite is given before the in-depth discussion. This synopsis includes the parasite genus, species, host (including other hosts the parasite may affect), location of the adult in the host, distribution (where available), derivation of the genus, transmission route, common name (where applicable), and zoonotic potential. Where applicable, reference to the organization determining the zoonotic potential (if in question) is provided. Treatments and preventive measures have been added to the sections on the major parasites seen in veterinary medicine. A chapter with a quick reference to the most common parasites has been provided, containing pictures of the most common parasite ova seen in diagnostic tests. We have also made a major improvement to this edition by replacing black-and-white photographs with color photographs. We have endeavored to use as many color photographs as possible to assist in the demonstration of key morphologic and diagnostic features needed for proper identification of all classes of parasites. Case studies have been added throughout the book to provide students with a chance to apply what they have learned. The end-of-chapter matching exercises have been reformatted so they are more user-friendly and reinforce student learning.

This latest edition of *Diagnostic Veterinary Parasitology* was prepared with the veterinary technician in mind. Parasitology is a large part of the technician's job in any veterinary clinic. Veterinary technicians are responsible for collecting, preparing, and examining fecal tests. In addition, the veterinary technician is responsible for client education in general and parasite education in particular. The information contained within this text will help veterinary technicians become familiar with the parasites seen in veterinary medicine. This includes case presentations and how the client was educated on the parasite in each case.

EVOLVE RESOURCES

New Case Questions have been created to accompany many of the pictures found throughout the text. The Case Questions will assist the student of parasitology in further learning the course material by using pictures of the parasites in different forms to answer the questions.

New Compare and Contrast Charts have been added to the Evolve Resources. These charts can be filled in and used to study the different major parasites. They list similarities as well as differences between the chosen parasites.

Listen and Spell Exercises have been added, instructing students to spell the pronounced word correctly.

The flash cards contain 10 categories that address/provide scientific name, common name, derivation of the name, audio pronunciation, type of parasite, adult morphology, immature stage morphology, location, clinical signs, infection route, diagnostic test, zoonosis, human disease, and a unique fact.

The flash cards will help the student of parasitology learn the important facts about each parasite in fun and interactive ways. They are an exciting new addition to this text that will help make learning and teaching parasitology fun.

Charles M. Hendrix
Ed Robinson

Contents

Parasites by Host Species

PARASITE	HOST	LOCATION OF ADULT	DISTRIBUTION	COMMON NAME	PAGE
CANINES AND FELINES					
Nematodes					
Gastrointestinal Tract					
Spirocerca lupi	Dogs and cats	Esophageal wall	Tropical and subtropical regions	Esophageal worm of dogs and cats	25
Physaloptera sp.	Dogs and cats	Lumen of stomach and small intestine	Worldwide	Stomach worm of dogs and cats	26
Aonchotheca putorii	Cats	Small intestine		Gastric capillarid of cats	27
Ollulanus tricuspis	Cats	Stomach		Feline trichostrongyle	27
Toxocara canis	Dogs	Small intestine	Worldwide	Canine roundworm	28
Toxocara cati	Cats	Small intestine	Worldwide	Feline roundworm	28
Toxascaris leonina	Dogs and cats	Small intestine	Worldwide	Roundworm of dogs and cats	28
Baylisascaris procyonis	Raccoons, dogs, cats, and other species	Small intestine	North America	Roundworm of raccoons	29
Ancylostoma caninum	Dogs	Small intestine	Worldwide	Canine hookworm	31
Ancylostoma tubaeforme	Cats	Small intestine	Worldwide	Feline hookworm	31
Ancylostoma braziliense	Dogs and cats	Small intestine	Worldwide	Hookworm of dogs and cats	31
Uncinaria stenocephala	Dogs	Small intestine	Northern regions of North America	Canine hookworm	31
Strongyloides stercoralis	Dogs, cats, and humans	Small intestine	Worldwide	Canine intestinal threadworm	34
Strongyloides tumefaciens	Dogs and cats	Small intestine	Worldwide	Canine intestinal threadworm	34

Continued

Parasites by Host Species—cont'd

PARASITE	HOST	LOCATION OF ADULT	DISTRIBUTION	COMMON NAME	PAGE
Trichuris vulpis	Dogs	Cecum and colon	Worldwide	Canine whipworm	35
Trichuris campanula	Cats	Cecum and colon	Worldwide but rare in North America	Feline whipworm	35
Trichuris serrata	Cats	Cecum and colon	Worldwide but rare in North America	Feline whipworm	35
Circulatory System					
Dirofilaria immitis	Dogs, cats, and humans	Right ventricle and pulmonary artery	Warm to temperate climates	Heartworm	38
Respiratory System					
Aelurostrongylus abstrusus	Cats	Bronchioles and alveolar ducts	Worldwide	Feline lungworm	44
Filaroides osleri	Dogs	Trachea	North America, Europe, and Japan	Canine lungworm	44
Filaroides hirthi	Dogs	Lung parenchyma	North America, Europe, and Japan	Canine lungworm	44
Filaroides milksi	Dogs	Bronchioles	North America, Europe, and Japan	Canine lungworm	44
Eucoleus aerophilus	Dogs and cats	Bronchi and trachea		Capillarid lungworm of dogs and cats	45
Eucoleus böehmi	Dogs	Nasal cavity and frontal sinuses		Capillarid respiratory worm of dogs	45
Urinary Tract					
Dioctophyma renale	Dogs	Right kidney	North America and Europe	Giant kidney worm of dogs	46
Capillaria plica	Dogs	Urinary bladder		Bladder worm of dogs	47
Capillaria feliscati	Cats	Urinary bladder		Bladder worm of cats	47
Skin					
Rhabditis strongyloides	Dogs	Superficial layers of the skin			47

Parasites by Host Species—cont'd

PARASITE	HOST	LOCATION OF ADULT	DISTRIBUTION	COMMON NAME	PAGE
Acanthocheilonema reconditum	Dogs	Subcutaneous tissues	Tropical and subtropical regions	Canine subcutaneous filarial worm	48
Dracunculus insignis	Dogs	Subcutaneous tissues		Guinea worm	49

Eye and Adnexa

Thelazia californiensis	Dogs and cats	Conjunctival sac and lacrimal duct	North America	Eyeworm of dogs and cats	50

Cestodes

Gastrointestinal Tract

Dipylidium caninum	Dogs and cats	Small intestine	Worldwide	Cucumber seed tapeworm or double-pored tapeworm	104
Taenia pisiformis	Dogs	Small intestine		Canine taeniid	106
Taenia hydatigena	Dogs	Small intestine		Canine taeniid	106
Taenia ovis	Dogs	Small intestine		Mutton tapeworm of dogs	106
Taenia taeniaeformis	Cats	Small intestine		Feline taeniid	110
Multiceps serialis	Dogs	Small intestine		Coenurus-producing tapeworm	112
Echinococcus granulosus	Dogs	Small intestine	Worldwide	Unilocular hydatid tapeworm	113
Echinococcus multilocularis	Cats	Small intestine	Countries in the Northern Hemisphere	Multilocular hydatid tapeworm	113
Mesocestoides sp.	Dogs, cats, and carnivores	Small intestine	North America, Asia, Europe, and Africa	Tetrathyridium tapeworm	115
Spirometra sp.	Dogs and cats	Small intestine	North America, South America, Far East, and Australia	Zipper tapeworm	119
Taenia multiceps	Dogs	Small intestine	Worldwide	Coenurus-producing tapeworm	112
Diphyllobothrium latum	Dogs, cats, and humans	Small intestine	North America, Scandinavian countries, and Ukraine	Broad fish tapeworm	120

Continued

Parasites by Host Species—cont'd

PARASITE	HOST	LOCATION OF ADULT	DISTRIBUTION	COMMON NAME	PAGE
Trematodes					
Platynosomum fastosum	Cats	Bile ducts	South America, southern United States, West Africa, Pacific Islands, Malaysia, and the Caribbean	"Lizard-poisoning fluke" of cats	134
Nanophyetus salmincola	Dogs	Small intestine	Pacific Northwest region of North America	"Salmon-poisoning fluke" of dogs	134
Alaria sp.	Dogs and cats	Small intestine	Northern United States and Canada	Intestinal fluke of dogs and cats	135
Paragonimus kellicotti	Dogs and cats	Lung parenchyma	North America	Lung fluke of dogs and cats	136
Heterobilharzia americana	Dogs	Mesenteric veins of small and large intestines and portal veins	North America	Schistosome of dogs	137
Protozoans					
Gastrointestinal Tract					
Flagellates					
Giardia sp.	Dogs, cats, horses, humans, exotic species	Intestinal mucosa	Worldwide	*Giardia*	154
Amoebae					
Entamoeba histolytica	Dogs, cats, primates, and humans	Large intestine	Worldwide	*Entamoeba*	156
Ciliates					
Balantidium coli	Dogs and pigs	Cecum and colon	Worldwide	*Balantidium*	157
Apicomplexans					
Cystoisospora sp.	Dogs, cats, and pigs	Small intestine		Coccidia	157
Toxoplasma gondii	Cats	Intestines	Worldwide	*Toxoplasma*	159
Cryptosporidium sp.	Dogs, cats, cattle, pigs, birds, guinea pigs, snakes, and mice	Small intestine		Cryptosporidia	160
Sarcocystis sp.	Dogs and cats	Small intestine	Worldwide	*Sarcocystis*	164

Parasites by Host Species—cont'd

PARASITE	HOST	LOCATION OF ADULT	DISTRIBUTION	COMMON NAME	PAGE
Circulatory System					
Flagellates					
Trypanosoma cruzi	Dogs and humans	Peripheral blood	Central and South America and southern United States	Trypanosomes	164
Leishmania sp.	Dogs	Reticuloendothelial cells of capillaries, spleen, and white blood cells (WBCs)	Worldwide	Leishmania	165
Apicomplexans					
Babesia canis	Dogs	Within red blood cells (RBCs)	Europe, Africa, Asia, North and South America	Babesia	165
Cytauxzoon felis	Cats	Within RBCs	Africa and United States		166
Hepatozoon canis	Dogs	Gamonts in WBCs; schizonts in spleen, bone marrow, and liver	United States, Africa, Asia, and southern Europe		166
Pentastomes					
Linguatula serrata	Dogs	Nasal passages and sinuses		Canine pentastome	269
Arthropods					
True Bugs					
Reduviid bugs	Dogs and humans	Periodic skin parasite		Kissing bugs	198
Rhodnius sp.	Dogs, humans, cats, guinea pigs, armadillos, rats, raccoons, and monkeys	Periodic skin of mouth and lips	South and Central America, southern and western United States	Kissing bugs	200
Panstrongylus sp.	Dogs, humans, cats, guinea pigs, armadillos, rats, raccoons, and monkeys	Periodic skin of mouth and lips	South and Central America, southern and western United States	Kissing bugs	200

Continued

Parasites by Host Species—cont'd

PARASITE	HOST	LOCATION OF ADULT	DISTRIBUTION	COMMON NAME	PAGE
Triatoma sp.	Dogs, humans, cats, guinea pigs, armadillos, rats, raccoons, and monkeys	Periodic skin of mouth and lips	South and Central America, southern and western United States	Kissing bugs	200
Lice					
Mallophagan order	Mammals and birds	Among hairs of host		Chewing lice	200
Anopluran order	Mammals and birds	Among hairs of host		Sucking lice	201
Dipterans					
Simulium sp.	Domesticated animals, poultry, and humans	Skin surface when feeding	Worldwide	Black flies or buffalo gnats	209
Lutzomyia sp.	Mammals, reptiles, avians, and humans	Skin surface when feeding	Worldwide	New World sand flies	209
Phlebotomus sp.	Mammals, reptiles, avians, and humans	Skin surface when feeding	Subtropical and Mediterranean regions	Sand flies	209
Culicoides sp.	Domestic animals and humans	Skin surface when feeding	Worldwide	No-see-ums, punkies, or sand flies	209
Anopheles quadrimaculatus	Mammals, reptiles, avians, and humans	Skin surface when feeding	Worldwide	Malaria mosquito	210
Aedes aegypti	Mammals, reptiles, avians, and humans	Skin surface when feeding	Worldwide	Yellow fever mosquito	210
Culex sp.	Mammals, reptiles, avians, and humans	Skin surface when feeding	Worldwide	Mosquito	210
Chrysops sp.	Large mammals, humans, and occasionally small mammals and birds	Skin surface when feeding	Worldwide	Deerflies	211
Tabanus sp.	Large mammals, humans, and occasionally small mammals and birds	Skin surface when feeding	Worldwide	Horseflies	211

Parasites by Host Species—cont'd

PARASITE	HOST	LOCATION OF ADULT	DISTRIBUTION	COMMON NAME	PAGE
Glossina sp.	Mammals, reptiles, birds, and humans	Skin surface when feeding	Africa	Tsetse fly	212
Musca domestica	Variety of animals and humans	Within the house	Worldwide	Housefly	216
Calliphora sp.	Domestic animals, wild animals, and humans	Free living in environment		Bottle flies or blowflies	218
Lucilia sp.	Domestic animals, wild animals, and humans	Free living in environment		Bottle flies or blowflies	218
Phormia sp.	Domestic animals, wild animals, and humans	Free living in environment		Bottle flies or blowflies	218
Phaenicia sp.	Domestic animals, wild animals, and humans	Free living in environment		Bottle flies or blowflies	218
Sarcophaga sp.	Domestic animals, wild animals, and humans	Free living in environment		Flesh fly	219
Hippelates sp.	Dogs and cattle	Mucocutaneous junction of eyes, lips, and penis		Dog penis gnats	219
Cochliomyia hominivorax	Domestic animals	Fresh, uncontaminated wounds	North America	Screw fly	221
Cuterebra sp.	Rabbits, squirrels, mice, rats, chipmunks, dogs, and cats	Larva around the head and neck		Warbles or wolves	222
Siphonaptera					
Ctenocephalides felis	Dogs and cats	Skin surface		Cat flea	226
Ctenocephalides canis	Dogs	Skin surface		Dog flea	226
Mites					
Sarcoptes scabiei variety canis	Dogs	Superficial layers of epidermis	Worldwide	Scabies mite of dogs	232
Sarcoptes scabiei variety felis	Cats	Superficial layers of epidermis	Worldwide	Scabies mite of cats	233
Notoedres cati	Cats and rabbits	Superficial layers of epidermis	Worldwide	Notoedric mange mite	234
Otodectes cynotis	Dogs, cats, and ferrets	External ear canal	Worldwide	Ear mites	240

Continued

Parasites by Host Species—cont'd

PARASITE	HOST	LOCATION OF ADULT	DISTRIBUTION	COMMON NAME	PAGE
Demodex canis	Dogs	Hair follicles and sebaceous glands	Worldwide	Demodectic mange mite of dogs	242
Demodex cati	Cats	Hair follicles and sebaceous glands	Worldwide	Demodectic mange mite of cats	242
Trombicula sp.	Domestic animals, wild animals, and humans	Larval stage on skin surface		Chiggers	244
Pneumonyssus caninum	Dogs	Nasal turbinates and nasal sinuses	Worldwide	Nasal mites	245
Cheyletiella parasitivorax	Dogs, cats, and rabbits	Surface of skin and hair coat	Worldwide	Walking dandruff	246
Lynxacarus radovskyi	Cats	Hair shafts on back, neck, thorax, and hind limbs	Tropical and warm regions of United States, Puerto Rico, Australia, and Fiji	Feline fur mite	248

Ticks

Otobius megnini	Dogs, horses, cattle, sheep, and goats	Larval and nymphal stages in the external ear canal	Arid and semiarid regions in southwestern United States	Spinose ear tick	255
Ixodes scapularis	Adult on dogs, horses, deer, and humans	Attached to skin when feeding	Eastern United States	Deer tick	257
Rhipicephalus sanguineus	Small mammals, dogs, and humans	Below hair coat attached to skin, especially ear canal and between toes	North America	Brown dog tick	257
Dermacentor variabilis	Small mammals, dogs, and humans	Attached to skin when feeding	Eastern two thirds of United States	Wood tick or American dog tick	258
Dermacentor andersoni	Adult on dogs, horses, cattle, goats, sheep, and humans	Attached to skin when feeding	Rocky Mountain regions	Rocky Mountain wood tick	259
Dermacentor occidentalis	Adult on large mammals	Attached to skin when feeding	Sierra Nevada Mountains	Pacific Coast dog tick	259
Amblyomma americanum	Adult on wide range of mammals and humans	Attached to skin when feeding	Southern United States, Midwest and Atlantic Coast of United States	Lone star tick	260

Parasites by Host Species—cont'd

PARASITE	HOST	LOCATION OF ADULT	DISTRIBUTION	COMMON NAME	PAGE
Amblyomma maculatum	Adult on cattle, sheep, horses, dogs, and humans	Attached to skin when feeding	Atlantic and Gulf coasts of United States	Gulf Coast tick	260
Haemaphysalis leporispalustris	Larval and nymphal stages on rabbits, birds, dogs, cats, and humans	Attached to skin when feeding	United States	Continental rabbit tick	261

RUMINANTS

Nematodes

Gastrointestinal Tract

PARASITE	HOST	LOCATION OF ADULT	DISTRIBUTION	COMMON NAME	PAGE
Gongylonema pulchrum	Sheep, goats, cattle, and occasionally pigs	Submucosa and mucosa of esophagus		Esophageal worm of ruminants	50
Bunostomum sp.	Cattle, sheep, and goats	Abomasum, small and large intestines	Worldwide	Trichostronglye of ruminants	51
Chabertia sp.	Cattle, sheep, and goats	Abomasum, small and large intestines	Worldwide	Trichostronglye of ruminants	51
Cooperia sp.	Cattle, sheep, and goats	Abomasum, small and large intestines	Worldwide	Trichostronglye of ruminants	51
Haemonchus sp.	Cattle, sheep, and goats	Abomasum, small and large intestines	Worldwide	Trichostronglye of ruminants	51
Oesophagostomum sp.	Cattle, sheep, and goats	Abomasum, small and large intestines	Worldwide	Trichostronglye of ruminants	51
Ostertagia sp.	Cattle, sheep, and goats	Abomasum, small and large intestines	Worldwide	Trichostronglye of ruminants	51
Trichostrongylus sp.	Cattle, sheep, and goats	Abomasum, small and large intestines	Worldwide	Trichostronglye of ruminants	51
Nematodirus sp.	Cattle, goats, and sheep	Abomasum, small and large intestines	Worldwide	Trichostrongyle of ruminants	51
Marshallagia sp.	Cattle, sheep, and goats	Abomasum, small and large intestines	Tropical and subtropical regions	Trichostronglye of ruminants	51
Strongyloides papillosus	Cattle	Small intestine	Worldwide	Bovine intestinal threadworm	53
Trichuris ovis	Cattle, sheep, and goats	Cecum and colon	Worldwide	Whipworms	53

Continued

Parasites by Host Species—cont'd

PARASITE	HOST	LOCATION OF ADULT	DISTRIBUTION	COMMON NAME	PAGE
Circulatory System					
Elaeophora schneideri	Sheep	Common carotid artery	Western and southwestern United States	Arterial worm of sheep	54
Respiratory System					
Dictyocaulus sp.	Cattle, sheep, and goats	Bronchi	Worldwide	Lungworms of ruminants	54
Muellerius capillaris	Sheep and goats	Bronchioles	Worldwide	Hair lungworm of sheep and goats	55
Protostrongylus sp.	Sheep and goats	Small bronchioles	Worldwide		
Skin					
Stephanofilaria stilesi	Cattle, goats, buffalo, and wild ruminants	Ventral midline		Skin worm of ruminants	56
Eye and Adnexa					
Thelazia rhodesii	Cattle, sheep, and goats	Conjunctival sac and lacrimal duct	Worldwide	Eyeworm of cattle, sheep, and goats	57
Thelazia gulosa	Cattle, sheep, and goats	Conjunctival sac and lacrimal duct	Worldwide	Eyeworm of cattle, sheep, and goats	57
Abdominal Cavity					
Setaria cervi	Cattle	Free within peritoneal cavity	Worldwide	Abdominal worm of cattle	57
Cestodes					
Gastrointestinal Tract					
Moniezia benedini	Cattle	Small intestine	Worldwide	Bovine tapeworm	96
Moniezia expansa	Cattle, sheep, and goats	Small intestine	Worldwide	Ruminant tapeworm	96
Thysanosoma actinoides	Cattle, sheep, and goats	Lumen of bile duct, pancreatic duct, and small intestine	North and South America	Fringed tapeworm of sheep and goats	99
Larval Stages in Musculature					
Taenia saginata	Cattle	Muscle	Worldwide	Beef tapeworm of humans	100
Larval Stages in Abdominal Cavity					
Taenia hydatigena	Cattle, sheep, and goats	Abdominal cavity	Worldwide	Canine taeniid	101

Parasites by Host Species—cont'd

PARASITE	HOST	LOCATION OF ADULT	DISTRIBUTION	COMMON NAME	PAGE
Trematodes					
Dicrocoelium dendriticum	Cattle, sheep, and goats	Bile ducts	Worldwide	Lancet fluke	130
Paramphistomum sp.	Cattle, sheep, and goats	Rumen and reticulum	Worldwide	Rumen flukes	131
Cotylophoron sp.	Cattle, sheep, and goats	Rumen and reticulum		Rumen flukes	131
Fasciola hepatica	Cattle, sheep	Bile duct	Worldwide	Liver fluke	131
Fascioloides magna	White-tailed deer	Liver parenchyma	North America, central and southwestern Europe	Liver fluke of wild ruminants	133
Protozoans					
Gastrointestinal Tract					
Apicomplexans					
Eimeria sp.	Ruminants	Cecum and colon	Worldwide	Coccidia of ruminants	167
Eimeria bovis	Ruminants	Cecum and colon	Worldwide	Coccidia of ruminants	167
Eimeria zuernii	Ruminants	Cecum and colon	Worldwide	Coccidia of ruminants	167
Cryptosporidium sp.	Dogs, cats, cattle, pigs, birds, guinea pigs, snakes, and mice	Small intestine		Cryptosporidia	167
Circulatory System					
Flagellates					
Trypanosoma sp.	Ruminants	Peripheral blood	Central and South America	Trypanosomes	168
Apicomplexans					
Babesia bigemina	Cattle	Within RBCs	Europe, Africa, Asia, South America, and North America	*Babesia*	169
Urogenital System					
Tritrichomonas foetus	Cattle	Prepuce in bull; cervix, uterus, and vagina in cow	Worldwide	*Trichomonas*	169

Continued

Parasites by Host Species—cont'd

PARASITE	HOST	LOCATION OF ADULT	DISTRIBUTION	COMMON NAME	PAGE
Arthropods					
Lice					
Mallophagan sp.	Mammals and birds	Among hairs of host		Chewing lice	200
Anopluran sp.	Mammals and birds	Among hairs of host		Sucking lice	201
Dipterans					
Simulium sp.	Domesticated animals, poultry, and humans	Skin surface when feeding	Worldwide	Black flies or buffalo gnats	208
Lutzomyia sp.	Mammals, reptiles, avians, and humans	Skin surface when feeding	Worldwide	New World sand flies	209
Phlebotomus sp.	Mammals, reptiles, avians, and humans	Skin surface when feeding	Subtropical and Mediterranean regions	Sand flies	209
Culicoides sp.	Domestic animals and humans	Skin surface when feeding	Worldwide	No-see-ums, punkies, or sand flies	209
Anopheles quadrimaculatus	Mammals, reptiles, avians, and humans	Skin surface when feeding	Worldwide	Malaria mosquito	210
Aedes aegypti	Mammals, reptiles, avians, and humans	Skin surface when feeding	Worldwide	Yellow fever mosquito	210
Culex sp.	Mammals, reptiles, avians, and humans	Skin surface when feeding	Worldwide	Mosquito	210
Chrysops sp.	Large mammals, humans, and occasionally small mammals and birds	Skin surface when feeding	Worldwide	Deerflies	211
Tabanus sp.	Large mammals, humans, and occasionally small mammals and birds	Skin surface when feeding	Worldwide	Horseflies	211
Glossina sp.	Mammals, reptiles, birds, and humans	Skin surface when feeding	Africa	Tsetse fly	212
Stomoxys calcitrans	Variety of animals and humans	Around large amounts of decaying vegetation	Worldwide	Stable fly	212

Parasites by Host Species—cont'd

PARASITE	HOST	LOCATION OF ADULT	DISTRIBUTION	COMMON NAME	PAGE
Haematobia irritans	Cattle and buffalo	Around horns, shoulders, back, side, and ventral abdomen	North America, Europe, and Australia	Horn fly	214
Melophagus ovinus	Sheep and goats	Deep within wool or fleece	Worldwide	Sheep ked	215
Musca domestica	Variety of animals and humans	Within the house	Worldwide	Housefly	216
Musca autumnalis	Predominantly cattle but also other large animals	Feeds around medial canthus of the eye	Worldwide	Face fly	217
Calliphora sp.	Domestic animals, wild animals, and humans	Free living in environment		Bottle flies or blowflies	218
Lucilia sp.	Domestic animals, wild animals, and humans	Free living in environment		Bottle flies or blowflies	218
Phormia sp.	Domestic animals, wild animals, and humans	Free living in environment		Bottle flies or blowflies	218
Phaenicia sp.	Domestic animals, wild animals, and humans	Free living in environment		Bottle flies or blowflies	218
Sarcophaga sp.	Domestic animals, wild animals, and humans	Free living in environment		Flesh fly	219
Hippelates sp.	Dogs and cattle	Mucocutaneous junction of eyes, lips, and penis		Dog penis gnats	219
Cochliomyia hominivorax	Domestic animals	Fresh, uncontaminated wounds	North America	Screw fly	221
Hypoderma sp.	Cattle, rarely in horses, sheep, and humans	Larva in large boil-like cyst on back	Northern and southern United States and Canada	Gadflies or cattle grubs	223
Oestrus ovis	Sheep and goats	Nasal passages	Worldwide	Nasal bot fly or grub	225

Mites

PARASITE	HOST	LOCATION OF ADULT	DISTRIBUTION	COMMON NAME	PAGE
Sarcoptes scabei variety bovis	Cattle	Superficial layers of epidermis	Worldwide	Scabies of cattle	233
Sarcoptes scabei variety ovis	Sheep and goats	Superficial layers of epidermis	Worldwide	Scabies of sheep and goats	233

Continued

Parasites by Host Species—cont'd

PARASITE	HOST	LOCATION OF ADULT	DISTRIBUTION	COMMON NAME	PAGE
Psoroptes cuniculi	Rabbits, horses, goats, and sheep	External ear canal	Worldwide	Rabbit ear mite	238
Psoroptes ovis	Sheep	Skin surface of body	Worldwide	Scabies of sheep	238
Psoroptes bovis	Cattle	Skin surface of withers, neck, and rump	Worldwide	Scabies of cattle	238
Chorioptes bovis	Cattle	Skin surface of lower hind legs, flanks, and shoulders	Worldwide	Foot and tail mite or itchy leg mite	239
Chorioptes caprae	Goats	Skin surface of lower hind legs, flanks, and shoulders	Worldwide	Foot and tail mite or itchy leg mite	239
Chorioptes ovis	Sheep	Skin surface of lower hind legs, flanks, and shoulders	Worldwide	Foot and tail mite or itchy leg mite	239
Demodex bovis	Cattle	Hair follicles and sebaceous glands	Worldwide	Demodectic mange mite of cattle	239
Demodex caprae	Goats	Hair follicles and sebaceous glands	Worldwide	Demodectic mange mite of goats	242
Trombicula sp.	Domestic animals, wild animals, and humans	Larval stage on skin surface		Chiggers	244

Ticks

PARASITE	HOST	LOCATION OF ADULT	DISTRIBUTION	COMMON NAME	PAGE
Otobius megnini	Dogs, horses, cattle, sheep, and goats	Larval and nymphal stages in the external ear canal	Arid and semiarid regions in southwestern United States	Spinose ear tick	255
Ixodes scapularis	Adult on dogs, horses, deer, and humans	Attached to skin when feeding	Eastern United States	Deer tick	257
Dermacentor andersoni	Adult on dogs, horses, cattle, goats, sheep, and humans	Attached to skin when feeding	Rocky Mountain regions	Rocky Mountain wood tick	259
Dermacentor occidentalis	Adult on large mammals	Attached to skin when feeding	Sierra Nevada Mountains	Pacific Coast dog tick	259
Amblyomma americanum	Adult on wide range of mammals and humans	Attached to skin when feeding	Southern United States, Midwest and Atlantic Coast of United States	Lone star tick	260

Parasites by Host Species—cont'd

PARASITE	HOST	LOCATION OF ADULT	DISTRIBUTION	COMMON NAME	PAGE
Amblyomma maculatum	Adult on cattle, sheep, horses, dogs, and humans	Attached to skin when feeding	Atlantic and Gulf coasts of United States	Gulf Coast tick	260
Rhipicephalus annulatus	Cattle	Attached to skin when feeding	Mexico and enzootic areas of United States	Texas cattle fever tick or North American tick	261

EQUINES

Nematodes

Gastrointestinal Tract

Habronema microstoma	Horses	Stomach mucosa	Worldwide	Stomach worm of horses	58
Habronema muscae	Horses	Stomach mucosa	Worldwide	Stomach worm of horses	58
Draschia megastoma	Horses	Stomach mucosa	Worldwide	Stomach worm of horses	58
Trichostrongylus axei	Horses, cattle, sheep, and pigs	Stomach	Worldwide	Stomach worm of horses and pigs	59
Parascaris equorum	Horses	Small intestine	Worldwide	Equine roundworm	59
Strongylus vulgaris	Horses	Large intestine	Worldwide	Strongyle of horses	61
Strongylus edentatus	Horses	Large intestine	Worldwide	Strongyle of horses	61
Strongylus equinus	Horses	Large intestine	Worldwide	Strongyle of horses	61
Strongyloides westeri	Horses	Small intestine	Worldwide	Intestinal threadworm of horses	62
Oxyuris equi	Horses	Cecum, colon, and rectum	Worldwide	Pinworm of horses	63

Respiratory System

Dictyocaulus arnfieldi	Horses, mules, and donkeys	Bronchi and bronchioles	Worldwide	Equine lungworm	65

Skin

Habronema microstoma	Horses	Larvae in skin	Worldwide	Stomach worm of horses	65
Habronema muscae	Horses	Larvae in skin	Worldwide	Stomach worm of horses	65

Continued

Parasites by Host Species—cont'd

PARASITE	HOST	LOCATION OF ADULT	DISTRIBUTION	COMMON NAME	PAGE
Draschia megastoma	Horses	Larvae in skin	Worldwide	Stomach worm of horses	65
Onchocerca cervicalis	Horses	Adult in ligamentum nuchae; larvae in dermis	Worldwide	Equine filarial worm	66
Eye and Adnexa					
Thelazia lacrymalis	Horses	Conjunctival sac and lacrimal duct	Worldwide	Eyeworm of the horse	67
Abdominal Cavity					
Setaria equina	Horses	Free within peritoneal cavity	Europe and North America	Abdominal worm of horses	67
Cestodes					
Gastrointestinal Tract					
Anoplocephala perfoliata	Horses	Small and large intestines and cecum	Worldwide	Lappeted equine tapeworm	102
Anoplocephala magna	Horses	Stomach and small intestine	Worldwide	Equine tapeworm with large scolex	102
Paranoplocephala mamillana	Horses	Stomach and small intestine	Worldwide	Equine tapeworm	102
Protozoans					
Gastrointestinal Tract					
Flagellates					
Giardia assemblage E	Horses, cattle, sheep, goats, and pigs	Small intestine	Worldwide	*Giardia*	170
Ciliates					
Eimeria leuckarti	Horses	Small intestine	Worldwide	Coccidia	170
Circulatory System					
Apicomplexans					
Babesia caballi	Horses	Within RBCs	Europe, Africa, Asia, North and South America	Equine piroplasm	171
Theileria equi	Horses	Within RBCs	Europe, Africa, Asia, North and South America	Equine piroplasm	171

Parasites by Host Species—cont'd

PARASITE	HOST	LOCATION OF ADULT	DISTRIBUTION	COMMON NAME	PAGE
Urogenital System					
Apicomplexans					
Klossiella equi	Horses	Kidneys			171
Nervous System					
Apicomplexans					
Sarcocystis neurona	Horses	Asexual stage in nervous system			172
Arthropods					
Lice					
Mallophagan sp.	Mammals and birds	Among hairs of host		Chewing lice	200
Anopluran sp.	Mammals and birds	Among hairs of host		Sucking lice	201
Dipterans					
Simulium sp.	Domesticated animals, poultry, and humans	Skin surface when feeding	Worldwide	Black flies or buffalo gnats	208
Lutzomyia sp.	Mammals, reptiles, avians, and humans	Skin surface when feeding	Worldwide	New World sand flies	209
Phlebotomus sp.	Mammals, reptiles, avians, and humans	Skin surface when feeding	Subtropical and Mediterranean regions	Sand flies	209
Culicoides sp.	Domestic animals and humans	Skin surface when feeding	Worldwide	No-see-ums, punkies, or sand flies	209
Anopheles quadrimaculatus	Mammals, reptiles, avians, and humans	Skin surface when feeding	Worldwide	Malaria mosquito	210
Aedes aegypti	Mammals, reptiles, avians, and humans	Skin surface when feeding	Worldwide	Yellow fever mosquito	210
Culex sp.	Mammals, reptiles, avians, and humans	Skin surface when feeding	Worldwide	Mosquito	210
Chrysops sp.	Large mammals, humans, and occasionally small mammals and birds	Skin surface when feeding	Worldwide	Deerflies	211

Continued

Parasites by Host Species—cont'd

PARASITE	HOST	LOCATION OF ADULT	DISTRIBUTION	COMMON NAME	PAGE
Tabanus sp.	Large mammals, humans, and occasionally small mammals and birds	Skin surface when feeding	Worldwide	Horseflies	211
Glossina sp.	Mammals, reptiles, birds, and humans	Skin surface when feeding	Africa	Tsetse fly	212
Stomoxys calcitrans	Variety of animals and humans	Around large amounts of decaying vegetation	Worldwide	Stable fly	212
Musca domestica	Variety of animals and humans	Within the house	Worldwide	Housefly	212
Musca autumnalis	Predominantly cattle but also other large animals	Feeds around medial canthus of the eye	Worldwide	Face fly	217
Calliphora sp.	Domestic animals, wild animals, and humans	Free living in environment		Bottle flies or blowflies	218
Lucilia sp.	Domestic animals, wild animals, and humans	Free living in environment		Bottle flies or blowflies	218
Phormia sp.	Domestic animals, wild animals, and humans	Free living in environment		Bottle flies or blowflies	218
Phaenicia sp.	Domestic animals, wild animals, and humans	Free living in environment		Bottle flies or blowflies	218
Sarcophaga sp.	Domestic animals, wild animals, and humans	Free living in environment		Flesh fly	219
Cochliomyia hominivorax	Domestic animals	Fresh, uncontaminated wounds	North America	Screw fly	221
Hypoderma sp.	Cattle, rarely in horses, sheep, and humans	Larva in large boil-like cyst on back	Northern and southern United States and Canada	Gadflies or cattle grubs	223
Gasterophilus sp.	Horses	Attached to gastric mucosa	Worldwide	Bot flies or horse bots	224

Parasites by Host Species—cont'd

PARASITE	HOST	LOCATION OF ADULT	DISTRIBUTION	COMMON NAME	PAGE
Mites					
Sarcoptes scabiei variety *equi*	Horses	Superficial layers of epidermis	Worldwide	Scabies of horses	233
Psoroptes cuniculi	Rabbits, horses, goats, and sheep	External ear canal	Worldwide	Rabbit ear mite	238
Psoroptes equi	Horses	Skin surface of mane and tail	Worldwide	Scabies of horses	238
Chorioptes equi	Horses	Skin surface of lower hind limbs, flanks, and shoulders	Worldwide	Foot and tail mite or itchy leg mite	239
Demodex equi	Horses	Skin of face and eyes	Worldwide	Demodectic mange mite of horses	242
Trombicula sp.	Domestic animals, wild animals, and humans	Larval stage on skin surface		Chiggers	244
Ticks					
Otobius megnini	Dogs, horses, cattle, sheep, and goats	Larval and nymphal stages in the external ear canal	Arid and semiarid regions in southwestern United States	Spinose ear tick	255
Ixodes scapularis	Adult on dogs, horses, deer, and humans	Attached to skin when feeding	Eastern United States	Deer tick	257
Dermacentor andersoni	Adult on dogs, horses, cattle, goats, sheep, and humans	Attached to skin when feeding	Rocky Mountain regions	Rocky Mountain wood tick	259
Dermacentor occidentalis	Adult on large mammals	Attached to skin when feeding	Sierra Nevada Mountains	Pacific Coast dog tick	259
Amblyomma americanum	Adult on wide range of mammals and humans	Attached to skin when feeding	Southern United States, Midwest and Atlantic Coast of United States	Lone star tick	260
Amblyomma maculatum	Adult on cattle, sheep, horses, dogs, and humans	Attached to skin when feeding	Atlantic and Gulf coasts of United States	Gulf Coast tick	260

Continued

Parasites by Host Species—cont'd

PARASITE	HOST	LOCATION OF ADULT	DISTRIBUTION	COMMON NAME	PAGE
SWINE					
Nematodes					
Gastrointestinal Tract					
Ascarops strongylina	Pigs	Stomach		Stomach worm of pigs	67
Physocephalus sexalatus	Pigs	Stomach		Stomach worm of pigs	67
Hyostrongylus rubidus	Pigs	Stomach	Worldwide	Red stomach worm of pigs	68
Trichostrongylus axei	Horses, sheep, cattle, and pigs	Stomach	Worldwide	Stomach worm of pigs	68
Ascaris suum	Pigs	Small intestine	Worldwide	Large intestinal roundworm of pigs	68
Strongyloides ransomi	Pigs	Small intestine	Worldwide	Intestinal threadworm of pigs	69
Oesophagostomum dentatum	Pigs	Large intestine	Worldwide	Nodular worm of pigs	69
Trichuris suis	Pigs	Cecum and colon	Worldwide	Whipworm	69
Trichinella spiralis	Pigs, definitive hosts	Small intestine	Worldwide except Denmark and Australia	Trichina worm	70
Respiratory System					
Metastrongylus elongatus	Pigs	Bronchi and bronchioles	Worldwide	Swine lungworm	71
Urinary Tract					
Stephanurus dentatus	Pigs	Cystic spaces around kidneys, ureters, and perirenal tissue		Swine kidney worm	71
Musculoskeletal System					
Trichinella spiralis	Pigs	Small intestine, larvae in muscle	Worldwide except Denmark and Australia	Trichina worm	72
Cestodes					
Larvae in Muscle					
Taenia solium	Pigs, intermediate host	Larvae in muscle tissue	Underdeveloped countries	Pork tapeworm of humans	100

Parasites by Host Species—cont'd

PARASITE	HOST	LOCATION OF ADULT	DISTRIBUTION	COMMON NAME	PAGE
Protozoans					
Gastrointestinal Tract					
Ciliates					
Balantidium coli	Pigs and dogs	Large intestine	Worldwide	*Balantidium*	172
Apicomplexans					
Cystoisospora suis	Pigs	Small intestine		Coccidia	172
Cryptosporidium sp.	Canines, felines, bovines, swine, avians, guinea pigs, snakes, and mice	Small intestine		*Cryptosporidium*	174
Arthropods					
Lice					
Mallophagan sp.	Mammals and birds	Among hairs of host		Chewing lice	200
Anopluran sp.	Mammals and birds	Among hairs of host		Sucking lice	201
Dipterans					
Simulium sp.	Domesticated animals, poultry, and humans	Skin surface when feeding	Worldwide	Black flies or buffalo gnats	208
Lutzomyia sp.	Mammals, reptiles, avians, and humans	Skin surface when feeding	Worldwide	New World sand flies	209
Phlebotomus sp.	Mammals, reptiles, avians, and humans	Skin surface when feeding	Subtropical and Mediterranean regions	Sand flies	209
Culicoides sp.	Domestic animals and humans	Skin surface when feeding	Worldwide	No-see-ums, punkies, or sand flies	209
Anopheles quadrimaculatus	Mammals, reptiles, avians, and humans	Skin surface when feeding	Worldwide	Malaria mosquito	210
Aedes aegypti	Mammals, reptiles, avians, and humans	Skin surface when feeding	Worldwide	Yellow fever mosquito	210
Culex sp.	Mammals, reptiles, avians, and humans	Skin surface when feeding	Worldwide	Mosquito	210
Chrysops sp.	Large mammals, humans, and occasionally small mammals and birds	Skin surface when feeding	Worldwide	Deerflies	211

Continued

Parasites by Host Species—cont'd

PARASITE	HOST	LOCATION OF ADULT	DISTRIBUTION	COMMON NAME	PAGE
Tabanus sp.	Large mammals, humans, and occasionally small mammals and birds	Skin surface when feeding	Worldwide	Horseflies	211
Glossina sp.	Mammals, reptiles, birds, and humans	Skin surface when feeding	Africa	Tsetse fly	212
Stomoxys calcitrans	Variety of animals and humans	Around large amounts of decaying vegetation	Worldwide	Stable fly	212
Musca domestica	Variety of animals and humans	Within the house	Worldwide	Housefly	216
Calliphora sp.	Domestic animals, wild animals, and humans	Free living in environment		Bottle flies or blowflies	218
Lucilia sp.	Domestic animals, wild animals, and humans	Free living in environment		Bottle flies or blowflies	218
Phormia sp.	Domestic animals, wild animals, and humans	Free living in environment		Bottle flies or blowflies	218
Phaenicia sp.	Domestic animals, wild animals, and humans	Free living in environment		Bottle flies or blowflies	218
Sarcophaga sp.	Domestic animals, wild animals, and humans	Free living in environment		Flesh fly	219
Cochliomyia hominivorax	Domestic animals	Fresh, uncontaminated wounds	North America	Screw fly	221
Mites					
Sarcoptes scabiei variety *suis*	Pigs	Superficial layers of epidermis	Worldwide	Scabies of pigs	233
Demodex phylloides	Pigs	Hair follicles and sebaceous glands	Worldwide	Demodectic mange mite	241
Trombicula sp.	Domestic animals, wild animals, and humans	Larval stage on skin surface		Chiggers	244
Ticks					
Amblyomma americanum	Adult on wide range of mammals and humans	Attached to skin when feeding	Southern United States, Midwest and Atlantic Coast of United States	Lone star tick	260

Parasites by Host Species—cont'd

PARASITE	HOST	LOCATION OF ADULT	DISTRIBUTION	COMMON NAME	PAGE
EXOTIC ANIMALS AND BIRDS					
Nematodes					
Gastrointestinal Tract					
Syphacia obvelata	Mice, rats, hamsters, and gerbils	Cecum and rectum		Pinworms of rodents	73
Aspiculuris tetraptera	Mice	Cecum and rectum		Pinworms of mice	73
Syphacia muris	Mice, rats, hamsters, and gerbils	Cecum and rectum		Pinworms of rodents	73
Dentostomella translucida	Gerbils	Stomach and proximal third of small intestine		Pinworm of gerbils	76
Paraspidodera uncinata	Guinea pig	Cecum and colon		Ascarid of guinea pigs	77
Passalurus ambiguus	Rabbits	Cecum and colon		Pinworm of rabbits	78
Obeliscoides cuniculi	Rabbits	Stomach		Trichostrongyle of rabbits	79
Trichostrongylus calcaratus	Rabbits	Small intestine		Trichostrongyle of rabbits	79
Ascaridia sp.	Birds	Small intestine	Worldwide	Ascarid of birds	80
Spiroptera incesta	Australian finches	Ventriculus		Spirurid of birds	80
Dispharynx nasuta	Finches	Ventriculus	Tropical and subtropical regions	Spirurid of birds	80
Tetrameres sp.	Pigeons	Proventriculus		Spirurid of birds	80
Capillaria sp.	Pheasants, peafowl, and poultry	Crop and upper alimentary tract	Worldwide	*Capillaria*	81
Urinary Tract					
Trichosomoides crassicauda	Rats	Urinary bladder		Bladder worm of rats	75
Cestodes					
Gastrointestinal Tract					
Hymenolepis nana	Mice, rats, gerbils, hamsters, dogs, and humans	Small intestine		Tapeworm of rodents	95
Hymenolepis diminuta	Mice, rats, gerbils, hamsters, dogs, and humans	Small intestine		Tapeworm of rodents	95

Continued

Parasites by Host Species—cont'd

PARASITE	HOST	LOCATION OF ADULT	DISTRIBUTION	COMMON NAME	PAGE
Trematodes					
Circulatory System					
Schistosoma sp.	Birds	Blood vasculature	North America	Avian schistosomes	139
Protozoans					
Gastrointestinal Tract					
Flagellates					
Giardia psittaci	Birds	Intestinal mucosa		*Giardia*	174
Histomonas meleagridis	Turkeys, peafowl, chickens, and pheasants	Liver	Worldwide	"Blackhead"	174
Trichomonas gallinae	Pigeons, doves, poultry, and raptors	Crop		Trichomonas	175
Tetratrichomonas microti	Mice	Small intestine		Flagellate of mice	180
Tritrichomonas muris	Mice	Cecum and colon		Flagellate of mice	180
Giardia assemblage G	Rodents	Proximal small intestine		*Giardia*	180
Spironucleus muris	Mice	Proximal small intestine		Flagellate of mice	180
Tritrichomonas caviae	Guinea pigs	Cecum		Flagellate of guinea pigs	183
Apicomplexans					
Eimeria irresidua	Rabbits	Small intestine		Coccidia of rabbits	178
Eimeria magna	Rabbits	Small intestine		Coccidia of rabbits	178
Eimeria media	Rabbits	Small intestine and large intestine		Coccidia of rabbits	178
Eimeria perforans	Rabbits	Small intestine		Coccidia of rabbits	178
Eimeria stiedae	Rabbits	Bile ducts		Coccidia of rabbits	179
Eimeria falciformis	Mice	Small intestine		Coccidia of mice	181
Eimeria ferrisi	Mice	Cecum		Coccidia of mice	181
Eimeria hansonorum	Mice	Small intestine		Coccidia of mice	181
Eimeria nieschultzi	Rats	Intestines		Coccidia of rats	182

Parasites by Host Species—cont'd

PARASITE	HOST	LOCATION OF ADULT	DISTRIBUTION	COMMON NAME	PAGE
Eimeria caviae	Guinea pigs	Large intestine		Coccidia of guinea pigs	184
Cryptosporidium wrairi	Guinea pigs	Tips of intestinal villi of the ileum			184
Amoeba					
Entamoeba caviae	Guinea pigs	Cecum		Amoeba of guinea pigs	183
Circulatory System					
Flagellates					
Trypanosoma sp.	Cockatoos	Peripheral blood	Worldwide	Trypanosomes of birds	176
Apicomplexans					
Haemoproteus sp.	Cockatoos, macaws, and conures	Within RBCs	Worldwide		176
Plasmodium sp.	Birds	Within RBCs	Worldwide		177
Leucocytozoon sp.	Raptors	Within RBCs	Worldwide		177
Aegyptianella sp.	Pet birds	Within RBCs			177
Respiratory System					
Apicomplexans					
Cystoisospora serini	Canaries and finches	Lung, liver, and spleen		Coccidia of birds or atoxoplasmosis	178
Urogenital System					
Apicomplexans					
Klossiella muris	Mice	Kidneys			181
Skin					
Ciliates					
Ichthyophthirius multifiliis	Freshwater and ornamental fish	Skin, gills, fins, and eyes		Ciliate of fish	185
Arthropods					
True Bugs					
Cimex lectularius	Humans, rabbits, poultry, and pigeons			Bedbugs	199
Rhodnius sp.	Dogs, humans, cats, guinea pigs, armadillos, rats, raccoons, and monkeys	Periodic skin of mouth and lips	South and Central America and southern and western United States	Kissing bugs	200

Continued

Parasites by Host Species—cont'd

PARASITE	HOST	LOCATION OF ADULT	DISTRIBUTION	COMMON NAME	PAGE
Panstrongylus sp.	Dogs, humans, cats, guinea pigs, armadillos, rats, raccoons, and monkeys	Periodic skin of mouth and lips	South and Central America and southern and western United States	Kissing bugs	200
Triatoma sp.	Dogs, humans, cats, guinea pigs, armadillos, rats, raccoons, and monkeys	Periodic skin of mouth and lips	South and Central America and southern and western United States	Kissing bugs	200
Lice					
Polyplax serrata	Mice	Within hair coat		Mouse louse	203
Polyplax spinulosa	Rat	Within hair coat		Rat louse	205
Hoplopleura meridionidis	Gerbil	Within hair coat		Gerbil louse	205
Gliricola porcelli	Guinea pig	Within hair coat		Guinea pig louse	206
Gyropus ovalis	Guinea pig	Within hair coat		Guinea pig louse	206
Hemodipsus ventricosus	Rabbit	Within hair coat		Rabbit louse	206
Dipterans					
Simulium sp.	Domesticated animals, poultry, and humans	Skin surface when feeding	Worldwide	Black flies or buffalo gnats	208
Lutzomyia sp.	Mammals, reptiles, avians, and humans	Skin surface when feeding	Worldwide	New World sand flies	208
Phlebotomus sp.	Mammals, reptiles, avians, and humans	Skin surface when feeding	Subtropical and Mediterranean regions	Sand flies	208
Anopheles quadrimaculatus	Mammals, reptiles, avians, and humans	Skin surface when feeding	Worldwide	Malaria mosquito	210
Aedes aegypti	Mammals, reptiles, avians, and humans	Skin surface when feeding	Worldwide	Yellow fever mosquito	210
Culex sp.	Mammals, reptiles, avians, and humans	Skin surface when feeding	Worldwide	Mosquito	210
Chrysops sp.	Large mammals, humans, and occasionally small mammals and birds	Skin surface when feeding	Worldwide	Deerflies	211

Parasites by Host Species—cont'd

PARASITE	HOST	LOCATION OF ADULT	DISTRIBUTION	COMMON NAME	PAGE
Tabanus sp.	Large mammals, humans, and occasionally small mammals and birds	Skin surface when feeding	Worldwide	Horseflies	211
Glossina sp.	Mammals, reptiles, birds, and humans	Skin surface when feeding	Africa	Tsetse fly	210
Lynchia sp.	Wild birds	Deep within feathers		Bird keds	216
Pseudolynchia sp.	Wild birds	Deep within feathers		Bird keds	216
Cuterebra sp.	Rabbits, squirrels, mice, rats, chipmunks, dogs, and cats	Larva around the head and neck		Warbles or wolves	22
Siphonaptera					
Cediopsylla simplex	Rabbits	On skin		Common eastern rabbit flea	226
Odontopsylla multispinosus	Rabbits	On skin		Giant eastern rabbit flea	226
Echidnophaga gallinacea	Poultry	On skin		Poultry flea	226
Mites					
Notoedres cati	Cats and rabbits	Superficial layers of epidermis	Worldwide	Notoedric mange mite	234
Notoedres muris	Rats	Superficial layers of epidermis		Scabies mite of rats	234
Cnemidocoptes pilae	Budgerigars and parakeets	Superficial epidermis of feet, cere, and beak	Worldwide	Scaly leg mite of parakeets	236
Cnemidocoptes mutans	Poultry	Superficial epidermis of feet	Worldwide	Scaly leg mite of chickens	236
Trixacarus caviae	Guinea pigs	Superficial layers of epidermis		Burrowing mite of guinea pigs	237
Psoroptes cuniculi	Rabbits, horses, goats, and sheep	External ear canal	Worldwide	Rabbit ear mite	238
Otodectes cynotis	Dogs, cats, and ferrets	External ear canal	Worldwide	Ear mites	240
Demodex aurati	Hamsters and gerbils	Hair follicles and sebaceous glands	Worldwide	Demodectic mange mite of hamsters and gerbils	243

Continued

Parasites by Host Species—cont'd

PARASITE	HOST	LOCATION OF ADULT	DISTRIBUTION	COMMON NAME	PAGE
Demodex criceti	Hamsters and gerbils	Hair follicles and sebaceous glands	Worldwide	Demodectic mange mite of hamsters and gerbils	243
Ornithonyssus sylviarum	Poultry	On skin	Worldwide in temperate zones	Northern fowl mite	246
Dermanyssus gallinae	Poultry	In environment	Worldwide	Red fowl mite	246
Ornithonyssus bacoti	Rats, mice, hamsters, and guinea pigs	On skin when feeding	Tropical and subtropical regions	Tropical rat mite	246
Cheyletiella parasitivorax	Dogs, cats, and rabbits	Surface of skin and hair coat	Worldwide	Walking dandruff	246
Myobia musculi	Mice	Hair shafts		Mouse fur mite	249
Myocoptes musculinus	Mice	Hair shafts		Mouse fur mite	249
Radfordia affinis	Mice	Hair shafts		Mouse fur mite	249
Radfordia ensifera	Rats	Hair shafts		Rat fur mite	251
Chirodiscoides caviae	Guinea pigs	Within pelt		Guinea pig fur mite	251
Listrophorus gibbus	Rabbits	Hair shafts		Rabbit fur mite	252

Ticks

PARASITE	HOST	LOCATION OF ADULT	DISTRIBUTION	COMMON NAME	PAGE
Argas persicus	Chickens, turkeys, and wild birds	Attached to skin when feeding		Fowl tick	256
Ixodes scapularis	Adult on dogs, horses, deer, and humans	Attached to skin when feeding	Eastern United States	Deer tick	257
Dermacentor andersoni	Adult on dogs, horses, cattle, goats, sheep, and humans	Attached to skin when feeding	Rocky Mountain regions	Rocky Mountain wood tick	259
Dermacentor occidentalis	Adult on large mammals	Attached to skin when feeding	Sierra Nevada Mountains	Pacific Coast dog tick	259
Amblyomma americanum	Adult on wide range of mammals and humans	Attached to skin when feeding	Southern United States, Midwest and Atlantic Coast of United States	Lone star tick	260
Amblyomma maculatum	Adult on cattle, sheep, horses, dogs, and humans	Attached to skin when feeding	Atlantic and Gulf coasts of United States	Gulf Coast tick	260
Haemaphysalis leporispalustris	Larval and nymphal stages on rabbits, birds, dogs, cats, and humans; adult stage on rabbits	Attached to skin when feeding	United States	Continental rabbit tick	261

1

The Language of Veterinary Parasitology

OUTLINE

LEARNING OBJECTIVES

After studying this chapter, the reader should be able to do the following:

- Briefly discuss the importance of veterinarians in public health.
- Briefly discuss the importance of veterinary parasitology.
- Describe the important types of symbiotic relationships.
- Become fluent in the language of veterinary parasitology.

- Utilize the Linnaean classification scheme within the discipline of veterinary parasitology.
- Define and describe terms associated with veterinary parasitology and give examples of parasites that exemplify these terms.

KEY TERMS

Aberrant parasite
Acaricides
Animalia
Anthelmintics
Antiprotozoals
Classification scheme
Commensalism
Common name
Definitive host
Ectoparasite
Ectoparasitism
Encysted
Endoparasite
Endoparasitism
Erratic parasite

Euryxenous parasite
Facultative parasite
Fungi
Genus name
Homoxenous parasite
Host
Incidental parasite
Infection
Infestation
Insecticides
Intermediate host
Life cycle
Monera
Monoxenous parasite
Mutualism

Obligatory parasite
Parasite
Parasitiasis
Parasiticides
Parasitism
Parasitology
Parasitosis
Paratenic host
Periodic parasite
Phoresis
Plantae
Predator
Predator-prey
  relationship
Prey

Protista
Pseudoparasite
Reservoir host
Scientific name
Specific epithet
Stenoxenous parasite
Symbiont
Symbiosis
Transport host
Veterinary
  parasitology
Zoonosis

Veterinary medicine continues to be one of the most rapidly evolving health care professions of the twenty-first century. Veterinarians are responsible for many aspects of human health promotion and disease prevention, especially in the areas of food safety, environmental health, prevention and control of zoonotic diseases, and the human-animal bond. To accomplish these important missions, successful veterinarians along with their professional associates must learn to communicate effectively with a variety of individuals, ranging from health care professionals in other disciplines to print and electronic journalists to the day-to-day clients who walk off the street into the veterinary practice.

> **TECHNICIAN'S NOTE** Veterinarians and technicians are responsible for many aspects of human health promotion and disease prevention.

One of the most important lines of communication, however, exists between veterinary practitioners and the members of their veterinary health care teams. Veterinary technicians serve as vital members of these health care teams. As such, these technicians must be able to understand and correctly use the nomenclature and terminology for almost every specialty discipline within veterinary medicine. This is especially true for the discipline of veterinary parasitology, the study of parasitic relationships affecting domesticated, wild, exotic, and laboratory animals and, to some extent, parasites that have the potential to be transmitted directly from animals to humans. If animal parasites are to be effectively treated and controlled, the veterinary technician must become "fluent" in the language of parasitology and be able to communicate effectively using the specialized terminology associated with these parasites and with the complex interactions between parasites and their animal hosts. This chapter assists the veterinary technician in acquiring fluency with regard to veterinary parasitology.

SYMBIOSIS

Planet Earth is home to millions of species of diverse, living organisms that include plants,

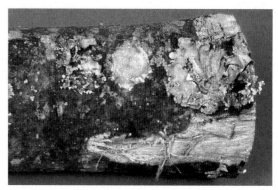

FIGURE 1-1 Lichen growing on the side of a tree is a symbiotic relationship between fungus and alga.

animals, fungi, algae, and unicellular organisms. Inevitably, there are millions of complex relationships taking place between and among these differing species. Many organisms live together in varied, intricate relationships. The term symbiosis (*sym* meaning "together" and *biosis* meaning "living," thus "living together") describes any association, either temporary or permanent, between at least two living organisms of different species. Each member of this association is called a symbiont. For example, lichen growing on the side of a tree (Figure 1-1) is actually a very complex symbiotic relationship between a fungus and an alga. Even the act of a human owning a dog and living with that dog is a type of symbiotic relationship. Two different living species cohabitate; the human "owner" and the "pet" dog are members of a very ancient symbiotic relationship.

> **TECHNICIAN'S NOTE** *Symbiosis* means living together between two different species or organisms. Some of these relationships are beneficial, some are indifferent, and others are detrimental to one or more of the organisms.

There are five types of symbiotic relationships: predator-prey, phoresis, mutualism, commensalism, and parasitism. A predator-prey relationship is an extremely short-term relationship in which one symbiont benefits at the expense of the other. For example, a lion (the predator) will kill a zebra (the prey). The prey pays with its life and serves as a food source for the predator.

In phoresis (*phore* meaning "to carry") the smaller member of the symbiotic relationship is mechanically carried about by the larger member. The bacterium *Moraxella bovis,* the etiologic agent of infectious bovine keratoconjunctivitis, or pinkeye of cattle, is mechanically carried from the eyes of one cow to those of another on the sticky footpads of the face fly, *Musca autumnalis* (Figure 1-2).

The term mutualism describes an association in which both organisms in a symbiotic relationship benefit. For example, within the liquid rumen environment of a cow are millions of microscopic, swimming, unicellular, ciliated protozoans. The cow provides these tiny creatures with a warm, liquid environment in which to live. In return, the rumen ciliates break down cellulose for the cow and aid in its digestion processes.

> **TECHNICIAN'S NOTE** In mutualistic symbiosis, both organisms benefit from the relationship.

The term commensalism describes an association in which one symbiont benefits and the other is neither benefited nor harmed. An example is the relationship between the shark and the remora, its "hitchhiker." The remora attaches to the underside of the shark and hitches a ride. The remora also eats the food scraps, or leftovers, after the shark's meals.

The remora benefits from this relationship, whereas the shark is neither benefited nor harmed.

In parasitism, an association exists between two organisms of different species in which one member (the parasite) lives on or within the other member (the host) and may cause harm. The parasite becomes metabolically dependent on the host.

This book discusses the host-parasite relationships between domesticated and wild animals and their parasites. Parasitology is the study of such parasitic relationships.

PARASITISM

Parasitism can occur in differing degrees. In parasitiasis the parasite is present on or within the host and is potentially pathogenic (harmful); however, the animal does not exhibit outward clinical signs of disease. For example, healthy cattle on pasture may harbor bovine trichostrongyles (roundworms) in their gastrointestinal tracts, but the cattle do not exhibit outward clinical signs of parasitism (Figure 1-3). Parasitiasis describes this type of parasitic relationship.

In parasitosis, the parasite is present on or within the host and does produce obvious injury or harm to the host animal. The host exhibits obvious outward signs of clinical parasitism (Figure 1-4). For example, an emaciated cow on pasture certainly harbors bovine trichostrongyles (roundworms) in

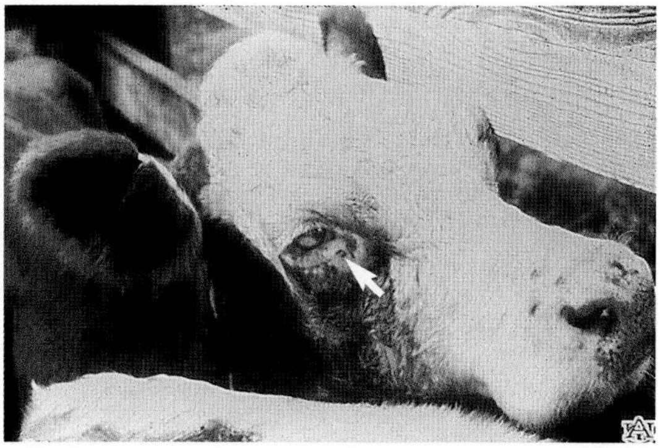

FIGURE 1-2 *Moraxella bovis,* etiologic agent of infectious bovine keratoconjunctivitis (pinkeye), is mechanically carried from the eyes of one cow to those of another on sticky foot pads of the face fly, *Musca autumnalis.*

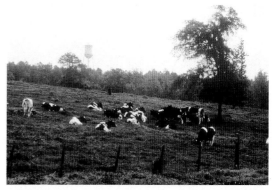

FIGURE 1-3 Healthy cattle on pasture may harbor bovine trichostrongyles (roundworms) in their gastrointestinal tracts but not exhibit outward clinical signs of parasitism. This condition is known as **parasitiasis**.

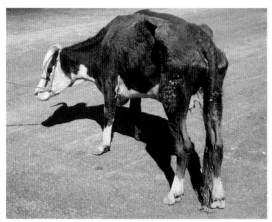

FIGURE 1-4 This emaciated cow probably harbors millions of bovine trichostrongyles (roundworms) in its gastrointestinal tract. As a result of this parasitism, the cow exhibits obvious outward clinical signs. This condition is referred to as **parasitosis**.

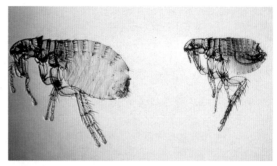

FIGURE 1-5 These cat fleas (*Ctenocephalides felis*) live within a dog's hair coat. They are ectoparasites and produce **ecto-parasitism**. Similarly, these fleas produce infestations in the host's hair coat.

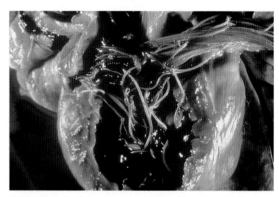

FIGURE 1-6 These heartworms (*Dirofilaria immitis*) live in a dog's heart. They are endoparasites and produce **endo-parasitism**. Heartworms produce infection within the host's heart. The dog is a definitive host for canine heartworm and harbors adult, sexual, or mature stages of the parasite.

its gastrointestinal tract. Parasitosis describes this type of parasitic relationship.

> **TECHNICIAN'S NOTE** A parasite can cause parasitiasis in some animals with a low parasite burden or number; however, it may also cause parasitosis with a high parasite burden.

In any parasitic relationship the parasite lives on or within the body of the host. If the parasite lives *on* the body of the host, it is called an ectoparasite. Cat fleas (*Ctenocephalides felis*) on a dog are ectoparasites (Figure 1-5). If a parasite lives *within* the body of the host, it is called an endoparasite. The dog heartworm (*Dirofilaria immitis*) is an endoparasite (Figure 1-6). Ectoparasitism is parasitism by an external parasite. Endoparasitism is parasitism by an internal parasite. Similarly, an ectoparasite will produce an infestation on the host, and an endo-parasite will produce an infection within that host.

> **TECHNICIAN'S NOTE** It is important to understand that an infection is a condition caused inside the host's body, whereas an infestation is a condition caused on the outside of the host's body.

Both endoparasitism and ectoparasitism in domestic animals can be treated by administering parasiticides, chemical compounds (both simple and complex) used to treat specific internal and external parasites. The different types of parasiticides include anthelmintics (or anthelminthics; compounds developed to kill roundworms, tapeworms, flukes, and thorny-headed worms), acaricides (compounds developed to kill mites and ticks), insecticides (compounds developed to kill insects), and antiprotozoals (compounds developed to kill protozoan organisms).

Sometimes a parasite will wander from its usual site of infection into an organ or location in which it does not ordinarily live. When this happens, the parasite is called an erratic parasite, or aberrant

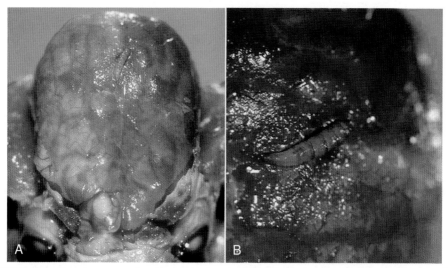

FIGURE 1-7 A, *Cuterebra* species (warbles, wolves) in the skin of dogs or cats may migrate into the cranial vault; *Cuterebra* is then an erratic (aberrant) parasite that has become "lost" on its migration path. **B,** Enlargement of a parasite in the cranial vault.

parasite. For example, *Cuterebra* species, called *warbles* or *wolves,* found in the skin of dogs or cats may accidentally "wander" or migrate into the cranial vault. When this happens, *Cuterebra* becomes an erratic (aberrant) parasite (Figure 1-7).

A parasite can be found in a host in which it does not usually live. When this occurs, the parasite is called an incidental parasite. For example, humans can become infected with larval stages of *D. immitis,* the canine heartworm. Because humans are not the usual host, the canine heartworm is an incidental parasite in people.

Organisms that are "free living" (nonparasitic) can become parasitic in certain hosts. These organisms are called facultative parasites. An example is *Pelodera strongyloides,* a free-living soil nematode (roundworm) that usually lives in the superficial layers of the soil as a "nonparasite." However, this roundworm is capable of penetrating the skin of many domesticated animals, particularly dogs lying in moist dirt and "downer cattle," and establishing a parasitic skin infection. *P. strongyloides* is therefore a facultative parasite.

An obligatory parasite, however, is a parasite that must lead a parasitic existence. These are not capable of leading a free-living existence. *D. immitis,*

the canine heartworm, is an obligatory parasite; most of the parasites that affect domesticated and wild animals are obligatory parasites.

> **TECHNICIAN'S NOTE**   Some parasites can have obligatory stages in their development when they need a host, and some life stages can be nonparasitic. In addition, with some parasites only the female adult is parasitic, whereas the free-living males and immature females are nonparasitic.

A parasite does not necessarily have to live on or within a host. It can make frequent short visits to its host to obtain nourishment or other benefits. Such a parasite is called a periodic parasite. The best example of a periodic parasite is the female mosquito, which sucks blood from the vertebrate host. The host's blood is required for her egg development; without a blood meal the female mosquito will not have sufficient protein to lay her eggs.

Living creatures or objects that are not parasitic may be mistaken for or erroneously identified as parasites. These are referred to as pseudoparasites. Sometimes, fecal flotation procedures reveal pollen grains from trees, such as pine pollen (Figure 1-8),

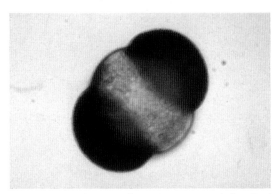

FIGURE 1-8 Pollen grains from a pine tree revealed on fecal flotation. A beginning veterinary student or technician may view this pollen on fecal flotation and erroneously assume the grains are parasites when they are actually pseudoparasites.

or from flowering plants. A novice veterinary student or veterinary technician may view these pollen grains on fecal flotation and erroneously identify them as parasites, but they are pseudoparasites.

> **TECHNICIAN'S NOTE** Novice veterinary students and veterinary technicians might mistake air bubbles on a fecal flotation slide for a parasite egg as well.

LIFE CYCLE

Each parasite has its own life cycle (Figure 1-9). The life cycle is the development of a parasite through its various life stages. Every parasite has at least one definitive host and may have one or more intermediate hosts. The definitive host is the host that harbors the adult, sexual, or mature stages of the parasite. For example, the dog is the definitive host for *D. immitis;* mature male and female heartworms (the sexual stages of the parasite) are found in the right ventricle and pulmonary arteries of the dog's heart (see Figure 1-6). The intermediate host is the host that harbors the larval, juvenile, immature, or asexual stages of the parasite. The female mosquito is the intermediate host for *D. immitis;* larval or immature heartworms (the developing stages of the parasite) are found in the Malpighian tubules and proboscis of the mosquito (Figures 1-10 and 1-11). The intermediate host transfers the parasite from

one definitive host to another. A parasite may have more than one intermediate host. In the life cycle of *Platynosomum concinnum,* the lizard-poisoning fluke of cats, a land snail is the first intermediate host and a lizard is the second intermediate host for the parasite. This liver fluke requires two intermediate hosts to infect the cat.

In a special type of intermediate host, a parasite does not undergo any development but instead remains arrested or encysted ("in suspended animation") within the host's tissues (either definitive host or intermediate host). This host is called the transport host, or paratenic host. The larvae remain in this suspended state until the definitive host eats the transport host. Once within the definitive host, the larvae "wake up," establish an infection, migrate to their predilection site, and grow to adult parasites within the definitive host.

A reservoir host is a vertebrate host in which a parasite or disease occurs in nature and is a source of infection for humans and domesticated animals. Heartworms may develop in the right ventricle and pulmonary artery of wild wolves and coyotes. Wolves and coyotes may be reservoir hosts for heartworm; the infection may be spread from the wolf or coyote to the family pet by the mosquito as intermediate host.

> **TECHNICIAN'S NOTE** Some parasites can serve as intermediate hosts for other parasites as well as being parasites themselves. For example, the mosquito feeds off animals and is thus a parasite but also acts as an intermediate host to the parasite that causes heartworm disease.

A homoxenous or monoxenous parasite is a parasite that infects only one type of host. For example, *Eimeria tenella,* a coccidian, infects only chickens. Similarly, a stenoxenous parasite is a parasite with a narrow host range. Because *E. tenella* will only infect chickens, it is a stenoxenous parasite. This protozoan parasite infects only the ceca of chickens (Figure 1-12). A euryxenous parasite is a parasite with a very broad host range. For example, *Toxoplasma gondii* infects more than 300 species of warm-blooded vertebrates; therefore it is a euryxenous parasite.

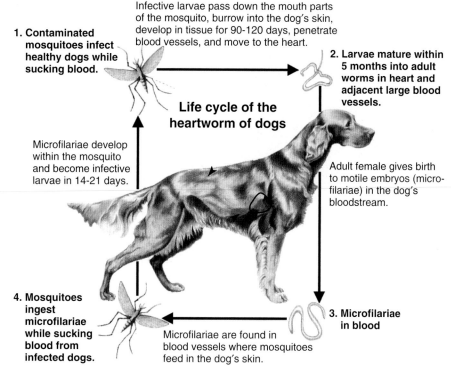

1. Contaminated mosquitoes infect healthy dogs while sucking blood.

Infective larvae pass down the mouth parts of the mosquito, burrow into the dog's skin, develop in tissue for 90-120 days, penetrate blood vessels, and move to the heart.

2. Larvae mature within 5 months into adult worms in heart and adjacent large blood vessels.

Life cycle of the heartworm of dogs

Microfilariae develop within the mosquito and become infective larvae in 14-21 days.

Adult female gives birth to motile embryos (micro-filariae) in the dog's bloodstream.

4. Mosquitoes ingest microfilariae while sucking blood from infected dogs.

Microfilariae are found in blood vessels where mosquitoes feed in the dog's skin.

3. Microfilariae in blood

FIGURE 1-9 Life cycle of *Dirofilaria immitis*. In this life cycle the dog is a definitive host and the mosquito is an intermediate host. Mature male and female heartworms (sexual stages of the parasite) are found in the right ventricle and pulmonary arteries of a dog's heart.

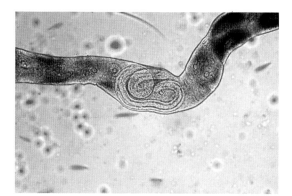

FIGURE 1-10 The mosquito is intermediate host for *Dirofilaria immitis;* larval or immature heartworms (developing stages of the parasite) are found in the mosquito's Malpighian tubules.

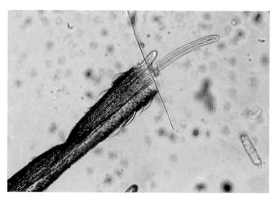

FIGURE 1-11 Larval or immature heartworms (developing stages of the parasite) may also be found in the mosquito's proboscis. The mosquito (intermediate host) transmits heartworm infection from one dog to another.

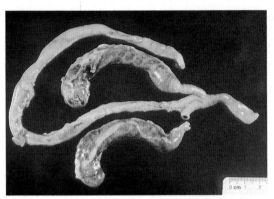

FIGURE 1-12 *Eimeria tenella* infects only the ceca of chickens; therefore it is a homoxenous or monoxenous parasite.

> **TECHNICIAN'S NOTE** It should be noted that *Toxoplasma gondii* infects more than 300 species of warm-blooded vertebrates; its sexual stages occur only in the feline.

A zoonosis is any disease or parasite that is transmissible from animals to humans. Examples of zoonotic parasites are *T. gondii*, *Trichinella spiralis*, *Ancylostoma caninum*, and *Toxocara canis*. Zoonotic parasites are discussed in later chapters.

THE LINNAEAN CLASSIFICATION SCHEME

In beginning biology, students must learn the classification scheme perfected by Carl Linnaeus, an early Swedish biologist. Every organism can be classified using the following classification scheme: kingdom, phylum, class, order, family, genus, and species (Figure 1-13). Students often remember this classification scheme with the simple mnemonic device "*King Philip came over for good spaghetti*," in which the first letter of each word in the sentence corresponds to the first letter in the Linnaean classification scheme.

The Linnaean classification scheme works in the following manner. Several million species of animals, plants, fungi, protozoans, and algae live on the earth. These creatures may have different common names in different regions of the world. A common name may refer to different organisms

in different places. The solution to this problem was to give each organism a scientific name composed of two Latin words, which is commonly written in italics. The first word is capitalized and is the genus name. The genus indicates the group to which a particular type of animal or plant belongs. The second word is not capitalized; it is the specific epithet and indicates the type of animal itself. Examples of common names of animals and their corresponding scientific names are the dog, *Canis familiaris;* the cat, *Felis catus;* the housefly, *Musca domestica;* and a bacterium normally found in the gut, *Escherichia coli.* Similar species are grouped together into the same genus. Similar genera (plural form of *genus*) are grouped together in the same family. Similar families are grouped together in the same order. Similar orders are grouped together in the same class. Similar classes are grouped together in the same phylum. Similar phyla are grouped together in the same kingdom. Therefore the classification scheme for the dog is as follows:

> **TECHNICIAN'S NOTE** For ease in finding particular parasites, this book is organized by phylum/class. Tables are provided showing the parasites by the hosts they affect along with the corresponding pages on which they are described.

Domain: Eukaryota
  Kingdom: Animalia
    Phylum: Chordata
      Subphylum: Vertebrata
        Class: Mammalia
          Order: Carnivora
            Family: Canidae
              Genus: *Canis*
                Species: *familiaris*

Every living creature has its own unique classification scheme. This text discusses many parasites that affect domesticated animals. It is important to learn the scientific names, the common names, the hosts, and the key identifying features for all of these parasites.

The domain has been added to the Linnaean classification scheme. There are three recognized domains in the scheme: bacteria, archaea, and

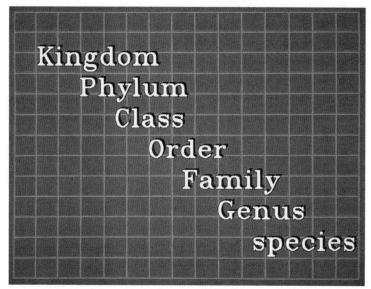

FIGURE 1-13 All organisms can be classified using the Linnaean classification scheme.

eukaryota. Eukaryota includes the kingdoms Plantae, Animalia, Protista, Monera, and Fungi.

The classification scheme contains the following five kingdoms: Plantae (plants), Animalia (animals), Protista (unicellular organisms), Monera (algae), and Fungi (fungi). Veterinary parasitology is concerned with only two of these kingdoms as true parasites of domesticated animals. The first is the kingdom Animalia, which contains platyhelminths (flatworms—trematodes [flukes] and cestodes [tapeworms]), nematodes (roundworms), acanthocephalans (thorny-headed worms), annelids (leeches), and arthropods (insects, mites, ticks, spiders, pentastomes, and other creatures with jointed appendages). The second is the kingdom Protista, which contains protozoans (unicellular organisms). The

following chapters present parasites from each of these groups and describe their significance in veterinary parasitology.

TECHNICIAN'S NOTE Most parasites of domestic animals belong to the kingdom Animalia.

Any student of veterinary parasitology must use the terms presented in this chapter and their definitions as the "framework" on which to build greater proficiency in this discipline. As with the veterinarians with whom they work, veterinary technicians must be encouraged to embrace continual improvement in their professional knowledge and competence.

CHAPTER ONE TEST

MATCHING—Match the term with the correct phrase or term.

A. Phoresis

B. Parasitology

C. Ectoparasite

D. Endoparasite

E. Erratic/aberrant parasite

F. Pseudoparasite

G. Incidental parasite

H. Periodic parasite

I. Zoonosis

J. Linnaean classification scheme

1. Parasite that wanders into an organ in which it does not normally live

2. Parasite in a host in which it does not usually live

3. Study of parasitic relationships

4. Creature or object that is mistaken for a parasite

5. Parasite that makes frequent visits to a host to obtain nourishment

6. Kingdom, phylum, class, order, family, genus, species

7. Face fly that carries the pinkeye bacterium from one cow to another

8. Disease or parasite that is transmissible from animals to humans

9. Parasitism by an internal parasite

10. Parasitism by an external parasite

QUESTIONS FOR THOUGHT AND DISCUSSION

1. Why is it important for a veterinary technician to know and understand the terminology associated with veterinary parasitology?

2. Compare and contrast the following terms. Why is it important to understand the difference between each pair of terms?
   - Intermediate host versus definitive host
   - Parasitosis versus parasitiasis
   - Infestation versus infection
   - Common name versus scientific name
   - Anthelmintic versus insecticide
   - Obligatory parasite versus facultative parasite
   - Stenoxenous parasite versus euryxenous parasite

3. Define three types of symbiotic relationships and give one example of each.

4. Briefly discuss the importance of the Linnaean classification scheme.

5. What are the five kingdoms within the Linnaean classification scheme? Which two are most important in veterinary parasitology?

2 Parasites That Infect and Infest Domestic Animals

OUTLINE

LEARNING OBJECTIVES

After studying this chapter, the reader should be able to do the following:

• Understand that many types of living "creatures" are capable of parasitizing domesticated, wild, exotic, and laboratory animals.

• Understand that the Linnaean classification scheme is an important tool for studying veterinary parasitology.

KEY TERMS

Acanthocephalans	Digenetic flukes	Parasitism	Toxins
Alimentary canal	Intermediate hosts	Pseudotapeworms	True tapeworms
Arthropoda	Leeches	Roundworms	Vectors
Causal agents	Monogenetic flukes	Tegument	Venomous substances

Chapter 1 describes parasitism as an association between two organisms of different species in which one member (the parasite) lives on or within the other member (the host) and may cause harm. The parasite is metabolically dependent on the host.

In parasitology, the study of parasitic relationships, parasitic groups are classified according to the Linnaean classification system. This chapter presents the parasites that infect and infest domesticated animals, indicating their important characteristics and their place in the Linnaean system.

MONOGENETIC TREMATODES (MONOGENETIC FLUKES)

Kingdom: Animalia (animals)
    Phylum: Platyhelminthes (flatworms)
        Class: Trematoda (flukes)
            Subclass: Monogenea (monogenetic flukes)

Monogenetic flukes are ectoparasites of fish, amphibians, and reptiles. They are rarely parasites of mammals. These flukes are seen most often as ectoparasites of the gills, skin, fins, and mouth of fishes and are rarely observed in a veterinary clinical situation. They might be seen by a veterinarian who specializes in diseases of aquarium fish. Also some veterinarians may specialize in fish farming or some aspect of aquaculture. Under these conditions, monogenetic flukes may be frequently observed.

> **TECHNICIAN'S NOTE** Monogenetic flukes are ectoparasites that parasitize fish, amphibians, and reptiles. They are rarely seen in a veterinary clinic setting.

DIGENETIC TREMATODES (DIGENETIC FLUKES)

Kingdom: Animalia (animals)
   Phylum: Platyhelminthes (flatworms)
      Class: Trematoda (flukes)
         Subclass: Digenea (digenetic flukes)

Digenetic flukes are important parasites of both large and small animals. These flattened, leaf-shaped flukes are primarily endoparasites of the gastrointestinal tract; however, digenetic flukes can also infect the lungs and blood vasculature. Regardless of the site of infection, the operculated eggs of these flukes can be identified in the feces of domestic animals.

> **TECHNICIAN'S NOTE** Digenetic flukes infect both large and small animals and are seen in the veterinary clinic setting.

EUCESTODES (TRUE TAPEWORMS)

Kingdom: Animalia (animals)
   Phylum: Platyhelminthes (flatworms)
      Class: Eucestoda (true tapeworms)

Adult true tapeworms are ribbonlike flatworms found in the gastrointestinal tract of their definitive hosts. True tapeworms lack a "gut" or alimentary canal; they absorb nutrients through their tegument (skin). The eggs of these tapeworms are frequently observed on fecal flotation. The larval stages of these true tapeworms may be found in a variety of extraintestinal tissue sites in domestic animals; the animals harboring the larval stages serve as the intermediate hosts. In these extraintestinal sites, the larval stages of these tapeworms may cause more pathology to the intermediate hosts than the adult tapeworm does to the definitive host in its intestinal sites.

> **TECHNICIAN'S NOTE** True tapeworms absorb nutrients from the host through their skin.

COTYLODA (PSEUDOTAPEWORMS)

Kingdom: Animalia (animals)
   Phylum: Platyhelminthes (flatworms)
      Class: Cotyloda (pseudotapeworms)

Similar to true tapeworms, adult pseudotapeworms are flattened and ribbonlike. They resemble true tapeworms and also are found in the gastrointestinal tract of their definitive hosts. Their egg stages may be diagnosed on fecal flotation; they produce operculated eggs. The larval stages of pseudotapeworms are found in microscopic aquatic crustaceans and in the musculature of fish and reptiles. These larval stages seldom produce pathology in domestic animals.

> **TECHNICIAN'S NOTE** Pseudotapeworms use microscopic aquatic crustaceans and the musculature of fish and reptiles as intermediate hosts for part of their life cycle.

NEMATODES (ROUNDWORMS)

Kingdom: Animalia (animals)
   Phylum: Nematoda (roundworms)

Nematodes, or roundworms, are elongated, unsegmented, cylindric worms. They are called *roundworms* because they are round when observed in cross section on histopathologic examination. Nematodes are the most numerous, complex, and variable among the helminth parasites of domesticated animals. They come in all sizes and shapes and can infect a variety of organs and organ systems.

They can produce significant pathology in domesticated animals. On planet Earth, nematodes are second only to arthropods with regard to their numbers and complexity of life cycles. The eggs and larvae of nematodes are most often diagnosed on fecal flotation, so it is important that veterinary technicians become proficient in their identification. Both adult and larval stages of nematodes can produce significant pathology in domesticated animals.

> **TECHNICIAN'S NOTE** The nematodes are the largest group of helminths that parasitize domesticated animals.

ACANTHOCEPHALANS (THORNY-HEADED WORMS)

Kingdom: Animalia (animals)
    Phylum: Acanthocephala (thorny-headed worms)

Acanthocephalans, or thorny-headed worms, are elongated, unsegmented, cylindric worms. They are different from nematodes, however, in that they possess a spiny proboscis on their anterior end. This spiny proboscis is used as an organ of attachment. Because of this anterior proboscis, acanthocephalans are often referred to as *thorny-headed worms*. As with the cestodes (tapeworms), thorny-headed worms lack a gut or alimentary tract; they also absorb nutrients through their tegument (skin). Adult acanthocephalans are very uncommon parasites and are most often found in the gastrointestinal tract. The eggs of these unusual parasites are diagnosed on fecal flotation.

> **TECHNICIAN'S NOTE** Acanthocephalans are referred to as *thorny-headed worms* because of the spiny proboscis on the anterior end, which is used as an organ of attachment.

HIRUDINEANS (LEECHES)

Kingdom: Animalia (animals)
    Phylum: Annelida (segmented worms)
        Class: Hirudinea (leeches)

Leeches are blood-feeding ectoparasites of both wild and domesticated animals. These annulated (ringed) worms are typically found in freshwater, although there may be marine and terrestrial varieties. Leeches may produce significant pathology in both wild and domesticated animals, or they may be beneficial when used after reconstructive surgical procedures in both animals and humans.

> **TECHNICIAN'S NOTE** Some species of leeches are used for medicinal purposes in reconstructive surgical procedures in humans and animals.

ARTHROPODS

Kingdom: Animalia (animals)
    Phylum: Arthropoda (animals with jointed legs)

The phylum Arthropoda is the largest phylum in the animal kingdom. This phylum is quite complex, containing pentastomes, crustaceans, centipedes, millipedes, insects, mites, ticks, scorpions, and spiders.

Arthropods are important in veterinary medicine for the following four reasons:
1. Arthropods may serve as causal agents themselves.
2. They may serve as intermediate hosts for certain helminths and protozoans.
3. They may serve as vectors for bacteria, viruses, spirochetes, and chlamydial agents.
4. They may produce toxins or venomous substances.

Arthropods may parasitize the host in both the adult and juvenile stages.

> **TECHNICIAN'S NOTE** Arthropoda is the largest phylum in the animal kingdom and includes most of the ectoparasites seen in the veterinary profession.

PROTISTA (PROTOZOANS)

Kingdom: Protista (protozoans—unicellular, or single-celled, organisms)

Trematodes, tapeworms, pseudotapeworms, roundworms, thorny-headed worms, leeches, and arthropods are all members of the animal kingdom. All the parasites described here are metazoan, or multicellular, organisms. The remaining parasites belong to the kingdom Protista, which is made up of all the unicellular organisms. The majority of protozoans on planet Earth are free living; however, those that are parasitic can cause significant pathology in domesticated animals. Within this kingdom are several phyla that include flagellates, amoebae, apicomplexans, and ciliates. These protozoans are the primary protozoans that cause significant pathology in domesticated animals. Despite their tiny size, protozoans have complex life cycles and may cause significant pathologic changes in the tissues and organs of domesticated animals.

TECHNICIAN'S NOTE The protozoans are single-celled endoparasites that include such organisms as *Giardia* species and the organisms that cause coccidiosis.

Each of these groups of parasites and its significance to veterinary parasitology are discussed in detail in the upcoming chapters.

CHAPTER TWO TEST

MATCHING—Match the term with the correct phrase or term.

A. Platyhelminthes	1. Thorny-headed worms
B. Protists	2. Pseudotapeworms
C. Eucestodes	3. Leeches
D. Cotyloda	4. True tapeworms
E. Nematodes	5. Roundworms
F. Acanthocephalans	6. Animals with jointed appendages
G. Metazoans	7. Flukes
H. Hirudineans	8. Unicellular or single-celled organisms
I. Arthropods	9. Flatworms
J. Trematodes	10. Multicellular organisms

QUESTION FOR THOUGHT AND DISCUSSION

1. Why is the Linnaean classification system so important in the study of veterinary parasitology? Can you think of a more efficient way to study, learn, and remember the various groups of parasites of domesticated, wild, exotic, and laboratory animals?

3 Introduction to the Nematodes

LEARNING OBJECTIVES

After studying this chapter, the reader should be able to do the following:

- Briefly discuss the importance of nematodes in veterinary practice.
- Describe the important external morphologic features for identifying nematodes.
- Name the important parts of the male nematode's reproductive system.
- Name the important parts of the female nematode's reproductive system.
- Determine which reproductive system (male or female) is more important in veterinary parasitology (diagnostically speaking).

- Describe the four types of nematode eggs.
- Determine the differences among these reproductive terms: oviparous, ovoviviparous, and larviparous.
- Describe the "typical life cycle" of a representative nematode.
- Explain the difference between a direct life cycle and an indirect life cycle.
- Integrate these terms with the nematode parasites covered in Chapter 4.

KEY TERMS

Ascaroid- or ascarid-
   type egg
Body cavity
Bursal rays
Cervical alae
Cloaca
Copulatory bursa
Dioecious
Direct life cycle
Hypodermis

Indirect life cycle
Infective third-stage
   larva
Larviparous
Leaf crown
Molts
Morula stage
Oviduct
Oviparous
Ovoviviparous

Papillae
Pseudocoelom
Pseudocoelomic
   membrane
Rectum
Seminal receptacle
Somatic muscular
   layer
Spicule pouch
Spicules

Spiruroid-type egg
Trichinelloid- or
   trichuroid-type
   egg
Trichostrongyle,
   strongyle-type egg
Tubular ovaries
Tubular testes
Vas deferens

Members of the phylum Nematoda, the nematodes, or roundworms, are the most numerous and most diverse group of animals on Earth. Approximately 10,000 species thrive in very diverse habitats. There are three basic types of nematodes: (1) the free-living nematodes residing in marine water, freshwater, and soil environments; (2) the nematodes that parasitize plants; and (3) the nematodes that parasitize domesticated and wild animals and humans. This chapter discusses the third category, nematodes that parasitize domesticated and wild animals and, to some extent, humans.

> **TECHNICIAN'S NOTE** Nematodes are collectively referred to as *roundworms* and are the most numerous and diverse group of animals on Earth.

NEMATODES OF IMPORTANCE IN VETERINARY MEDICINE

Nematodes in domesticated farm animals in the United States alone cause the loss of billions of dollars in animal agriculture resulting from veterinary bills and death. Plant nematodes cause approximately 10% of cultivated crops to be lost each year. It is impossible to determine similar monetary losses in the pet or companion animal "industry."

KEY MORPHOLOGIC FEATURES

Protozoans, discussed in Chapters 10 and 11, are unicellular organisms; nematodes, however, are multicellular organisms. Whereas trematodes (leaflike in form) and cestodes (chainlike or boxcarlike in form) are dorsoventrally flattened in cross section, nematodes are unsegmented, elongate, rounded on both ends, circular in cross section, and bilaterally symmetric (Figure 3-1); thus they are often referred to as *roundworms*. Nematodes come in a variety of sizes from *Strongyloides stercoralis*, a tiny parasitic female worm only 2 mm in length and about 35 μm wide (Figure 3-2), to *Dioctophyma renale*, "the giant kidney worm" measuring 100 cm (1 m) in length and 1.2 cm wide (Figure 3-3). As mentioned previously, most nematodes are cylindric and rounded on both ends; however, nematodes come in a wide variety of shapes from

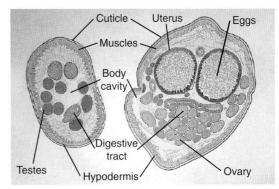

FIGURE 3-1 Cross section of male *(left)* and female *(right)* *Ascaris suum,* the pig roundworm. Whereas flukes and tapeworms are dorsoventrally flattened, roundworms are usually round in cross section.

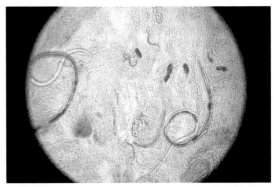

FIGURE 3-2 Numerous parasitic female *Strongyloides stercoralis* (approximately 2 mm in length and about 35 μm wide) recovered from mucosal scrapings from a canine small intestine. Also note the presence of eggs and first-stage larvae. This is an unusual nematode in that parasitic males do not exist.

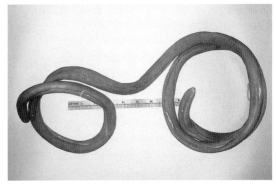

FIGURE 3-3 Largest nematode known to parasitize domesticated animals, *Dioctophyma renale,* the "giant kidney worm" of dogs. This largest of parasites measures 100 cm (1 m) in length and is approximately 1.2 cm wide.

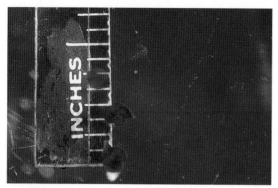

FIGURE 3-4 Nematodes come in a variety of shapes. Some are spherical, such as *Tetrameres* species, which parasitize the gizzard of domesticated and wild birds.

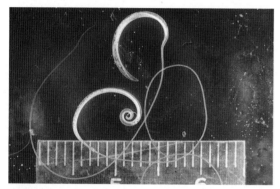

FIGURE 3-5 Whiplike *Trichuris* species parasitize every domesticated animal except the horse.

spherical (definitely not cylindric), such as *Tetrameres* species, parasites of the gizzard of domesticated and wild birds (Figure 3-4), to the whiplike *Trichuris* species, which parasitize every domesticated animal except the horse (Figure 3-5).

> **TECHNICIAN'S NOTE** Nematodes are referred to as *roundworms* because they are circular in cross section, rounded at both ends, unsegmented, elongate, and bilaterally symmetric.

External Morphologic Features

Nematodes are covered by a thin cuticle (see Figure 3-1). This cuticle covers the exterior body surface of the nematode and extends into all its body openings, that is, the mouth, esophagus, and rectal and genital openings. On the external surface the cuticle has a variety of modifications. There may be lateral

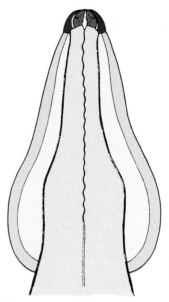

FIGURE 3-6 Diagrammatic representation of lateral flattened expansion of the cuticle on the anterior end of *Toxocara cati,* the feline ascarid. These expansions are called *cervical alae.*

flattened expansions of the cuticle in the region of the anterior end; these expansions are called **cervical alae** (Figure 3-6). There also may be lateral flattened expansions of the cuticle in the region of the posterior end of some male nematodes; this posterior lateral expansion is called the **copulatory bursa** and serves to hold on to or to grasp the female nematode during the mating process (Figure 3-7). The copulatory bursa is composed of fingerlike projections called **bursal rays**. Between each adjacent bursal ray are thin membranes. The male's highly chitinous and pigmented **spicules** (see Figure 3-7) (the intromittent organs, or "penis") are associated with the copulatory bursa. The cervical alae and the copulatory bursa are only two of the many modifications of the external cuticle of nematodes. The nematode's cuticle is secreted, or formed, by the thin layer directly beneath it, the **hypodermis** (see Figure 3-1).

Just beneath the hypodermis lies the **somatic muscular layer**, the layer of muscles that enables the nematode to move about (see Figure 3-1, *muscles*). These muscle fibers are spindle-shaped and lie along the edge of the hypodermis. Nematodes also possess specialized muscles that aid in

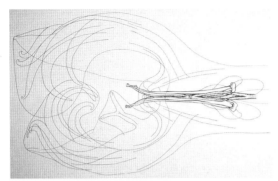

FIGURE 3-7 Diagrammatic representation of lateral flattened expansion of the cuticle on the posterior end of male *Haemonchus contortus*, the "barberpole worm" of ruminants. This expansion is called the *copulatory bursa* and serves to hold on to or grasp the female nematode during the mating process. The copulatory bursa is composed of fingerlike projections called *bursal rays*. Between each adjacent bursal ray are thin membranes. Male spicules (or intromittent organs) are associated with the copulatory bursa.

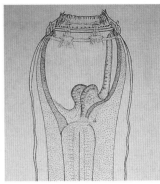

FIGURE 3-8 Fingerlike projections, or bumps, called *papillae* on the anterior end of *Strongylus vulgaris*. Collectively, these papillae may number as many as 40 and are referred to as the *leaf crown*. The mouth connects to a buccal cavity, which connects to the esophagus, which eventually connects to the long, winding intestine.

feeding and reproductive activities. The muscles line the nematode's body cavity (see Figure 3-1). Unlike trematodes (flukes) and cestodes (tapeworms), which lack a body cavity, nematodes (roundworms) do have a body cavity. The body cavity of a typical nematode is not considered a true coelom; it is a pseudocoelom lined by a pseudocoelomic membrane.

> **TECHNICIAN'S NOTE** The nematode has a pseudocoelom, which lies between the middle and inner layers of the three body-tissue layers, rather than a true coelom (or true body cavity).

Internal Morphologic Features

The most important of the nematode's organ systems are the digestive and reproductive systems.

The digestive tract of the typical nematode is a long, straight tube that extends from the mouth to the anus. On cross section the digestive tract resembles a tube within a tube (see Figure 3-1, *digestive tract*).

The mouth may be surrounded by lips, numbering two to eight. In some nematodes the lips are replaced by fingerlike projections, or bumps, called papillae. Collectively, these papillae may number as

many as 40 and are referred to as the leaf crown (Figure 3-8). The mouth connects to a buccal cavity, which connects to the esophagus, which connects to a long, winding intestine. The intestine ends with an opening to the outside. Female nematodes have a rectum, and male nematodes have a cloaca. Remember that the cloaca and the rectum are lined with cuticle and open to the outside through an anus. The part of the nematode's body posterior to the anus is the tail.

> **TECHNICIAN'S NOTE** The most important organ systems of the nematode are the reproductive system and the digestive system.

Whereas trematodes (flukes) and cestodes (tapeworms) are hermaphroditic (or monoecious), nematodes are dioecious; that is, they have separate sexes. There are both male nematodes and female nematodes.

The male reproductive organs consist of one or two tubular testes (see Figure 3-1). Usually, a vas deferens leads from the testes to the cloaca. There may be a spicule pouch, which contains two spicules. Remember that the male nematode's spicules (or intromittent organs) are associated with the copulatory bursa and serve to open the female nematode's vulva during copulation to allow sperm to enter the vagina.

The female reproductive organs consist of one or two tubular ovaries (see Figure 3-1, *ovary*). Usually an oviduct leads from the ovary to the uterus. A seminal receptacle for sperm storage may be present. The uterus leads to the vagina, which opens to the outside through the vulva. The uterus may contain thousands of eggs or larvae (see Figure 3-1, *uterus* and *eggs*). Parasitic nematodes are very prolific; a single female nematode may produce several thousand eggs (or larvae) each day. The reproductive system is important because it allows for the production of eggs (and eventually offspring). A veterinary diagnostician confronted with an unrecognized type of nematode can dissect it, and if the nematode is a female, characteristic eggs (or larvae) may be released. When examined microscopically, these eggs or larvae provide a valuable clue as to the type (or species) of nematode.

> ⓘ **TECHNICIAN'S NOTE** A female nematode can produce thousands of eggs or larvae each day; however, whipworms tend to produce fewer eggs and release them only every third day.

Female nematodes produce several egg types: (1) the ascaroid, or ascarid, type (e.g., *Toxocara canis*) (Figure 3-9); (2) the trichostrongyle or strongyle type (e.g., *Haemonchus contortus* of ruminants, *Strongylus vulgaris* of horses, *Ancylostoma caninum*

of dogs) (Figure 3-10); (3) the spiruroid, or spirurid, type (e.g., *Spirocerca lupi* of dogs, *Physaloptera* spp. of dogs and cats) (Figure 3-11); and (4) the trichinelloid or trichuroid type (e.g., *Trichuris vulpis*, the whipworm of dogs, *Capillaria* spp.) (Figure 3-12). In addition, some adult female nematodes produce characteristic larval stages: (1) the microfilaria, or prelarval, stage (e.g., *Dirofilaria immitis* of dogs) (Figure 3-13); (2) the lungworm, or kinked-tail, larvae (e.g., *Aelurostrongylus abstrusus* of cats, *Filaroides osleri* of dogs) (Figure 3-14); and (3) the dracunculoid, or long-tailed, larvae

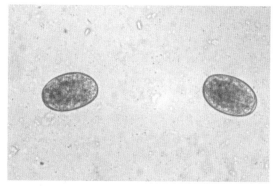

FIGURE 3-10 Trichostrongyle or strongyle, or hookworm, type of nematode egg is best represented by that of *Ancylostoma caninum*, the hookworm of dogs. The adult female nematode producing this egg type is oviparous. This nematode egg contains a morula stage within the eggshell.

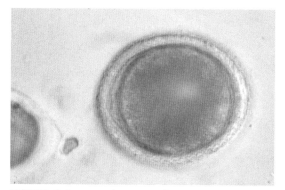

FIGURE 3-9 Ascaroid, or ascarid, type of nematode egg is best represented by that of *Toxocara canis*, the canine roundworm. The adult female nematode producing this egg type is oviparous. This nematode egg contains a single-cell stage within the eggshell.

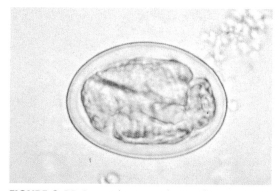

FIGURE 3-11 Spiruroid, or spirurid, type of nematode egg is best represented by that of *Spirocerca lupi*, the esophageal worm of dogs. The adult female nematode producing this egg type is ovoviviparous. This nematode egg contains a first-stage larva within the eggshell.

(e.g., *Dracunculus insignis* of dogs) (Figure 3-15). Nematode eggs (and larvae) vary greatly in size and composition. This fact is very important when attempting to render a diagnosis.

> **TECHNICIAN'S NOTE** Nematodes produce one of four types of characteristic eggs and can produce one of three types of characteristic larvae; however, the size and composition vary greatly.

Some female nematodes are oviparous; that is, the eggs produced by these nematodes contain a single-cell stage (see Figures 3-9 and 3-12) or a morula stage within the eggshell (see Figure 3-10). Some female nematodes are ovoviviparous; that is, the eggs produced by these nematodes contain a first-stage larva within the eggshell (see Figure 3-11). Finally, some female nematodes are larviparous; that is, they retain their eggs within the uterus and incubate them, then give birth to live larvae (see Figures 3-13, 3-14, and 3-15).

LIFE CYCLE OF THE NEMATODE

Compared with the complex life cycles of trematodes (flukes) and cestodes (tapeworms), the typical nematode life cycle is quite simple (Figure 3-16).

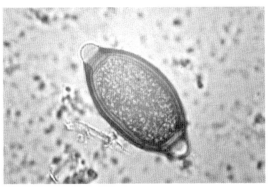

FIGURE 3-12 Trichinelloid type of nematode egg is best represented by that of *Trichuris vulpis*, the whipworm of dogs. The adult female nematode producing this egg type is oviparous. This nematode egg contains a single-cell stage within the eggshell.

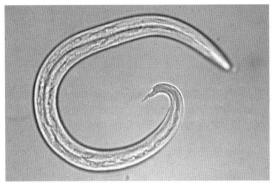

FIGURE 3-14 The first-stage, kinked-tail larvae of *Aelurostrongylus abstrusus*, the lungworm of cats, are characteristic of lungworm larvae. The adult female nematode producing this larval type is larviparous. She produces live offspring.

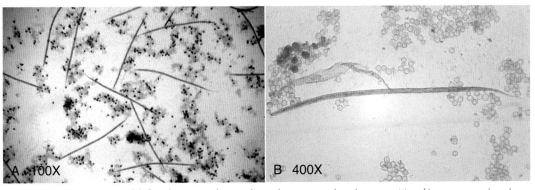

FIGURE 3-13 Some adult female nematodes produce characteristic larval stages. Microfilariae, or prelarval, stages of *Dirofilaria immitis*, the heartworm of dogs and cats, are characteristic of filarial parasites. The adult female nematode producing this larval type is larviparous. She produces live offspring.

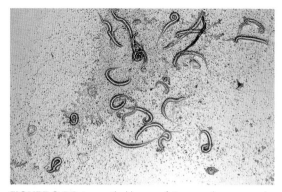

FIGURE 3-15 Long-tailed larvae of *Dracunculus insignis,* the guinea worm of dogs, are also characteristic larvae. The adult female nematode producing this larval type is larviparous. She produces live offspring.

The adult female nematode produces an egg, which is a single-cell stage within the eggshell. The original cell divides into two cells, two cells divide into four, four cells divide into eight, and so on. The original single-cell stage eventually develops into a morula stage, which in turn develops into a tadpole stage. The tadpole stage develops into a fully formed first-stage larva within the eggshell. This first-stage larva is ready to hatch. The larva emerges from the eggshell, molts (sheds its external cuticle), and develops into a second-stage larva. The second-stage larva eventually molts into the third-stage larva. This stage is often referred to as the infective third-stage larva because it is infective for the definitive host.

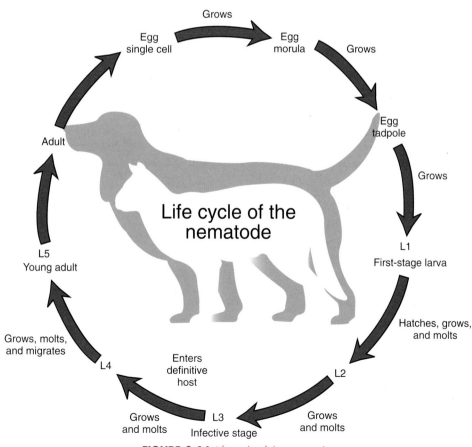

FIGURE 3-16 Life cycle of the nematode.

The first three larval stages can develop in the external environment or within the intermediate host. The intermediate host serves as the means of transmission to the definitive host. Once the infective third larval stage has been reached, it must return to the definitive host to survive. It infects the host either by direct penetration or by intervention of the intermediate host. The intermediate host serves as a means of transmission to the definitive host. Once within the definitive host, the third larval stage molts to the fourth larval stage, which subsequently molts to the fifth larval stage. The fifth larval stage is actually the immature, or preadult, nematode. This stage eventually migrates to its organ or system predilection site and develops into the sexually mature adult stage. The male and female nematodes breed, and the cycle begins again.

> **TECHNICIAN'S NOTE** The general nematode life cycle is a simple life cycle compared with the trematode and cestode life cycles.

Nematodes may or may not use an intermediate host. If there is no intermediate host, the life cycle is said to be a direct life cycle. For example, canine hookworms (*Ancylostoma* spp.) develop to the infective third stage in the external environment. They penetrate the dog's skin and migrate to the small intestine, where they mature to adults. The canine hookworm's life cycle is said to be "direct."

If the nematode uses an intermediate host, the life cycle is said to be an indirect life cycle. For example, a female mosquito ingests microfilariae of the canine heartworm, *D. immitis*, along with her blood meal. The mosquito incubates the microfilariae, and they eventually develop into infective third-stage larvae within the proboscis (mouthparts) of the mosquito. When the mosquito takes a blood meal from an uninfected dog, the infective third-stage larvae emerge from the mouthparts and migrate into the puncture wound made by the mosquito. Within the dog, the third-stage larvae molt to fourth-stage larvae and then molt again to fifth-stage larvae (immature, or preadult, heartworms). These larvae migrate to the right ventricle and pulmonary artery of the dog's heart, where they mature to adults. The adults breed, and the females produce microfilariae. The life cycle begins again. (See Figure 1-10.) The canine heartworm's life cycle is said to be *indirect*.

> **TECHNICIAN'S NOTE** The nematode can develop by a direct life cycle with no intermediate host, or it can develop through an indirect life cycle where an intermediate host is necessary to complete the life cycle.

A few nematodes produce eggs that do not hatch in the external environment. Within this egg the larva develops to the second stage but does not hatch from the egg. It remains within the egg; the infective stage for these nematodes is the egg containing the second-stage larva.

It is important to remember that there are many variations for this typical nematode life cycle. For every nematode there is a distinct life cycle and the detailed life cycles of the most commonly seen nematodes are typified within this chapter.

CHAPTER THREE TEST

MATCHING—Match the term with the correct phrase or term.

A. Direct life cycle

B. Indirect life cycle

C. Spicules

D. Cervical alae

E. Copulatory bursa

F. Bursal rays

G. Larviparous

H. Third-stage larva

I. Molt

J. Dioecious

1. Fingerlike projections of a copulatory bursa

2. The infective stage for many nematodes

3. The "penis" of a male nematode

4. A nematode life cycle that does not utilize an intermediate host

5. A female nematode that gives "birth" to live larvae

6. Having separate sexes—both male and female nematodes

7. The shedding of the cuticle ("skin") of a nematode

8. Morphologic feature on the anterior end of an adult nematode

9. Morphologic feature on the posterior end of a male nematode

10. A nematode life cycle that utilizes an intermediate host

QUESTIONS FOR THOUGHT AND DISCUSSION

1. Diagnostically speaking, which reproductive system (male or female) is more important in veterinary practice? Would you rather use a male nematode for diagnosis or a female nematode for diagnosis of a parasite problem? Why?

2. Compare and contrast the following types of nematode eggs. You may use drawings with labels to illustrate the differences. Give examples of nematodes that typify these egg types (see Chapter 4 for examples).
   - Ascaroid- or ascarid-type egg
   - Trichostrongyle or strongyle-type egg
   - Spiruroid-type egg
   - Trichinelloid- or trichuroid-type egg

3. Define the terms *direct life cycle* and *indirect life cycle*. Give an example of a genus of nematode that utilizes each type of life cycle.

4. What are some external morphologic features used to identify intact adult nematodes?

5. Describe the "typical nematode life cycle."

6. Define the following terms that are commonly used in veterinary practice:
   - Infective third-stage larva
   - Trichinelloid- or trichuroid-type egg
   - Oviparous nematode

4 Nematodes That Infect Domestic Animals

OUTLINE

LEARNING OBJECTIVES

After studying this chapter, the reader should be able to do the following:

- Remember the scientific names and corresponding common names for major parasites affecting domestic and laboratory animals.
- Recognize the pathology produced by nematodes of domesticated and laboratory animals.
- Recognize ova and distinctive larval stages of major parasites affecting domestic and laboratory animals.
- Understand the life cycles of the following parasites:

- Canine roundworm (*Toxocara canis*)
- Canine hookworm (*Ancylostoma caninum*)
- Canine whipworm (*Trichuris vulpis*)
- Canine heartworm (*Dirofilaria immitis*)
- Feline heartworm (*Dirofilaria immitis*)
- Ruminant lungworm (*Dictyocaulus viviparus*)
- Equine roundworm (*Parascaris equorum*)
- Equine large and small strongyles (*Strongylus vulgaris*)

KEY TERMS

Adulticides	Cutaneous	Oxyurids	Strongyles
Ascarids	onchocerciasis	Parthenogenesis	Summer sores
Asymptomatic	Facultative parasites	Prepatent period	Thumps
Benzimidazoles	L2 larvae	Probenzimidazoles	Vermicide
Cutaneous draschiasis	Microfilariae	Rhabditiform	Vermifuge
Cutaneous	Microfilaricide	esophagus	
habronemiasis	Neotenic		

This chapter includes brief descriptions of many of the common nematode parasites of domesticated (and wild) animals in the United States. The discussions include information on the tissue, organ, or organ system parasitized in the host. Where appropriate, information is also provided on the prepatent period (time from the point of infection until a specific diagnostic stage can be recovered), the diagnostic stage (life cycle stage) most often identified, a morphologic description of this diagnostic stage (e.g., eggs, larvae, or adult), and treatment for the most common parasites.

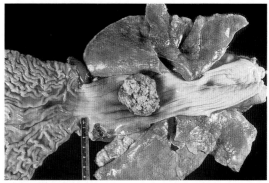

FIGURE 4-1 *Spirocerca lupi*, the esophageal worm, is a nematode usually associated with formation of nodules in the esophageal wall of dogs and cats.

NEMATODES OF DOGS AND CATS

GASTROINTESTINAL TRACT

Parasite: *Spirocerca lupi*
Host: Canines and felines
Location of Adult: Esophageal wall
Distribution: Tropical and subtropical regions
Derivation of Genus: Coiled tail
Transmission Route: Ingestion of eggs
Common Name: Esophageal worm
Zoonotic: No

Spirocerca lupi, the esophageal worm, is a nematode usually associated with the formation of nodules in the esophageal wall of dogs and cats. Occasionally this roundworm may be found in granulomas or nodules in the stomach wall of both dogs and cats (Figure 4-1). Adult worms reside in tunnels deep within these nodules and expel their eggs through the fistulous (tractlike) openings in the nodules. These nodules can cause obstruction of the gastrointestinal tract, esophagus, or stomach. Eggs are

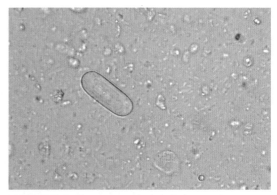

FIGURE 4-2 Characteristic thick-shelled eggs of *Spirocerca lupi* with a unique paper clip shape.

passed down the esophagus and out in the feces. The thick-shelled eggs of *S. lupi* are 30 to 37 μm × 11 to 15 μm and contain a larva when laid. These eggs have a unique "paper clip" shape (Figure 4-2). An animal is infected by ingesting the eggs of this parasite. Eggs usually can be observed on fecal flotation but may also be recovered from vomitus that has been subjected to standard fecal flotation procedures. Radiographic or endoscopic examination may reveal a characteristic nodule or granuloma within the esophagus or stomach. The prepatent period for this roundworm is 6 months.

> **TECHNICIAN'S NOTE** Adult *Spirocerca lupi* reside inside nodules, which can cause esophageal obstruction.

Parasite: 🅩 *Physaloptera* species
Host: Canines and felines
Location of Adult: Lumen of the stomach or small intestine, more commonly attached to the stomach mucosa
Distribution: Worldwide
Derivation of Genus: Bladder wing
Transmission Route: Ingestion of eggs
Common Name: Canine and feline stomach worms
Zoonotic: Yes, however rarely seen in humans per the American Association of Veterinary Parasitologists (AAVP)

Physaloptera species are stomach worms of both the dog and the cat. Although occasionally found in the lumen of the stomach or small intestine, *Physaloptera* species are usually firmly attached to the mucosal surface of the stomach where they suck blood. When an endoscope is used, these nematodes can be observed in their attachment sites (Figure 4-3). Their diet consists of blood and tissue derived from the host's gastric mucosa. The feeding habits of these worms may expose their attachment sites, which often continue to bleed after the parasite has detached. Vomiting, anorexia, and dark, tarry stools are often observed in infected animals. The adults are creamy white, sometimes tightly coiled, and 1.3 to 4.8 cm long (Figure 4-4). They may also be recovered in the pet's vomitus; when this happens, *Physaloptera* species can easily be confused with ascarids. A quick way to differentiate the

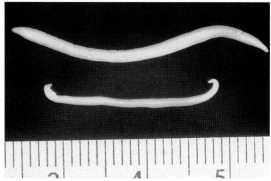

FIGURE 4-4 Adult of *Physaloptera* is creamy white, sometimes tightly coiled, and 1.3 to 4.8 cm long.

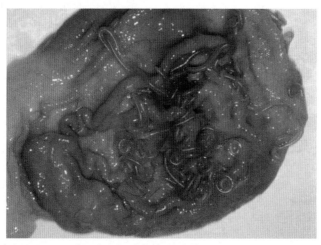

FIGURE 4-3 *Physaloptera praeputialis* in the stomach of a cat. (From Bowman: *Georgis' Parasitology for Veterinarians*, ed 10, 2013, Elsevier.)

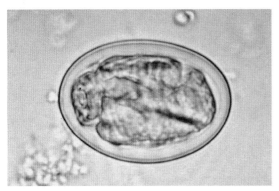

FIGURE 4-5 Characteristic smooth, thick-shelled, embryonated (larvated) eggs of *Physaloptera* species. Eggs usually can be recovered on standard fecal flotation using solutions with a specific gravity greater than 1.25.

two parasites is to break open an adult specimen and (if the specimen is female) examine the eggs microscopically.

The eggs of *Physaloptera* species are small, smooth, thick shelled, and embryonated (larvated) when passed in the feces. These eggs are quite similar in appearance to the eggs of *S. lupi*. They are 30 to 34 μm × 49 to 59 μm and contain a larva when laid. (See Figure 4-5 for the characteristic egg of *Physaloptera* species.) This parasite infects animals that ingest the larvated eggs. Eggs can usually be recovered on standard fecal flotation of either feces or vomitus using solutions with a specific gravity greater than 1.25. The prepatent period for this nematode is 56 to 83 days.

> **TECHNICIAN'S NOTE** The eggs of *Physaloptera* species can be confused with ascarids.

Parasite: *Aonchotheca putorii*
Host: Felines and minks
Location of Adult: Small intestine
Distribution: Tropic and temperate countries, worldwide
Derivation of Genus: Sheath diminished in bulk
Transmission Route: Ingestion of eggs
Common Name: Gastric capillarid of cats
Zoonotic: No

Aonchotheca putorii is commonly referred to as the *gastric capillarid of cats*. This nematode was once known by another scientific name, *Capillaria putorii*. This capillarid frequently parasitizes minks but has also been reported in cats. *A. putorii* is rarely reported in North America. The adult parasites can be found in the small intestine where they suck blood. The eggs of *A. putorii* are easily confused with those of other trichuroid nematodes. (See the following section on identification of feline whipworms.) The eggs of *A. putorii* are 53 to 70 μm × 20 to 30 μm and exhibit a netlike surface similar to the eggs of *Eucoleus aerophilus*, another capillarid found in the upper respiratory system. The eggs of *A. putorii* are dense and less delicate than those of *E. aerophilus*; they have flattened sides and contain a one- or two-cell embryo that fills the egg. This parasite is passed to new hosts by ingestion of the embryonated egg. The eggs can be detected on fecal flotation.

Parasite: *Ollulanus tricuspis*
Host: Felines
Location of Adult: Stomach
Distribution: Worldwide
Derivation of Genus: Small feline hair
Transmission Route: Ingestion of larvae from vomitus
Common Name: Feline trichostrongyle
Zoonotic: No

Ollulanus tricuspis is the feline trichostrongyle. As a group, the trichostrongyles are considered to be parasites of the gastrointestinal tract of ruminants such as cattle, sheep, and goats; it is quite unusual for the cat to serve as a host for a trichostrongyle. *O. tricuspis* is often diagnosed in cats that exhibit chronic vomiting. These nematodes are usually identified by examining the cat's vomitus under a dissecting or compound microscope. Feline vomitus can also be examined with a standard fecal flotation procedure. The best flotation solution for identification is a modified Sheather flotation solution. Adult female *O. tricuspis* are tiny, only 0.8 to 1 mm long, and possess three major tail cusps, or toothlike processes, on the tip of the tail (thus the specific epithet *tricuspis*). Adult male nematodes are 0.7 to 0.8 mm long and possess a copulatory bursa. The female worms are larviparous and release infective third-stage larvae (500 × 22 μm), which mature to adults in the cat's stomach. This feline trichostrongyle also is unusual in that these third-stage larvae are immediately infective for any cat that may ingest vomitus containing them. Free-living stages in the external environment are not required for completion of the life cycle.

> **TECHNICIAN'S NOTE** *Ollulanus tricuspis* females release third-stage infective larvae that are immediately infective to cats.

Parasites: *Toxocara canis, Toxocara cati,* and *Toxascaris leonina*
Host: Canines and felines
Location of Adults: Small intestine
Distribution: Worldwide
Derivation of Genus: *Toxocara*—arrowhead; *Toxascaris*—arrow ascaris
Transmission Route: Ingestion of egg with infective larva
Common Name: Canine and feline roundworms
Zoonotic: *T. canis* and *T. cati:* Yes; *T. leonina:* No

Toxocara canis, Toxocara cati, and *Toxascaris leonina* are the ascarids, or large roundworms, of dogs and cats. These roundworms may be found in the small intestine of dogs and cats in most areas of the world. All young puppies and kittens presenting to a veterinary clinic should be examined for the presence of these large, robust nematodes. Adult ascarids may vary in length from 3 to 18 cm and, when passed in the feces, are usually tightly coiled, similar to a coiled bedspring (Figure 4-6). Ascarids in young puppies and kittens may produce vomiting, diarrhea, constipation, and other nonspecific clinical signs. The adult worm does not attach to the host but rather uses an undulating motion to remain in the small intestine. Therefore adult worms may "swim" into the stomach and cause vomiting. The worm may then be present in the vomitus. Because of the presence of the adult worm in the vomitus, the owner may describe the vomitus as having "spaghetti" in it. An accumulation of adults can cause gastrointestinal obstruction.

The eggs of *Toxocara* species are unembryonated and spherical and have a deeply pigmented center

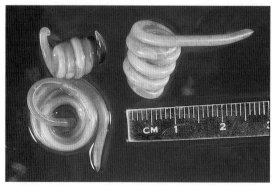

FIGURE 4-6 Adult ascarids may vary in length from 3 to 18 cm and when passed in feces are usually tightly coiled.

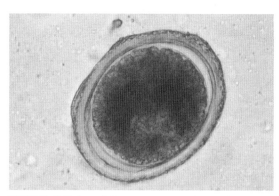

FIGURE 4-7 Egg of *Toxocara canis* with unembryonated, spherical form with deeply pigmented center and rough, pitted outer shell.

and rough, pitted outer shell. The eggs of *T. canis* are 75 to 90 μm in diameter (Figure 4-7), whereas those of *T. cati* are smaller, 65 to 75 μm in diameter (Figure 4-8). The eggs of *T. leonina* are spherical to ovoid, with dimensions of 75 × 85 μm. In contrast to the eggs of *Toxocara* species, the eggs of *T. leonina* have a smooth outer shell and a hyaline, or "ground glass," central portion (Figure 4-9). The prepatent period for *T. canis* is 21 to 35 days, whereas that of *T. leonina* is 74 days. Ascarids are among the most frequently diagnosed nematodes in young puppies and kittens.

> **TECHNICIAN'S NOTE** Adult ascarids are commonly seen in vomitus and may be described by pet owners as "spaghetti-like" worms.

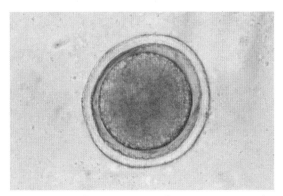

FIGURE 4-8 Characteristic egg of *Toxocara cati* is similar in structure to that of *Toxocara canis* but smaller in diameter.

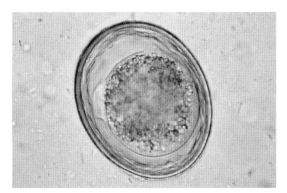

FIGURE 4-9 Eggs of *Toxascaris leonina* are spherical to ovoid, with dimensions of 75 × 85 μm. In contrast to eggs of *Toxocara* species, these eggs have a smooth outer shell and hyaline, or ground glass, central portion.

Adult roundworms are present in the small intestine, where they mate. The female produces unembryonated eggs that are passed in the host's feces. The eggs embryonate on the ground to the point that they contain L2 larvae. They are ingested by a host, and the L2 larvae are released from the eggs. The L2 larvae may go into dormancy in an adult host, but they grow and migrate to various tissues in the young host. Finally, the L2 larvae migrate to the young host's lungs, where they are coughed up and swallowed by the host. They grow to adulthood in the host's small intestine and begin a new life cycle (Figure 4-10).

In the adult female host the infective larvae remain dormant until the female host mates and produces hormones during pregnancy. At this time the larvae become active once more and migrate through the female host's body. The larvae (with the exception of *T. cati*) can cross the placental barrier to infect the host's offspring. The most common symptoms of a roundworm infection are diarrhea, vomiting, and a potbellied appearance.

The most common way of identifying an infection by *T. canis*, *T. cati*, or *T. leonina* is through the fecal flotation technique. Usually the pregnant female will have feces tested for these parasites to determine the chances of her puppies or kittens becoming infected. Puppies and kittens are routinely dewormed during their first few visits to the veterinary office.

Several types of anthelmintics can be used to treat a roundworm infection. A vermifuge (anthelmintic that paralyzes the parasite so it passes out in the feces) such as piperazine or pyrantel is often used to treat this type of parasite. A vermicide (anthelmintic that kills the parasite and allows the parasite to be broken down by the body) such as thiabendazole or mebendazole can also be used to treat a roundworm infection.

> **TECHNICIAN'S NOTE** The best way to identify a roundworm infection is through the fecal flotation technique.

T. canis, although primarily a parasite of the dog, can also infect humans (visceral larva migrans), as discussed in Chapter 16. The best way to prevent infection to humans and other animals is cleaning up feces in the yard daily. Also, children should be prevented from playing in the yard and placing their contaminated hands on their mouths.

Parasite: 🅩 *Baylisascaris procyonis*
Host: Raccoon, but also seen in many species
Location of Adult: Small intestine
Distribution: North America (Mississippi-Ohio River basin)
Derivation of Genus: Named after a renowned parasitologist, Dr. H.A. Baylis
Transmission Route: Ingestion of eggs
Common Name: Raccoon roundworm
Zoonotic: Yes

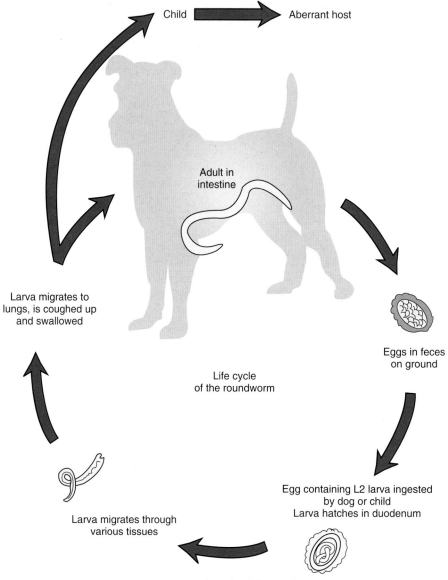

Child → Aberrant host

Adult in intestine

Larva migrates to lungs, is coughed up and swallowed

Life cycle of the roundworm

Eggs in feces on ground

Egg containing L2 larva ingested by dog or child
Larva hatches in duodenum

Larva migrates through various tissues

FIGURE 4-10 Life cycle of the roundworm.

Baylisascaris procyonis is the roundworm of the raccoon. *B. procyonis* is common in North America and is a zoonotic parasite. The adult resides in the small intestine of the raccoon. The ova are found in the feces. The ova are unembryonated and spherical with a deeply pigmented center and a rough/pitted outer shell. They are slightly smaller than the ova of *T. canis* (Figure 4-11). An accumulation of adults in the small intestine can cause a gastrointestinal obstruction in the natural host.

B. procyonis is diagnosed by finding the ova on fecal flotation. The ova can be found anywhere that raccoons defecate and in naturally infected canines. Although the raccoon is the natural host, *B. procyonis*

CASE PRESENTATION 4-1

Setting Up the Scenario

Ms. Eliot presented Julius, a 3-month-old male Labrador, for a first puppy visit. Ms. Eliot also noted that Julius had diarrhea. A fecal centrifugation was performed, and *Toxocara canis* was found. Dr. Wright informed Ms. Eliot that Julius had roundworms and would be treated with three doses of pyrantel pamoate. The technician then educated Ms. Eliot on *T. canis.*

What Information Must the Veterinary Technician Convey to Ms. Eliot?

Technician: "Ms. Eliot, because Julius has been diagnosed as having roundworms, let me give you some information on that intestinal parasite. Roundworms are commonly found in puppies because they are passed from the mother through her milk when the puppies are nursing. The adult worms produce eggs that are released with the puppy's stool. Although these eggs can infect other dogs, it is also important to know that they can cause a disease in humans called *visceral larva migrans*, which means the baby worms can travel through the organs of the human body and cause problems. It is important to clean up the puppy's stools from the yard. In addition to cleaning up the stools, you and any family member or guest should wash your hands thoroughly after handling the puppy. If you experience any abnormalities, please see your family physician and let him or her know that Julius was diagnosed as having roundworms. Dr. Wright has given a first deworming to Julius, and you will give another dose in 2 weeks and again 2 weeks later. You may see long white "spaghetti-like" worms in Julius's stool or in some vomit after the deworming. This is normal and should not worry you. Do you have any questions for me at this point?"

The technician also noted in the patient record that Ms. Eliot was given education on the zoonotic parasite diagnosed in Julius.

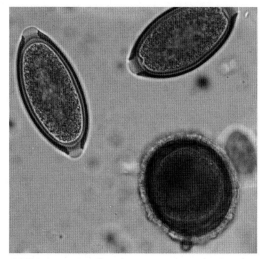

FIGURE 4-11 Egg of *Baylisascaris procyonis* and two eggs of *Trichuris vulpis.* (From Bowman: *Georgis' Parasitology for Veterinarians,* ed 10, 2013, Elsevier.)

can cause zoonotic disease in many species. Because the larvae migrate to the central nervous system, this is a very pathogenic parasite in the incidental host (Bowman, 2009), producing a zoonotic condition known as *neurologic larva migrans.*

> **TECHNICIAN'S NOTE** *Baylisascaris procyonis* is a very pathogenic zoonotic parasite that can infect humans.

Parasites: *Ancylostoma caninum, Ancylostoma tubaeforme, Ancylostoma braziliense,* and *Uncinaria stenocephala*

Host: *A. caninum,* canine; *A. tubaeforme,* feline; *A. braziliense,* canine and feline; and *U. stenocephala,* canine

Location of Adult: Small intestine

Distribution: *Ancylostoma* species (worldwide), *U. stenocephala* (northern regions of North America)

Derivation of Genus: *Ancylostoma*—curved mouth and straight trumpet shape; *Uncinaria*—hooked nose and narrow head

Transmission Route: Ingestion of eggs, through the skin, across the placenta, and through mammary milk

Common Name: Canine and feline hookworm

Zoonotic: Yes

Ancylostoma caninum, the canine hookworm; *Ancylostoma tubaeforme,* the feline hookworm;

Ancylostoma braziliense, the canine and feline hookworm; and *Uncinaria stenocephala,* the northern canine hookworm, are nematodes that infect the small intestine. Hookworms are found throughout the world but are most often found in tropical and subtropical areas of North America. Hookworms attach to the small intestinal mucosa. *A. caninum* demonstrates a frightful buccal cavity—it has three pairs of ventral teeth with which it attaches to the mucosa of the small intestine (Figure 4-12). These parasites may change feeding sites and reattach elsewhere in the small intestine. Because this hookworm feeds on blood, it secretes an anticoagulant from its mouth, which causes the former attachment sites to continue to bleed. Thus the hookworm's voracious feeding activity and the secondary hemorrhage produced can cause significant anemia. Because this bleeding occurs within the small intestine, the blood is often digested by the host and often appears as black, tarry stool. The resulting anemia can be quite severe in young kittens and puppies. Hookworms often produce serious problems in kennels and catteries. The prepatent period depends on the species of hookworm. Animals are usually infected through percutaneous, prenatal, and transmammary routes.

The male and female worms attach to adjacent villi of the intestinal wall. The male and female mate continuously, and therefore the female continually produces eggs that are laid in the feces. The egg contains the morula stage as it is passed out of the host's body in the feces. These eggs embryonate into L1 larvae in the external environment. The L1 larvae hatch, feed, grow, and molt to L2 larvae. The L2 larvae feed, grow, and molt to L3 larvae but do not release the cuticle of the L2 larvae. They are ensheathed L3 larvae that do not feed. They are the infective-stage larvae. The L3 larvae can be ingested, or they can penetrate the host's intact skin and migrate through the tissues of the body until they reach the lungs. Once in the lungs, the larvae are coughed up and swallowed by the host (Figure 4-13).

> **TECHNICIAN'S NOTE** Hookworms can cause a black, tarry stool in the host as a result of the attachment and reattachment of the parasite and the digestion of free blood in the intestinal tract.

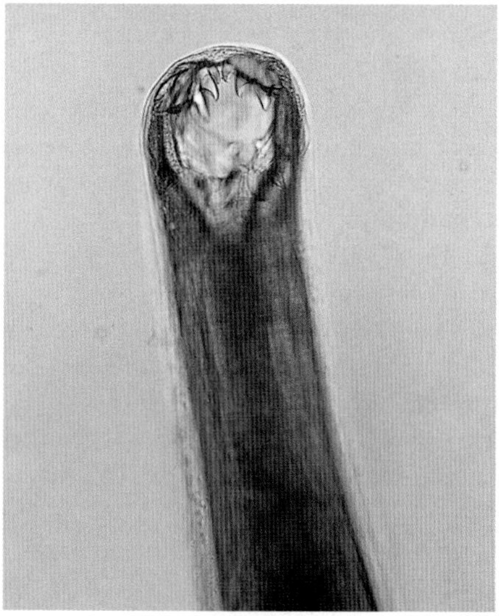

The larvae of this parasite are able to cross the placenta and also can be passed from mother to offspring through the colostrum. Therefore the pregnant host should be checked several times during pregnancy for the presence of these parasites. Because these parasites can penetrate intact skin, they can also enter the skin of humans (cutaneous larva migrans), as discussed in Chapter 16

Eggs of all hookworm species are oval or ellipsoidal and thin walled and contain an 8- to 16-cell morula when passed in feces. Because these eggs embryonate, or larvate, rapidly in the external environment (as early as 48 hours), fresh feces are needed for diagnosing hookworm infections. Eggs of *A. caninum* are 56 to 75 μm $\times$ 34 to 47 μm; those of *A. tubaeforme* are 55 to 75 μm $\times$ 34.4 to 44.7 μm; those of *A. braziliense* are 75 $\times$ 45 μm; and those of *U. stenocephala* are 65 to 80 μm $\times$ 40 to 50 μm. These eggs can be easily recovered on standard fecal flotation (Figure 4-14).

FIGURE 4-12 *Ancylostoma caninum* demonstrates a frightful buccal cavity, with three pairs of ventral teeth with which it attaches to the mucosa of the small intestine of dogs.

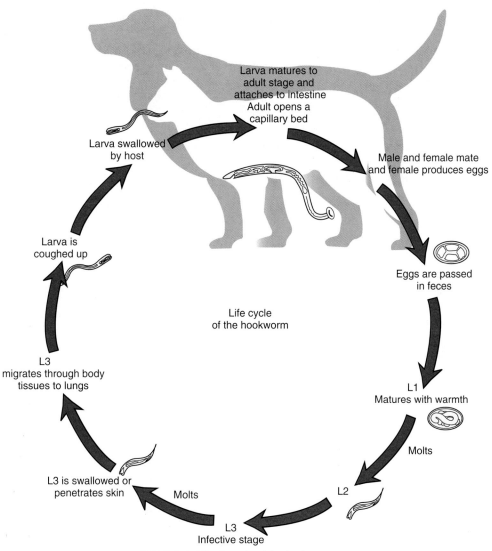

FIGURE 4-13 Life cycle of the hookworm.

Treatment for the hookworm species can take two forms. The first is prevention with the use of once-a-month heartworm preventive agents; Interceptor™ and Heartgard Plus™ are the most common brands, although other brands of heartworm preventatives also work against hookworms. Many of these preventive medications are also labeled for the prevention of hookworms. If the parasite eggs are found on fecal flotation or other techniques, the veterinarian may choose a vermicide such as mebendazole or fenbendazole.

The best way to prevent hookworm species from infecting animals or humans is removing the feces after defecation by the host. Removal during warm weather should take place immediately after

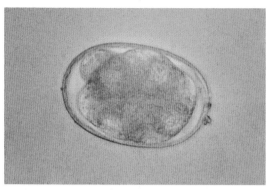

FIGURE 4-14 Eggs of all hookworm species are oval or ellipsoidal and thin-walled and contain an 8- to 16-cell morula when passed in feces. These eggs may represent one of several genera that parasitize dogs and cats: *Ancylostoma caninum, Ancylostoma tubaeforme, Ancylostoma braziliense,* and *Uncinaria stenocephala.*

defecation, whereas removal during cold months can take place every other day.

> *TECHNICIAN'S NOTE* The best way to prevent hookworm infections is to remove feces from the yard on a daily basis before the larvae hatch from the ova.

Parasites: *Strongyloides stercoralis* and *Strongyloides tumefaciens*
Host: Dogs, cats, and humans
Location of Adult: Small intestine
Distribution: Worldwide
Derivation of Genus: Roundlike shape
Transmission Route: Through the skin and in mammary milk
Common Name: Intestinal threadworms
Zoonotic: *S. stercoralis:* Yes; *S. tumefaciens:* No

Because parasitic males do not exist, the female worms are capable of producing viable ova without fertilization from a male worm. This process is called parthenogenesis.

Strongyloides stercoralis and *Strongyloides tumefaciens* are often referred to as *intestinal threadworms.* These nematodes are unique in that only a parthenogenetic female is parasitic in the host and resides in the small intestine. The female has an approximately cylindric esophagus that is one

CASE PRESENTATION 4-2

Setting Up the Scenario:
Mr. Watson presented Cleo, a 6-year-old female-spayed, who has been vomiting and has had diarrhea for 3 days. A fecal centrifugation was run, and *Ancylostoma caninum* was found. Dr. Whitney informed Mr. Watson that his dog had hookworms. A course of fenbendazole was prescribed for Cleo. The technician then educated Mr. Watson on *A. caninum.*

What Information Must the Veterinary Technician Convey to Mr. Watson?
Technician: "Mr. Watson, Cleo has been diagnosed as having hookworms. This adult intestinal parasite produces eggs that are passed in Cleo's stool. When the eggs hatch, they produce a baby worm called a *larva* that can enter your dog and even humans through the skin. In humans, this parasite causes a disease called *cutaneous larva migrans,* which means the infective larvae travel through the skin. In your dog they will travel through the skin and end up in the intestines, where they will grow to adults. In humans they tend to die in most cases; however, in rare cases they can reach the intestines and become adults. Because humans can be infected, it is important to clean up Cleo's stool after defecation no less than once a day to prevent reinfection to Cleo, as well as to prevent infection of you and your family. Dr. Whitney has prescribed a dewormer that you need to mix with Cleo's food once a day for 3 days. If you have any itching with wormlike lesions, you should see your physician."

The technician also noted in the patient record that the owner was educated on this zoonotic parasite.

quarter the length of the parasite's body. These females produce embryonated or larvated eggs, but in dogs the eggs hatch in the intestine, releasing first-stage larvae that may be observed in fresh feces. (Figure 4-15 shows the parasitic adult females, eggs, and first-stage larvae of *Strongyloides* species.) The larval *Strongyloides* species are 280 to 310 μm long and possess a rhabditiform esophagus with a club-shaped anterior corpus, a narrow median isthmus, and a caudal bulb. The larvae go through a free-living stage in the environment before

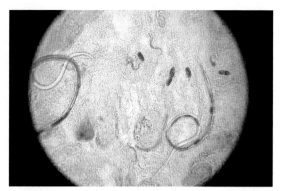

FIGURE 4-15 Parasitic adult females, eggs, and first-stage larvae of *Strongyloides stercoralis*, intestinal threadworms.

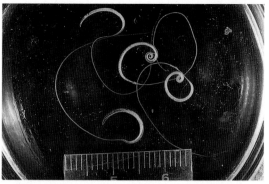

FIGURE 4-16 *Trichuris vulpis*, the canine whipworm, derives its common name from the fact that adults possess a thin, filamentous anterior end ("lash" of the whip) and a thick posterior end ("handle" of the whip).

becoming infective third-stage larvae that can penetrate the skin and cause migratory damage in the host. In the dog the major method of transmission is from mother to pups through the mammary glands. The prepatent period is 8 to 14 days. These nematodes are frequently associated with moderate to severe diarrhea in young puppies, particularly in kennel environments during the summer months. Because humans can also be infected with *S. stercoralis*, there is the potential of zoonosis called *strongyloidiasis*.

> **TECHNICIAN'S NOTE** In dog feces you will commonly find the larvae (rather than the ova) of *Strongyloides* species.

Parasites: *Trichuris vulpis, Trichuris campanula,* and *Trichuris serrata*
Host: *T. vulpis,* canine; *T. campanula* and *T. serrata,* feline
Location of Adult: Cecum and colon
Distribution: Worldwide, but *T. campanula* and *T. serrata* are rare in North America
Derivation of Genus: Hair tail
Transmission Route: Ingestion of eggs
Common Name: Whipworm
Zoonotic: No

Trichuris vulpis, the canine whipworm, and *Trichuris campanula* and *Trichuris serrata*, the feline whipworms, reside in the cecum and colon of their respective definitive hosts. Whipworms are a

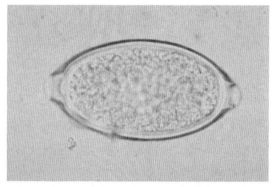

FIGURE 4-17 Characteristic egg of *Trichuris vulpis* is described as *trichinelloid* or *trichuroid*; it has a thick, yellow-brown, symmetric shell with polar plugs at both ends. Eggs are unembryonated (not larvated) when laid.

common clinical occurrence in dogs; however, it is important to remember that feline whipworms are quite rare in North America and have been diagnosed only sporadically throughout the world. Whipworms derive their name from the fact that the adults have a thin, filamentous anterior end (the "lash" of the whip) and a thick posterior end (the "handle" of the whip) (Figure 4-16). The thin end of the whipworm was once thought to be the tail of the parasite. The egg of the whipworm is described as *trichuroid* or *trichinelloid*; it has a thick, yellow-brown, symmetric shell with prominent polar plugs at both ends. The eggs are unembryonated (not larvated) when laid. Eggs of *T. vulpis* are 70 to 89 μm × 37 to 40 μm. (Figure 4-17 shows the characteristic egg of *T. vulpis*.) The prepatent period for *T. vulpis* is 70 to 90 days.

Adult *Trichuris* species are attached to the wall of the cecum or colon where they suck blood and produce eggs. The eggs are passed out in the feces of the host every third day. Once in the environment, the eggs go through a period of development to become an L1 (infective) larva within the egg. Unlike the hookworm species, the whipworm species must be ingested by the host. The L1 larva hatches from the egg once in the host's small intestine. The larva molts several times in the small and large intestines before becoming an adult. The new adult migrates back through the colon to the cecum and attaches to the intestinal wall (Figure 4-18). The most common symptoms seen in infected animals are diarrhea, anemia, and mucus-coated stool.

> **TECHNICIAN'S NOTE** The eggs of *Trichuris* species are passed in the stool only every third day rather than every day like the eggs of most nematodes.

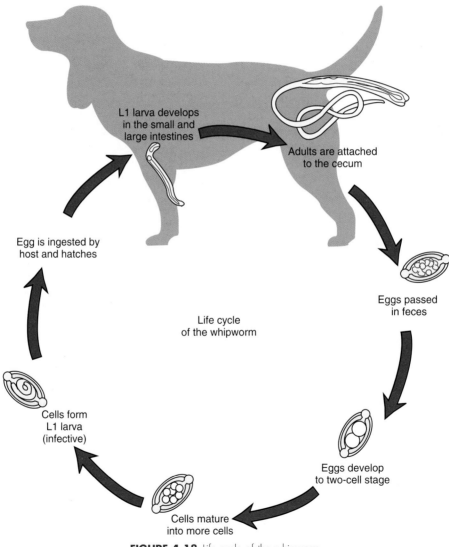

L1 larva develops in the small and large intestines

Adults are attached to the cecum

Egg is ingested by host and hatches

Eggs passed in feces

Life cycle of the whipworm

Cells form L1 larva (infective)

Eggs develop to two-cell stage

Cells mature into more cells

FIGURE 4-18 Life cycle of the whipworm.

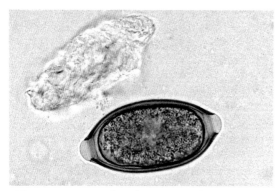

FIGURE 4-19 Egg of *Trichuris campanula* (pictured) and *Trichuris serrata*, the feline whipworms, may be easily confused with *Aonchotheca putorii*, *Eucoleus aerophilus*, and *Pearsonema feliscati*, parasites of the feline stomach, respiratory tract, and urinary system, respectively. Eggs of *T. campanula* average 63 to 85 μm × 34 to 39 μm.

The eggs of *T. campanula* and *T. serrata,* the feline whipworms, may be easily confused with those of *A. putorii, E. aerophilus,* and *Pearsonema feliscati,* parasites of the feline stomach, respiratory tract, and urinary system, respectively. The eggs of *T. campanula* average 63 to 85 μm × 34 to 39 μm (Figure 4-19). When examining a cat's feces for trichurids, the diagnostician must remember that pseudoparasites, that is, the eggs of trichurids or capillarids, may parasitize nonfeline hosts such as mice, rabbits, or birds (an outdoor cat's prey). The eggs of trichurids or capillarids from a cat's prey may pass undigested and unaltered through the cat's gastrointestinal system, remaining intact and unembryonated.

Fecal flotation is the most common way of identifying the eggs of this parasite; however, whipworm eggs do not float well in most common fecal flotation media. Therefore it is imperative that the eggs be allowed to float for a minimum of 15 minutes before viewing under the microscope. Once identified, the veterinarian will most often use the vermicides mebendazole or fenbendazole for treatment of these worms. Prevention involves daily feces removal to remove the uninfective eggs from the host's environment.

Parasite: *Enterobius vermicularis*
Host: Humans

CASE PRESENTATION 4-3

Setting Up the Scenario
Ms. Swanson presented Bruno, a 2-year-old male-neutered corgi with mucus-coated stool and diarrhea. A fecal centrifugation was performed, and *Trichuris vulpis* was found. Dr. Williams told Ms. Swanson that Bruno had whipworms. Dr. Williams prescribed fenbendazole for 3 days, to be repeated in 3 weeks and 3 months.

What Information Must the Veterinary Technician Convey to Ms. Swanson?
Technician: "Ms. Swanson, Bruno has been diagnosed as having whipworms. Dr. Williams is sending you home with three sets of deworming medication. You will give one dose on 3 consecutive days then repeat the dosing 3 weeks after finishing the first 3 days and again 3 months after finishing the first three doses. Repeated doses are necessary because whipworms are resilient parasites, so we need to make sure all of the adults are treated. You will also need to keep your yard clean of stools to prevent Bruno from being reinfected. Although Bruno can be reinfected, humans do not get infected with canine whipworms, so you do not have to worry about an infection."

The technician also noted in the patient record that the owner was educated on this parasite.

Distribution: Worldwide
Derivation of Genus: Intestinal life
Transmission Route: Ingestion of eggs
Common Name: Human pinworm
Zoonotic: No

Dogs and cats may often be blamed for serving as hosts for certain parasites of humans. *Enterobius vermicularis* is the pinworm found in humans, often in young children. This pinworm *does not* parasitize dogs or cats. Nevertheless, the family pet is often falsely incriminated by physicians, family practitioners, and pediatricians as a source of pinworm infection in young children. The veterinary diagnostician should remember this rule: Pinworms are parasites of omnivores (mice, rats, monkeys, and humans) and herbivores (rabbits and horses) but *never* carnivores (dogs and cats).

CASE PRESENTATION 4-4

Ms. Peterson phoned the clinic asking about a treatment for Scruffles, her 5-year-old spayed Yorkshire terrier. Ms. Peterson had taken her son, Jeremy, to the family physician because of a pruritic rectum. The physician diagnosed Jeremy as having *Enterobius vermicularis*, the human pinworm. The physician intimated that Jeremy was infected by the family dog.

Upon taking Ms. Peterson's call, the technician educated her on pinworms. "Ms. Peterson, there are two important things you need to know about pinworms. The first is that dogs and cats are two species of animals that do not get infected with pinworms; therefore Scruffles could not have infected Jeremy with pinworms. The second important fact is that pinworms are species specific, so a family pet with pinworms could infect only another of its own species. This means that Jeremy could be infected only by another human with pinworms. If you need me to discuss this further with your family physician, please have her call me."

The technician noted the discussion in the patient record.

TECHNICIAN'S NOTE Because whipworm ova are heavy and hard to float, they require at least 15 minutes with a standard fecal flotation technique before viewing under a microscope. Ideally, centrifugal flotation should be used to better float the whipworm ova.

CIRCULATORY SYSTEM

Parasite: **Z** *Dirofilaria immitis*
Host: Canine, feline, and ferret; has been observed in humans as an incidental parasite
Intermediate Host: Female mosquito
Location of Adult: Right ventricle and pulmonary arteries of the heart
Distribution: Warm-temperate climates around the world
Derivation of Name: Dread thread and inexorable
Transmission Route: Bite of infective mosquito
Common Name: Heartworm
Zoonotic: Yes (incidental host)

Dirofilaria immitis is often referred to as the *canine heartworm* (Figure 4-20); however, this nematode has been known to parasitize cats and ferrets as well (Figure 4-21). The definitive host for *D. immitis* is the canine. Although cats and ferrets have been parasitized by this parasite, they rarely serve as a source for transmission. Heartworms are long, slender parasites (Figure 4-22). As adults, these parasites are found within the right ventricle and the pulmonary arteries and its fine branches. The offspring of filarial worms such as *D. immitis* are known as microfilariae.

Among the nematodes of small animals, *D. immitis* is perhaps the one nematode that may be found in sites other than its normal predilection

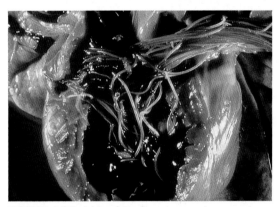

FIGURE 4-20 Adults of *Dirofilaria immitis*, the canine heartworm, are found within the right ventricle and pulmonary artery and its fine branches.

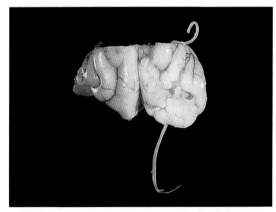

FIGURE 4-21 Canine heartworms may be found in sites other than the heart and in hosts other than the dog. These heartworms were recovered from the brain of a ferret.

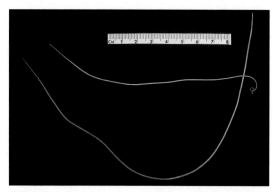

FIGURE 4-22 Heartworms are long, slender parasites, evolved for fitting into the fine branches of pulmonary arteries.

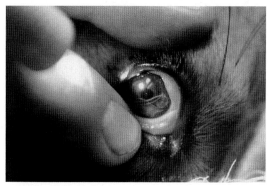

FIGURE 4-23 *Dirofilaria immitis*, the canine heartworm, may also be recovered from a variety of aberrant sites, such as the anterior chamber of the eye.

sites. This parasite is often recovered in a variety of aberrant sites such as the brain, anterior chamber of the eye (Figure 4-23), and subcutaneous sites. The prepatent period in dogs is approximately 6 months.

> **TECHNICIAN'S NOTE** *Dirofilaria immitis* is the parasite that causes heartworm disease in dogs and cats. It has a prepatent period of 6 months before it can be diagnosed in the dog.

The life cycle of *D. immitis* requires the mosquito intermediate host to be transmitted from animal to animal. The adults live in the right ventricle and pulmonary arteries, where they can obstruct the blood vasculature. The male and female adults mate, and the female produces microfilariae. The

microfilariae are released into the host's bloodstream, where they are ingested by feeding female mosquitoes. The microfilariae grow and molt in the mosquito until they reach the infective stage. Once they become infective, they enter a new host the next time the mosquito feeds (Figure 4-24). Once in the new host, the larvae migrate and molt through various body tissues on their way to the heart. It is at this time that the larvae may grow and molt to become adults in sites other than the heart.

> **TECHNICIAN'S NOTE** *Dirofilaria immitis* larvae must develop to an infective stage within a mosquito before they can be transferred to a new host.

In microfilaremic dogs, diagnosis is made by observing microfilariae in blood samples using one of several concentration techniques, such as the modified Knott test (Figures 4-25 and 4-26) or commercially available filter techniques (Figure 4-27). For dogs (amicrofilaremic or microfilaremic) infection can also be diagnosed using one of the commercially available enzyme-linked immunosorbent assay (ELISA) tests (Figure 4-28). It is important to remember that *Acanthocheilonema* (formerly known as *Dipetalonema*) *reconditum*, a subcutaneous filariid of dogs, also produces microfilariae in the peripheral blood (Figures 4-29 and 4-30). The microfilariae of this nonpathogenic nematode must be differentiated from those of *D. immitis* (see Figures 4-25 and 4-26).

The damage that *D. immitis* causes to the heart will cause the hallmark symptoms of heartworm disease in dogs. The symptoms are a decrease in exercise tolerance, right-sided heart enlargement, and abdominal ascites (fluid accumulation in the abdomen). These symptoms are caused by the parasite's location in the heart and pulmonary arteries, which reduces blood flow on the right side of the heart and causes inflammation to the lining of the blood vessels.

> **TECHNICIAN'S NOTE** The classic symptoms of heartworm disease are exercise intolerance, right-sided heart enlargement, and abdominal ascites caused by reduced blood flow on the right side of the heart.

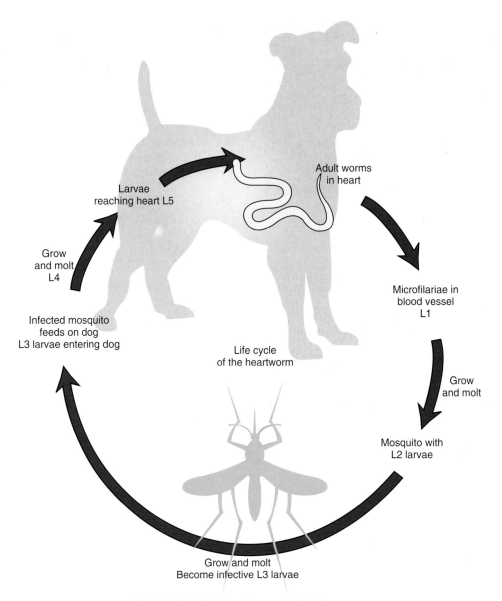

Adult worms
in heart

Larvae
reaching heart L5

Grow
and molt
L4

Microfilariae in
blood vessel
L1

Infected mosquito
feeds on dog
L3 larvae entering dog

Life cycle
of the heartworm

Grow
and molt

Mosquito with
L2 larvae

Grow and molt
Become infective L3 larvae

FIGURE 4-24 Life cycle of the canine *Dirofilaria immitis.*

The treatment for heartworm disease involves pretreatment testing, treatment, and posttreatment rest. The first step in treatment involves determining the canine's ability to withstand the treatment by performing blood work; this determines the status of the internal organs. Radiographs are taken to determine the status of the heart and the stage of the disease. After testing, the canine is treated for the adult heartworms. **Adulticides** (drugs that kill the adult stages of the parasite) such as Immiticide™ are used to kill adult heartworms. As the adults die, they move with the flow of blood toward the lungs. This could cause problems for the canine if it is allowed to exercise after the adulticide

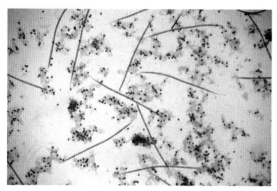

FIGURE 4-25 Microfilariae of *Dirofilaria immitis* subjected to the modified Knott test. Microfilariae of this pathogenic nematode must be differentiated from those of *Acanthocheilonema reconditum*.

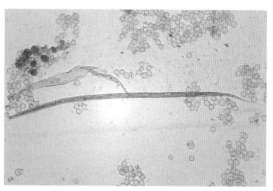

FIGURE 4-26 Microfilaria of *Dirofilaria immitis* subjected to the modified Knott test. Note the tapering anterior end and straight tail. This microfilaria measures approximately 310 μm in length.

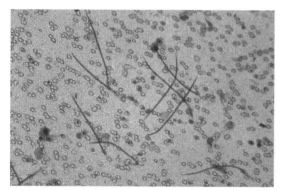

FIGURE 4-27 Microfilariae of *Dirofilaria immitis* subjected to a commercially available filter technique.

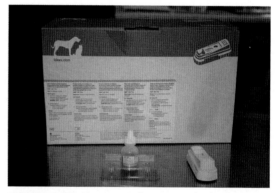

FIGURE 4-28 Heartworm infection can also be diagnosed using commercially available enzyme-linked immunosorbent assay (ELISA) tests.

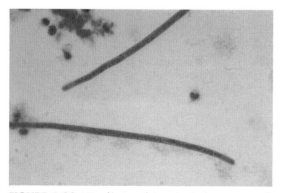

FIGURE 4-29 Microfilariae of *Acanthocheilonema reconditum* subjected to the modified Knott test. Note the broomhandle anterior end. This microfilaria measures approximately 280 μm in length. Microfilariae of this nonpathogenic nematode must be differentiated from those of *Dirofilaria immitis*.

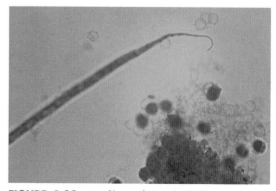

FIGURE 4-30 Microfilaria of *Acanthocheilonema reconditum* subjected to the modified Knott test. Note the buttonhook posterior end, which is an artifact of formalin fixation used in the modified Knott procedure.

treatment. The canine must be kept quiet for several weeks after treatment while the body resorbs the dead adults. Once the adults have been treated and resorbed by the body, the canine is treated with a microfilaricide (usually ivermectin) to clear the blood of any microfilariae. The final part of the treatment is heartworm testing. This usually involves a microfilariae test and an ELISA test to confirm that the microfilariae and adults have been cleared from the canine's body.

The treatment for canine heartworm disease can be very stressful on a dog's body. Therefore prevention is recommended so that the dog does not contract the parasite. The various preventive regimens include daily preventive medications, monthly medications, and an injection every 6 months. Recent studies have shown that there is resistance by *D. immitis* to the macrocyclic lactone (monthly) preventatives. The studies further showed the preventatives have better efficacy with consistent use (monthly) rather than a single dose given infrequently. Only moxidectin has been shown to be 100% effective as a single-dose preventative.

Resistance has been seen in other preventatives, which may be attributed to client compliance. It is recommended that all dogs receive a preventative year-round; however, studies have shown only about 50% of dogs are on year-round prevention.

Feline hosts for *D. immitis* occur in the same areas in which canines are infected. Cats are susceptible to the parasite but tend to be very resistant to infection. Therefore it takes a greater exposure to the microfilariae from the mosquito to infect a cat than it does to infect a dog. Whereas *D. immitis* causes enough damage to produce hallmark symptoms in dogs, cats do not show specific symptoms of the infection. Cats tend to show signs similar to those seen with respiratory disease.

The life cycle of *D. immitis* in cats begins as it does in dogs. The adults live in the right ventricle and pulmonary arteries of the dog. The adults mate, and the female produces microfilariae, which are present in the vessels of the dog. Mosquitoes feed on the infected canine and ingest the microfilariae. The microfilariae grow and molt to infective L3 larvae. Once infective, the mosquito feeds on a cat, and the larvae are transferred to the cat. The larvae grow, molt, and migrate in the cat on their way to the heart (Figure 4-31).

> *TECHNICIAN'S NOTE* Feline heartworm diseases do not produce the hallmark symptoms observed in canine heartworm disease. The symptoms are similar to those seen with respiratory disease.

Identification of the parasite in the cat is difficult. The adults do not produce many microfilariae in the cat, so the microfilarial tests produce negative results in most cases. Tests developed for dogs are not sensitive enough for the infection in cats, so ELISA tests have been developed for detection of *D. immitis* in cats. Two types of tests are available for in-clinic use: antigen tests and antibody tests. The antigen test is the definitive test, although a negative result does not rule out a heartworm infection. The antibody test can detect a reaction by the cat's body to the microfilariae, but the microfilariae may die before becoming adults. Therefore a positive antibody test result does not positively detect an active infection. A positive antigen or antibody test result in the presence of clinical respiratory symptoms indicates an active infection (https://www.heartwormsociety.org/images/pdf/2014-AHS-Feline-Guidelines.pdf).

At this time there are no approved treatments for feline heartworm disease. Therefore the best treatment is prevention. Preventive options available for cats include once-a-month pills or a single topical monthly application for the prevention of feline heartworm disease.

Setting Up the Scenario

Mr. and Mrs. Milton presented Wilma, a 3-month-old female boxer, for her first puppy visit. After getting a weight for Wilma, the technician asked Mr. and Mrs. Milton if they knew anything about canine heartworm disease. Mr. and Mrs. Milton replied, "No."

What Information Must the Veterinary Technician Convey to Mr. and Mrs. Milton?

The technician replied, "Let me give you some information on canine heartworm disease. Canine heartworm disease is caused by a parasite called *Dirofilaria immitis*. The adult worms reside in the right side of the heart, as you can see in this model. The adults produce babies called *microfilariae*. The

microfilariae are found in the blood, where they are picked up by the mosquito when it bites a canine heartworm–infected dog. The microfilariae or babies then incubate an infective larva. At this stage the mosquito bites Wilma and transfers the infective larvae to her. The microfilariae travel through Wilma's tissues to her heart. Once in the heart, they mature to adults. We have monthly heartworm preventatives to help keep Wilma from developing heartworm disease. The preventatives kill the larvae before they can reach the heart and become adults. We are going to give you a puppy kit for Wilma that includes the first dose of heartworm prevention. Our hospital recommends using the preventative year-round."

The technician noted in the patient record that heartworm disease and prevention were discussed.

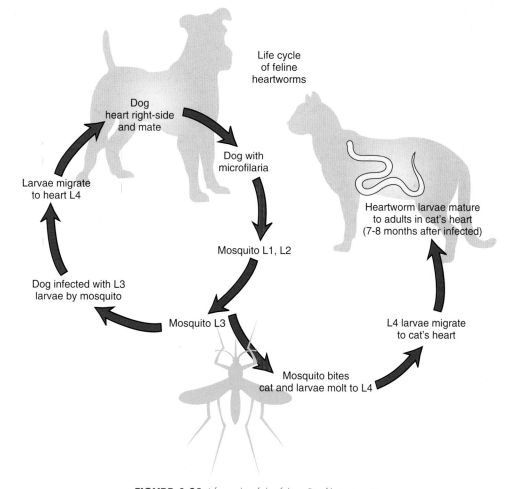

FIGURE 4-31 Life cycle of the feline *Dirofilaria immitis*.

RESPIRATORY SYSTEM

Parasite: *Aelurostrongylus abstrusus*
Host: Feline
Location of Adult: Respiratory bronchioles and alveolar ducts
Distribution: Worldwide
Derivation of Genus: Cat strongyle
Transmission Route: Ingestion of larvae
Common Name: Feline lungworm
Zoonotic: No

Aelurostrongylus abstrusus is the feline lungworm. The adults live in the terminal respiratory bronchioles and alveolar ducts, where they form small egg nests or nodules where they can obstruct the bronchioles. Initially this parasite lays embryonated (larvated) eggs. The eggs of this parasite are forced into the lung tissue, where they hatch to form characteristic first-stage larvae, approximately 360 mm long. These larvae are quite distinct; each has a tail with a unique S-shaped bend with a dorsal spine (Figure 4-32). These larvae are coughed up by the cat, swallowed, and passed out in the feces. Diagnosis is made by finding these characteristic larvae on fecal flotation or by the Baermann technique (see Chapter 17). It is also possible to recover the larvae using a tracheal wash (Figure 4-33). The prepatent period for the feline lungworm is approximately 30 days.

Parasite: *Oslerus osleri, Oslerus hirthi,* and *Oslerus milksi* (*Oslerus* was formerly known as *Filaroides*)
Host: Canine
Location of Adult: Trachea, lung parenchyma, and bronchioles, respectively
Distribution: North America, Europe, and Japan
Derivation of Genus: Threadlike shape
Transmission Route: Ingestion of infected L1 larvae
Common Name: Canine lungworm
Zoonotic: No

Oslerus osleri, Oslerus hirthi, and *Oslerus milksi,* the canine lungworms, are found in the trachea, lung parenchyma, and bronchioles, respectively. The larva is 232 to 266 μm in length and has a tail with a short S-shaped appendage. *Oslerus* (formerly *Filaroides*) species are unique among nematodes in that their first-stage larvae are immediately infective for the canine definitive host. No period of development is required outside the host. These parasites are transmitted from the dam to her offspring as she licks and cleans her puppies. Diagnosis is made by finding these characteristic

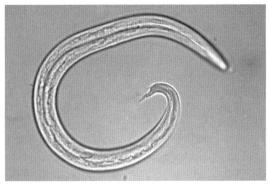

FIGURE 4-32 First-stage larva of *Aelurostrongylus abstrusus,* the feline lungworm. Each larva has a tail with an S-shaped bend and a dorsal spine. Diagnosis is made by finding these characteristic larvae on fecal flotation or by the Baermann technique.

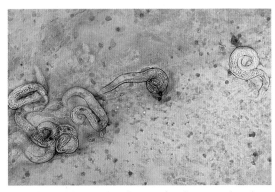

FIGURE 4-33 First-stage larvae of *Aelurostrongylus abstrusus* recovered on tracheal wash.

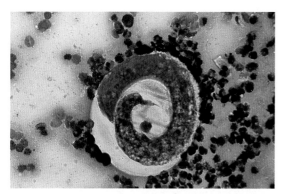

FIGURE 4-34 Tracheal wash revealing the characteristic first-stage larva of *Filaroides osleri,* the canine lungworm, which has a tail with a short S-shaped appendage. *Filaroides* species are unique among nematodes in that their first-stage larvae are immediately infective for the canine definitive host. No period of development is required outside the host.

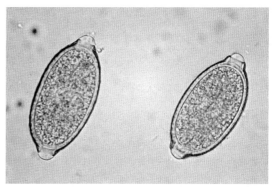

FIGURE 4-36 Egg of *Eucoleus aerophilus (Capillaria aerophila),* a capillarid nematode found in the trachea and bronchi of dogs and cats. The eggs are smaller than whipworm eggs and more broadly barrel-shaped and lighter in color. The eggs have a rough outer surface with a netted appearance.

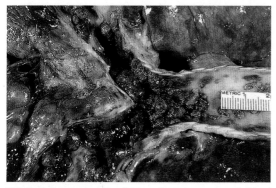

FIGURE 4-35 Nodules of *Filaroides osleri* are usually found at the bifurcation of the trachea, where they can be easily observed at necropsy.

larvae on fecal flotation or by the Baermann technique. (Figure 4-34 shows the unique infective larvae of *O. osleri.*) Nodules of *O. osleri* are usually found at the bifurcation of the trachea, where they can cause obstruction of the airway and be easily observed at necropsy (Figure 4-35). The prepatent period for *O. osleri* is approximately 10 weeks.

Parasite: 🅩 *Eucoleus aerophilus* and *Eucoleus böehmi*
Host: Canines/felines and canines, respectively
Location of Adult: Bronchi and trachea, nasal cavity and frontal sinuses, respectively

Distribution: North America, South America, and Europe
Derivation of Genus: Good sheath
Transmission Route: Ingestion of ova from feces or mucoid discharge
Common Name: Respiratory capillarid
Zoonotic: *E. aerophilus:* Yes (per AAVP); *E. böehmi:* No

Eucoleus aerophilus (Capillaria aerophila) is a capillarid nematode found in the trachea and bronchi of both dogs and cats, where it can cause an inflammatory response by the host. The prepatent period is approximately 40 days. The ova are passed through the feces or mucoid discharge from coughing them up in sputum. The ova are ingested by the host. During standard fecal flotation, eggs of *Eucoleus* species are often confused with those of *Trichuris* species (whipworms). Eggs of *E. aerophilus* are smaller (59 to 80 μm × 30 to 40 μm), more broadly barrel-shaped, and lighter in color than whipworm eggs. The egg has a rough outer surface with a netted appearance (Figure 4-36). *E. böehmi* is found in the nasal cavity and frontal sinuses of dogs, where it can cause obstruction of the nasal cavity and sinuses. Its eggs are smaller and have a smoother outer surface than those of *E. aerophilus.* Its shell has a pitted appearance. *E. böehmi* can be diagnosed by standard fecal flotation.

TECHNICIAN'S NOTE *Eucoleus aerophilus* and *Eucoleus böehmi* ova are easily confused with *Trichuris* ova on fecal flotation.

URINARY TRACT

Parasite: ⓩ *Dioctophyma renale*
Host: Canine
Location of Adult: Right kidney
Distribution: North America (primarily Canada) and Europe (but not Britain)
Derivation of Genus: Distended growth
Transmission Route: Ingestion of infected larvae within an annelid
Common Name: Canine giant kidney worm
Zoonotic: Yes but rare in humans (per *The Merck Veterinary Manual*)

Dioctophyma renale is the giant kidney worm of dogs. This largest of the parasitic nematodes that affect domestic animals (Figure 4-37) frequently infects the right kidney of dogs and ingests the parenchyma, leaving only the capsule of the kidney (Figure 4-38). The eggs from the canine urine are ingested by an annelid worm and mature into an infective larva. Ingestion of the annelid worm with an infective larva spreads the parasite to a new canine host. Eggs may be recovered by centrifugation and examination of the urine sediment. They are characteristically barrel-shaped, bipolar, and yellow-brown. The shell has a pitted

appearance. Eggs measure 71 to 84 μm × 46 to 52 μm. (Figure 4-39 shows the characteristic egg of *D. renale*.) *D. renale* is also known for its wandering activity; it often "gets off course" during its migration to the kidney. This nematode also may occur freely within the peritoneal cavity. When the kidney worm is in an aberrant site, its eggs cannot be passed to the external environment. The prepatent period for this largest of nematodes is approximately 18 weeks.

TECHNICIAN'S NOTE *Dioctophyma renale* is the largest parasitic nematode of domestic animals and can ingest the parenchyma of the right kidney.

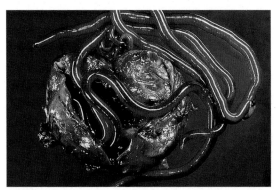

FIGURE 4-38 *Dioctophyma renale* frequently infects the right kidney of dogs and ingests the entire parenchyma, leaving only the capsule of the kidney.

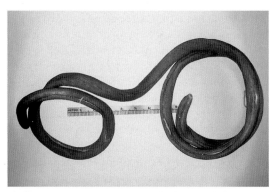

FIGURE 4-37 *Dioctophyma renale*, the giant kidney worm of dogs, is the largest of the parasitic nematodes that affect domestic animals.

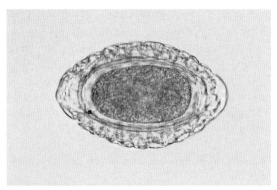

FIGURE 4-39 Egg of *Dioctophyma renale* with its characteristic barrel-shaped, bipolar, yellow-brown appearance. The shell has a pitted appearance.

Parasite: *Pearsonema plica* and *Pearsonema feliscati*
Host: Canines and felines, respectively
Location of Adult: Urinary bladder
Distribution: Southeastern United States
Transmission Route: Ingestion of infective intermediate host, earthworm; ingestion of earthworm containing infected L3 larvae
Common Name: Bladder worm of canines and felines, respectively
Zoonotic: No

Pearsonema plica and *P. feliscati* (formerly *Capillaria*) are nematodes of the urinary bladder of dogs and cats, respectively. Their eggs may be found in urine or in feces contaminated with urine. Eggs are clear to yellow, measure 63 to 68 μm × 24 to 27 μm, and have flattened, bipolar end plugs. The outer surface of the shell is roughened (Figure 4-40). These eggs may be confused with eggs of the respiratory and gastric capillarids and those of the whipworms. The eggs are ingested by an earthworm where they mature to infective larvae. If the earthworm is ingested by a new host, the larvae will migrate to the urinary bladder.

> ⬛TECHNICIAN'S NOTE *Pearsonema* species can be found in urine sediment or in fecal samples contaminated with urine, but the eggs can be easily confused with other capillarid ova of the respiratory and intestinal tract and with *Trichuris* species ova.

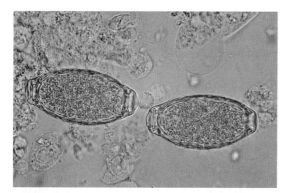

FIGURE 4-40 Egg of *Pearsonema plica*, the urinary capillarid. The eggs are clear to yellow and have flattened bipolar end plugs and a rough outer surface. The eggs may be confused with those of respiratory and gastric capillarids and whipworms.

SKIN

Parasite: *Rhabditis strongyloides*
Host: Canine
Location of Adult: Superficial layers of the skin
Distribution: Worldwide
Derivation of Genus: Rod-shaped
Transmission Route: First-stage larvae enter directly through the skin (percutaneous)
Common Name: Free-living soil nematodes
Zoonotic: No

Rhabditis strongyloides (formerly *Pelodera*) are free-living saprophytic nematodes that normally live in moist soil. These roundworms are facultative parasites; that is, they are normally free-living but under certain circumstances invade mammalian skin and develop to a parasitic mode of existence. Male and female adult *R. strongyloides* are found in soil mixed with moist organic debris such as straw or hay. The females produce eggs that hatch into first-stage larvae. These larvae invade the superficial layers of damaged or scarified skin, producing a mild dermatitis. The skin may become reddened, denuded, and covered with a crusty material. Occasionally, a pustular dermatitis develops. Because dogs acquire the infection by lying on contaminated bedding or soil, these lesions are usually observed on the ventral, or inner, surface of the limbs. Larvae of *R. strongyloides* also can be recovered from the skin of almost any domesticated animal, particularly downer cattle when these cows come in direct contact with soil containing larval *R. strongyloides.*

Larval (and adult) stages can be identified after superficial skin scrapings of the affected areas on the ventral, or inner, surface of the thighs where the larvae have a distinctive esophagus (Figure 4-41). Larvae of *P. strongyloides* are 596 to 600 μm long. These larvae must be differentiated from the microfilariae of the canine heartworm, *D. immitis* (Figures 4-25 and 4-26), the microfilariae of *A. reconditum* (Figures 4-29 and 4-30), and the first-stage larvae of *Dracunculus insignis* (Figure 4-42).

As discussed earlier, *D. immitis,* the canine heartworm, normally resides in the right ventricle and pulmonary arteries of the canine definitive host. This parasite tends to wander aberrantly and may be found in a variety of extravascular sites,

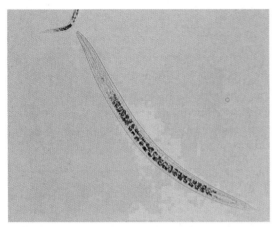

FIGURE 4-41 Larval and adult stages of *Rhabditis strongyloides* can be identified after the superficial skin scrapings of affected areas that have come in contact with infected soil.

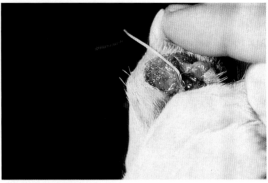

FIGURE 4-43 Aberrant adult *Dirofilaria immitis* in a subcutaneous interdigital cyst. Heartworms found aberrantly are usually single, immature, isolated worms lost en route to the heart.

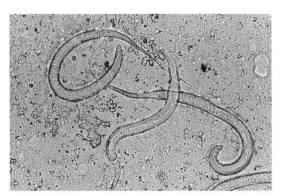

FIGURE 4-42 Unique first-stage larvae of *Dracunculus insignis* with the characteristic long, pointed tail.

including cystic spaces in subcutaneous sites. Figure 4-43 shows an aberrant adult *D. immitis* in a subcutaneous interdigital cyst. When heartworms are found aberrantly, they are usually single, immature, isolated worms that have become "lost" en route to the heart. If the worm within the cyst is female, she will not have been fertilized by a male heartworm. Therefore she will not be gravid and will not produce microfilariae.

> **TECHNICIAN'S NOTE** Although *Rhabditis strongyloides* can cause inflammation of the skin in animals, it is usually a free-living organism.

However, other adult male and female heartworms may be in their predilection sites, the right ventricle and pulmonary arteries. It is possible for these adult females to produce microfilariae. These microfilariae occasionally may be recovered in deep skin scrapings that draw blood.

Aberrant *D. immitis* within cystic spaces in the skin can be removed surgically. When subjected to the modified Knott procedure, the microfilariae of *D. immitis* are 310 to 320 μm long, with straight tails and tapering anterior ends. They must be differentiated from microfilariae of *A. reconditum* (Figures 4-29 and 4-30), the first-stage larvae of *R. strongyloides* (Figure 4-41), and the first-stage larvae of *D. insignis* (Figure 4-42).

Parasite: *Acanthocheilonema reconditum*
Host: Canine
Location of Adult: Subcutaneous tissues
Distribution: Tropical and subtropical regions
Derivation of Genus: Thorny-lipped worm
Transmission Route: Bite from infected flea
Common Name: Canine subcutaneous filarial worm
Zoonotic: No

Adult *A. reconditum*, the subcutaneous filarial worm, is a nonpathogenic nematode residing in the subcutaneous tissues of the dog. The adult filarial parasites are seldom found (Figure 4-44). (See Figures 4-29 and 4-30 for the frequently seen

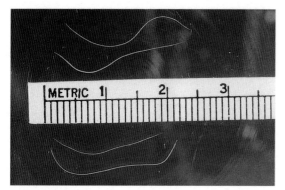

FIGURE 4-44 Adults of *Acanthocheilonema reconditum*, the subcutaneous filarial worm, are nonpathogenic. They reside in subcutaneous tissues of the dog and are seldom recovered at necropsy.

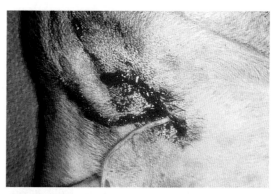

FIGURE 4-45 Adult female *Dracunculus insignis*, the guinea worm, is often found in subcutaneous tissues of the dog. The guinea worm causes a draining, ulcerous lesion in the skin, usually on the limb.

microfilariae.) These parasites may also be found within the body cavity. Occasionally, subcutaneous abscesses and ulcerated areas have been associated with *A. reconditum*. The intermediate host for this parasite is the cat flea, *Ctenocephalides felis*. Because this parasite is found in enzootic areas where *D. immitis* is present, it is necessary to differentiate the microfilariae of these two filarial parasites.

> **TECHNICIAN'S NOTE** *Acanthocheilonema reconditum* is transmitted to the dog by ingestion of the cat flea, *Ctenocephalides felis*.

Adult *A. reconditum* are rarely recovered from subcutaneous sites. More often, their microfilariae are recovered in peripheral blood samples. These microfilariae may be rarely recovered in deep skin scrapings that draw blood. On examination of microfilaremic peripheral blood subjected to the modified Knott procedure, the microfilariae of *A. reconditum* average about 285 μm in length and have "buttonhook" tails and blunt (broom handle–shaped) anterior ends (Figures 4-29 and 4-30). It is important to differentiate these microfilariae from the microfilariae of *D. immitis* (Figures 4-25 and 4-26), the first-stage larvae of *R. strongyloides* (Figure 4-41), and the first-stage larvae of *D. insignis* (Figure 4-42).

> **TECHNICIAN'S NOTE** *Acanthocheilonema reconditum* larvae are often confused with *Dirofilaria immitis* in a Knott test or heartworm filter test.

Parasite: *Dracunculus insignis*
Host: Canine
Location of Adult: Subcutaneous tissues
Distribution: North America
Derivation of Genus: Small dragon
Transmission Route: Ingestion of intermediate host, small aquatic crustaceans
Common Name: Guinea worm
Zoonotic: No

D. insignis, the guinea worm, is a nematode found in the subcutaneous tissues of the dog. The adult female nematode may be extremely long, up to 120 cm. In comparison, the male is quite short, only 2 to 3 cm in length; however, it is rarely seen. The female resides subcutaneously and produces a draining, ulcerous lesion in the skin usually on the dog's limb (Figure 4-45). The anterior end of the female worm extends from this ulcer. If the female worm within the lesion comes in contact with water, her uterus will prolapse through her anterior end and rupture, releasing a mass of first-stage larvae into the water. These larvae are 500 to 750 μm in length and have long tails that are quite distinct. (See Figure 4-42 for the first-stage larvae of *D. insignis.*) Larvae are ingested by tiny crustaceans in the water; within the crustaceans, the larvae develop to the infective third stage. Dogs become infected with *D. insignis* by drinking water containing these infected crustaceans.

If *D. insignis* is observed in an ulcerous lesion, the ulcer with its associated worm should be dipped in cool water. The cool water is a stimulus for the female worm to expel her larvae. The water containing expelled larvae should be collected and centrifuged; the sediment must then be examined for the presence of the characteristic first-stage larvae. Larvae of *D. insignis* must be differentiated from the microfilariae of *D. immitis* (Figures 4-25 and 4-26), the microfilariae of *A. reconditum* (Figures 4-29 and 4-30), and the first-stage larvae of *R. strongyloides* (Figure 4-41). Once diagnosed, the adult female worm must be surgically removed.

> **TECHNICIAN'S NOTE** *Dracunculus insignis* larvae can be found on a deep skin scraping and therefore must be differentiated from larvae of *Dirofilaria immitis* and *Acanthocheilonema reconditum*.

EYE AND ADNEXA

Parasite: Ⓩ *Thelazia californiensis*
Host: Canine and feline
Location of Adults: Conjunctival sac and lacrimal duct of the eye
Distribution: North America
Derivation of Genus: Nipple saliva
Transmission Route: Infection by infective larvae from intermediate host, *Musca autumnalis*
Common Name: Eyeworm of canines and felines
Zoonotic: Yes, but rare in humans (per *The Merck Veterinary Manual*)

Thelazia californiensis is the eyeworm of dogs and cats. Adult parasites can be recovered from the conjunctival sac and lacrimal duct (Figure 4-46). Examination of the lacrimal secretions may also reveal eggs or first-stage larvae. The cat or dog is infected with *T. californiensis* by larvae passed to the animal by the face fly, *Musca autumnalis*.

As mentioned previously, *D. immitis* can be recovered from a variety of aberrant sites, including the anterior chamber of the eye (Figure 4-43). As with aberrant parasites that occur in the skin, those found in the eye are usually single, immature,

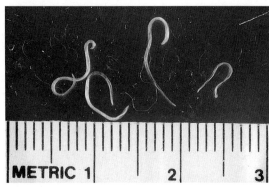

FIGURE 4-46 *Thelazia californiensis* is the eyeworm of dogs and cats. Adult parasites can be recovered from the conjunctival sac and lacrimal duct. Examination of lacrimal secretions may also reveal eggs or first-stage larvae.

isolated worms that have become lost en route to the heart. If the worm within the anterior chamber is female, she will not have been fertilized by a male heartworm. Therefore she will not be gravid and will not produce microfilariae. This nematode can be surgically removed from the eye.

> **TECHNICIAN'S NOTE** *Thelazia californiensis* adults are seen in the conjunctival sac and lacrimal ducts of the dog or cat, whereas ova can be recovered from lacrimal secretions.

NEMATODES OF RUMINANTS

GASTROINTESTINAL TRACT

Parasite: *Gongylonema pulchrum*
Host: Sheep, goats, cattle, and occasionally pigs and horses
Location of Adult: Submucosa and mucosa of the esophagus
Distribution: Worldwide
Intermediate Host: Dung beetle or cockroach
Derivation of Genus: Worms with bumps
Transmission Route: Ingestion of infective intermediate host, dung beetle, or cockroach
Common Name: Esophageal worm of ruminants
Zoonotic: No

Gongylonema pulchrum inhabits the esophagus of sheep, goats, cattle, and occasionally pigs and

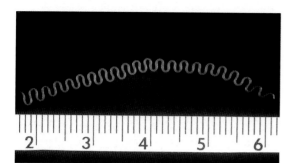

FIGURE 4-47 *Gongylonema pulchrum* inhabits the esophagus of sheep, goats, cattle, and occasionally pigs and horses. The parasite lies embedded within the submucosa or mucosa of the esophagus; it has a unique appearance in that it lies in a zigzag fashion.

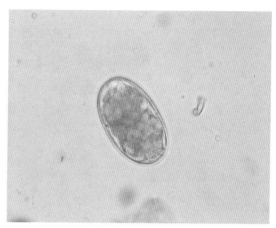

FIGURE 4-48 Oval, thin-shelled eggs that typify the eggs of ruminant trichostrongyles. Eggs contain a morula with four or more cells. Some eggs can be identified to their respective genera; however, identification is usually difficult because mixed infections are common. Identification of these should be recorded as "trichostrongyle types of eggs," and no attempt should be made to identify them to individual genus names.

horses. This parasite lies embedded within the submucosa or mucosa of the esophagus; it has a unique appearance in that it lies in a zigzag fashion within the tissues (Figure 4-47). Its eggs are 50 to 70 µm × 25 to 37 µm. *G. pulchrum* requires an intermediate host in which to develop before it can be transmitted to the ruminant host. A dung beetle or cockroach is required as an intermediate host. The ova can be identified by standard fecal flotation.

Parasite: (Z) *Bunostomum* species, *Trichostrongylus* species, *Chabertia* species, *Cooperia* species, *Haemonchus* species, *Oesophagostomum* species, and *Ostertagia* species

Host: Cattle, sheep, and goats

Location of Adult: Abomasum, small and large intestines

Distribution: Worldwide

Derivation of Genus: Mound mouth—*Bunostomum*, blood spear—*Haemonchus*, esophagus mouth—*Oesophagostomum*, and hair round—*Trichostrongylus*

Transmission Route: Ingestion of infective larvae

Common Name: Trichostrongyles of cattle and sheep

Zoonotic: *Bunostomum* species and *Trichostrongylus* species: Yes (per *The Merck Veterinary Manual*); *Chabertia* species, *Cooperia* species, *Haemonchus* species, *Oesophagostomum* species, and *Ostertagia* species: No

TECHNICIAN'S NOTE Trichostrongyle ova of any genera are too similar in appearance to accurately identify them by specific genus and species.

The bovine trichostrongyles comprise several genera of nematodes within the abomasum and the small and large intestines of cattle and other ruminants. The genera that can be classified as producing the trichostrongyle type of eggs are *Bunostomum*, *Chabertia*, *Cooperia*, *Haemonchus*, *Oesophagostomum*, *Ostertagia*, and *Trichostrongylus* species. These seven genera (there are many others) produce oval, thin-shelled eggs. The bovine trichostrongyles have a similar life cycle. The adults live in the abomasum and intestines where they feed on blood from the host. The female passes eggs in the feces. The eggs have a morula that contains four or more cells and are 70 to 120 µm in length (Figure 4-48). Some of these eggs can be identified to their respective genera; however, identification is usually difficult because mixed infections are quite common. On identification of the characteristic eggs, the veterinary diagnostician should record the identification as "trichostrongyle type of egg" and should not attempt to identify them to the individual genus names. Identification to genus and species is usually performed by fecal culture and larval identification. (Figure 4-49 shows representative examples of trichostrongyle

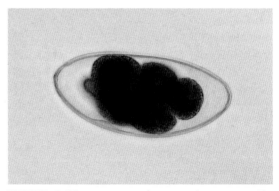

Trichostrongyle type of ovum

Monezia species

Eimeria species

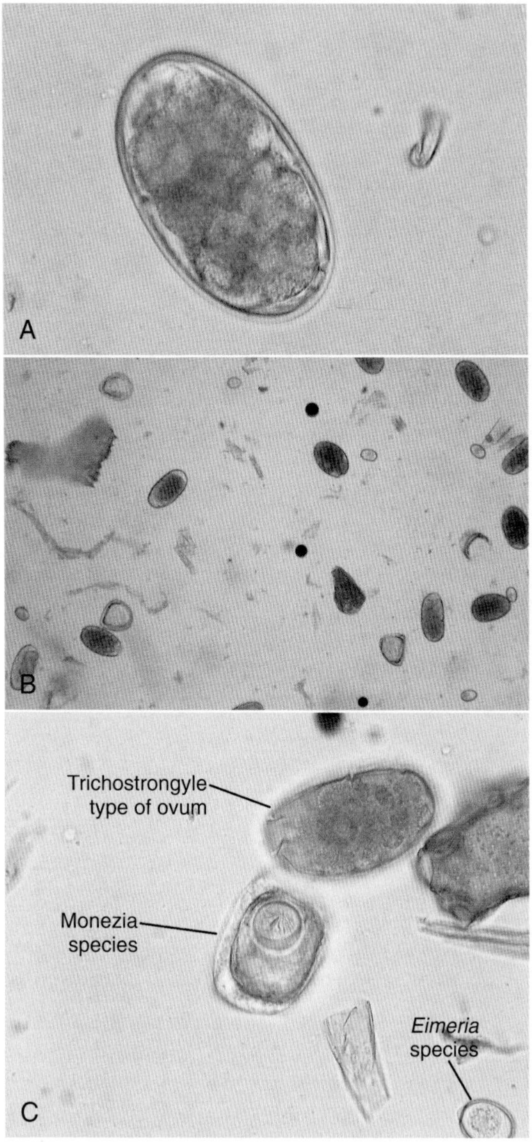

FIGURE 4-49 Representative examples of the trichostrongyle types of eggs. Trichostrongyles are perhaps the most common nematodes diagnosed on fecal flotation of ruminants. **A,** 400× close-up of trichostrongyle type of egg. **B,** 100× normal magnification. **C,** Trichostrongyle type of egg with other species of parasite eggs.

types of eggs.) The trichostrongyles are perhaps the most common nematodes diagnosed on fecal flotation of ruminants.

The most common dewormers used for the trichostrongyles are fenbendazole, levamisole, and ivermectin.

TECHNICIAN'S NOTE The most common dewormers used for trichostrongyles are fenbendazole, levamisole, and ivermectin.

Parasite: *Nematodirus* species and *Marshallagia* species
Host: Cattle, goats, and sheep
Location of Adult: Abomasum, small and large intestines
Distribution: Worldwide (*Nematodirus*) and tropical/subtropical regions (*Marshallagia*)
Derivation of Genus: Terrible nematode—*Nematodirus*, parasite studied by Dr. Marshall
Transmission Route: Ingestion of infective larvae
Common Name: Trichostrongyles with very large eggs
Zoonotic: No

Nematodirus species and *Marshallagia* species are also ruminant trichostrongyles; however, the eggs of these nematodes are much larger than those of the genera just mentioned and are the largest in the trichostrongyle family. The prepatent period is 15 to 26 days. Figure 4-50 shows the eggs of *Nematodirus* species. In standard fecal flotation, the eggs of

FIGURE 4-50 Large eggs of *Nematodirus* species. The eggs are the largest of the ruminant trichostrongyle eggs and have tapering ends and a morula with four to eight cells.

Nematodirus species are large, 150 to 230 μm × 80 to 100 μm, and have tapering ends and a four- to eight-cell morula. The eggs of *Marshallagia* species are also large, 160 to 200 μm × 75 to 100 μm, and have parallel sides and a rounded end and contain a 16- to 32-cell morula. Infected animals may have diarrhea, anorexia, dehydration, and a dull hair coat.

> **TECHNICIAN'S NOTE** *Nematodirus* species and *Marshallagia* species have ova similar to those of other trichostrongyle species except the eggs are the largest of the trichostrongyles.

Parasite: *Strongyloides papillosus*
Host: Cattle
Location of Adult: Small intestine
Distribution: Worldwide
Derivation of Genus: Roundlike shape
Transmission Route: Ingestion of infective larvae or penetration of skin by infective larvae
Common Name: Bovine intestinal threadworm
Zoonotic: No

Strongyloides papillosus is the intestinal thread-worm of cattle. These nematodes are unique in that only a parthenogenetic female is parasitic in the bovine host. Parasitic male *Strongyloides* do not exist. The female worms produce larvated eggs with a rhabditiform esophagus measuring 40 to 60 μm × 20 to 25 μm. Eggs are usually recovered in the flotation of fresh feces. (See Figure 4-15 for the parasitic adult females, eggs, and first-stage larvae of *Strongyloides* species.) The eggs grow and molt as they pass through the feces to the environment. Once the eggs hatch, the larvae become free-living adults or infective-stage female larvae. The infective-stage larvae can enter the host by penetration of the skin (usually between the hooves) or by ingestion. The larval *Strongyloides* species are 280 to 310 μm long and possess a rhabditiform esophagus with a club-shaped anterior corpus, narrow median isthmus, and caudal bulb. The larvae migrate to the lungs through the circulatory system, are coughed up, and are swallowed. Once in the intestines, they mature to adults and feed on the host's blood. The larvae can be passed to the ruminant neonate through the colostrum. The prepatent period is 5 to 7 days. Light infections may be asymptomatic, but heavy infections produce diarrhea, anorexia, blood and mucus in the feces, and weight loss.

The most common anthelmintics for *S. papillosus* are the benzimidazoles (e.g., fenbendazole, oxfendazole, albendazole), the probenzimidazoles (e.g., thiophanate, febantel, netobimin), and ivermectin. Because most ruminants spend part or all of their lives in pasture, the animals are subject to constant reinfection. Treatment with dewormers is only part of the treatment for ruminant parasites. Prevention plays a major role in the treatment procedure. Pasture rotation with nonruminant animals, such as horses, mules, and donkeys, reduces the infective larvae in the pasture.

> **TECHNICIAN'S NOTE** Only the parthenogenetic female *Strongyloides papillosus* is parasitic to the bovine host. Parasitic males do not exist. The female worm is commonly treated with benzimidazoles, probenzimidazoles, and ivermectin.

Parasite: *Trichuris ovis*
Host: Cattle, sheep, and goats
Location of Adult: Cecum and colon
Distribution: Worldwide
Derivation of Genus: Hair tail
Transmission Route: Ingestion of infective ova
Common Name: Whipworms
Zoonotic: No

Trichuris ovis parasites are commonly called *whipworms* and infect the cecum and colon of ruminants. (See the discussion of nematode parasites of the gastrointestinal tract of dogs and cats for details of gross morphology of adult whipworms.) The egg of the whipworm is described as trichinelloid or trichuroid; it has a thick, yellow-brown, symmetric shell with polar plugs at both ends. The eggs are unembryonated (not larvated) when laid. Eggs of bovine whipworms measure 50 to 60 μm × 21 to 25 μm. (See Figure 4-17 for the characteristic egg.) Symptoms are usually not apparent with *T. ovis* but can include dark feces, anorexia, and anemia. As with whipworms of dogs and cats, ruminant whipworms are diagnosed with the standard fecal flotation technique. The most common anthelmintics are the benzimidazoles, probenzimidazoles, and ivermectin.

> **TECHNICIAN'S NOTE** Trichurids of ruminants pass ova intermittently. Whipworm ova may be hard to find, so daily collection is recommended.

CIRCULATORY SYSTEM

Parasite: *Elaeophora schneideri*
Host: Sheep
Location of Adult: Common carotid artery
Distribution: Western and southwestern United States
Derivation of Genus: Bearing oil
Transmission Route: Bite of an infective horse fly, *Tabanus* species
Common Name: Arterial worms of sheep
Zoonotic: No

Elaeophora schneideri, the arterial worm, is found in the common carotid arteries of sheep in the western and southwestern United States. Although the adults are found in these predilection sites where they can cause obstruction of the arteries, their microfilariae are restricted to the skin. Microfilariae are 270 μm in length × 17 μm in thickness, bluntly rounded anteriorly, and tapering posteriorly. In the skin the microfilariae usually reside in the capillaries of the forehead and face. In sheep, filarial dermatitis is seen on the face, poll region, and feet.

Diagnosis of *E. schneideri* is by observation of characteristic lesions and identification of microfilariae in the skin. The most satisfactory means of diagnosis is to macerate a piece of skin in warm saline and examine the fluid for microfilariae after about 2 hours. In sheep, microfilariae are rare and may not be found in the skin of affected animals. Postmortem examination may be necessary to confirm the diagnosis of adult parasites within the common carotid arteries. The prepatent period for *E. schneideri* is 4½ months or longer.

> **TECHNICIAN'S NOTE** Filarial dermatitis caused by *Elaeophora schneideri* is found on the face, poll region, and feet of sheep.

RESPIRATORY SYSTEM

Parasite: *Dictyocaulus* species
Host: Cattle, sheep, and goats
Location of Adult: Bronchi
Distribution: Worldwide
Derivation of Genus: Netlike stalk
Transmission Route: Ingestion of infective larvae
Common Name: Lungworms of ruminants
Zoonotic: No

Dictyocaulus species are the lungworms of cattle *(Dictyocaulus viviparus)*, sheep, and goats *(Dictyocaulus filaria)*. Adult parasites are found in the bronchi of infected hosts. The prepatent period varies between the species but is approximately 28 days. The female worm lays her eggs in the lungs. The eggs are usually coughed up, are swallowed, and hatch in the intestine, producing larvae that may be recovered in the feces. Larvae of *D. filaria* have brown food granules in their intestinal cells, a blunt tail, and an anterior cuticular knob. These larvae are from 550 to 580 μm in length. Larvae of *D. viviparus* also have brown food granules in their intestinal cells, but they have a straight tail. They are from 300 to 360 μm in length but lack the anterior cuticular knob. (Figure 4-51 shows representative examples of eggs and larvae of *D. viviparus*.) The larvae pass out of the host through the feces to

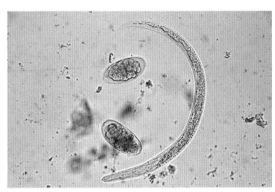

FIGURE 4-51 Representative examples of the eggs and larvae of *Dictyocaulus viviparus*, the lungworms of cattle. Eggs are usually coughed up and swallowed and hatch in the intestine, producing larvae that may be recovered in feces. Larvae of *D. viviparus* have brown food granules in their intestinal cells, a straight tail, and an anterior cuticular knob.

grow and molt from L2 to L3 larvae in the environment. The L3 infective larvae are ingested by the host and migrate through the tissues to the lymph vessels. The larvae grow and molt to L4 larvae and follow the lymph vessels to the heart. From the heart, the larvae follow the circulatory system to the lungs where they mature into adults (Figure 4-52). The adult worms are white with a small buccal cavity and short, dark, and granular spicules with the vulva in the center of the body. The most common symptom is coughing. The eggs can be found in mucus discharge or coughed-up sputum.

Benzimidazoles, probenzimidazoles, and ivermectin are the most common anthelmintics used in ruminants.

> *TECHNICIAN'S NOTE* The ova of *Dictyocaulus* species hatch in the host's intestines, and the larvae are present in the feces. Therefore diagnosis is made by finding the larvae on standard fecal flotation or flotation of the sputum-mucus discharge or by use of the Baermann technique.

Parasite: *Muellerius capillaris*
Host: Sheep and goats

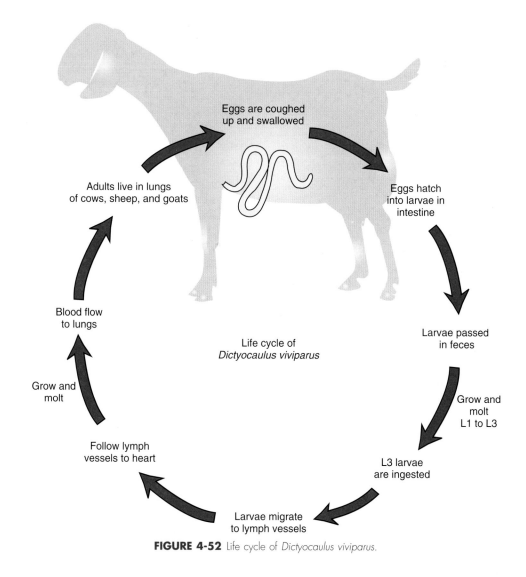

FIGURE 4-52 Life cycle of *Dictyocaulus viviparus*.

Location of Adult: Bronchioles
Distribution: Worldwide
Derivation of Genus: A parasite named for Dr. Mueller
Transmission Route: Ingestion of infective larvae
Common Name: Hair lungworm of sheep and goats
Zoonotic: No

Muellerius capillaris is often called the *hair lungworm* of sheep and goats. Adults are found within the bronchioles, mostly in nodules in the lung parenchyma where they can obstruct the bronchioles. The eggs develop in the lungs of the definitive host, and first-stage larvae are coughed up, swallowed, and passed out with the feces. The larvae are from 230 to 300 µm long. The larval tail has an undulating tip and a dorsal spine. Figure 4-53 shows representative examples of eggs and larvae of *M. capillaris*.

> *TECHNICIAN'S NOTE* *Muellerius capillaris* is best diagnosed by finding the first-stage larvae in the feces on a standard fecal flotation.

Parasite: *Protostrongylus* species
Host: Sheep and goats
Location of Adult: Small bronchioles
Distribution: Worldwide

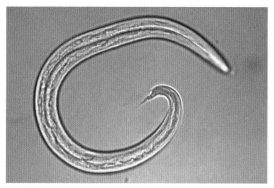

FIGURE 4-53 Representative examples of the eggs and larvae of *Muellerius capillaris*, the hair lungworm of sheep and goats. Eggs develop in the lungs of the definitive host, and first-stage larvae are coughed up, swallowed, and passed out with feces. The larval tail has an undulating tip and dorsal spine.

Derivation of Genus: First round
Transmission Route: Ingestion of infective larvae
Zoonotic: No

Adult *Protostrongylus* species occur in the small bronchioles of sheep and goats where the adults can cause obstruction of the bronchioles. The eggs develop in the lungs of the definitive host. First-stage larvae are coughed up, swallowed, and passed out with the feces. These larvae are 250 to 320 µm long. This nematode's larval tail has an undulating tip but lacks the dorsal spine.

The Baermann technique is used to diagnose lungworm infection in ruminants (see Chapter 17).

> *TECHNICIAN'S NOTE* The ova of *Protostrongylus* species develop in the lungs of the host, and larvae are passed in the feces where they can be found by using the Baermann technique.

SKIN

Parasite: *Stephanofilaria stilesi*
Host: Cattle, goats, buffalo, and wild ruminants
Location of Adult: Ventral midline skin
Distribution: United States
Derivation of Genus: Crown thread
Transmission Route: Bite by the infective horn fly, *Haematobia irritans*
Common Name: Skin worm of ruminants
Zoonotic: No

Stephanofilaria stilesi parasites are small nematodes found in the skin of cattle, goats, buffalo, and other wild ruminants. In the United States they typically produce a dermatitis along the ventral midline of cattle (Figure 4-54). The infective larvae are transmitted by the bite of the horn fly, *Haematobia irritans*. The skin lesions are thought to be caused by both adult and microfilarial stages of this parasite.

The lesions caused by *S. stilesi* are located at or near the umbilicus and consist initially of small red papules. Later the lesions develop into large pruritic areas (up to 25 cm) of alopecia, with thick, moist crusts. Both the adults (6 mm) and microfilariae may be found in deep skin scrapings after the crusts have been removed from the lesions.

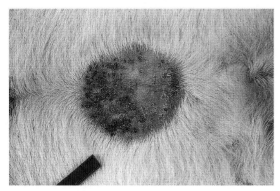

FIGURE 4-54 *Stephanofilaria stilesi* are small nematodes found in the skin of cattle, goats, buffalo, and other wild ruminants. They typically produce dermatitis, a plaque-like lesion, along the ventral midline of cattle in the United States.

> **TECHNICIAN'S NOTE** *Stephanofilaria stilesi* adults and microfilariae cause skin lesions in the host that can be found on deep skin scraping. Remember that other parasite larvae can also be recovered from the skin of many animals.

Although *E. schneideri*, the arterial worm, is found in the common carotid arteries of sheep in the western and southwestern United States, the microfilariae are restricted to the skin (see earlier discussion under Circulatory System).

It is important that the veterinary diagnostician remember that larvae of *R. strongyloides* also can be recovered from the skin of almost any domesticated animal, particularly downer cattle that come in contact with moist soil containing larvae of the genus *Rhabditis*. The larvae actively penetrate the skin and can produce a severe dermatitis (Figure 4-41).

EYE AND ADNEXA

Parasite: *Thelazia rhodesii* and *Thelazia gulosa*
Host: Cattle, sheep, and goats
Location of Adult: Conjunctival sac and lacrimal duct
Intermediate Host: *Musca autumnalis*
Distribution: Worldwide
Derivation of Genus: Nipple saliva
Transmission Route: Infective larvae in face fly (*M. autumnalis*) feces around the eyes
Common Name: Eyeworms of cattle, sheep, and goats
Zoonotic: No

Thelazia rhodesii and *Thelazia gulosa* are the eyeworms of cattle, sheep, and goats. Adult parasites can be recovered from the conjunctival sac and lacrimal duct. Examination of lacrimal secretions may reveal eggs or first-stage larvae. The larvae require an intermediate host, *M. autumnalis*, the face fly, to develop into an infected larva. The infected larvae are deposited by the face fly when it feeds around the eyes of the definitive host. The larvae and adults can cause inflammation of the conjunctival sacs and lacrimal ducts. Microscopic evaluation of lacrimal secretions is used for diagnosis by finding ova or first-stage larvae.

> **TECHNICIAN'S NOTE** *Thelazia rhodesii* and *Thelazia gulosa* are diagnosed by finding the ova or first-stage larvae in lacrimal secretions.

ABDOMINAL CAVITY

Parasite: *Setaria cervi*
Host: Cattle
Location of Adult: Free within the peritoneal cavity
Intermediate Host: Female mosquito
Distribution: Worldwide
Derivation of Genus: Bristles
Transmission Route: Bite by an infective mosquito
Common Name: Abdominal worm of cattle
Zoonotic: No

Setaria cervi is the abdominal worm of cattle. Large white adults are usually observed on postmortem examination and are found free within the peritoneal cavity (Figure 4-55). The sheathed microfilariae are approximately 250 × 7 μm. Antemortem diagnosis is by demonstration of microfilariae in peripheral blood smears. Damage to the cow may occur because of the migration of the microfilariae to the peritoneal cavity through the tissues.

> **TECHNICIAN'S NOTE** *Setaria cervi* may be found free in the abdomen when performing abdominal surgery. During routine abdominal surgery, adult *S. cervi* may be found free within the abdominal cavity.

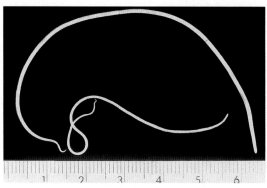

FIGURE 4-55 *Setaria cervi* is the abdominal worm of cattle. Adults are usually observed on postmortem examination and are found free within the peritoneal cavity.

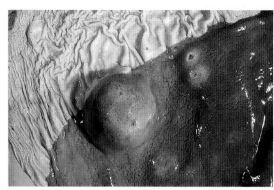

FIGURE 4-56 *Draschia megastoma* is often associated with the formation of large, thickened, fibrous nodules within the stomach mucosa of horses.

NEMATODES OF EQUIDS

GASTROINTESTINAL TRACT

Parasite: *Habronema microstoma, Habronema muscae,* and *Draschia megastoma*

Host: Horses

Location of Adult: Stomach mucosa

Intermediate Host: Muscidae fly

Distribution: Worldwide

Derivation of Genus: Delicate thread—*Habronema*; worm named for Dr. Drasch

Transmission Route: Ingestion of infective Muscidae fly

Common Name: Stomach worms of horses

Zoonotic: No

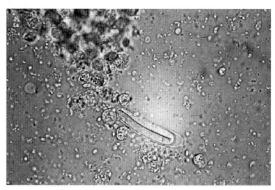

FIGURE 4-57 Larvated eggs or larvae of *Habronema* and *Draschia* species may be recovered on standard fecal flotation. Eggs of both genera are elongate and thin walled and often contain first-stage larvae.

Habronema microstoma, Habronema muscae, and *Draschia megastoma* are nematodes found in the stomach of horses. *H. microstoma* and *H. muscae* reside on the mucosa of the stomach, just beneath a thick layer of mucus. *D. megastoma* is often associated with the formation of large, thickened fibrous nodules within the stomach mucosa (Figure 4-56). Larvae of both *Habronema* and *Draschia* species may also parasitize skin lesions, causing a skin condition of horses known as *summer sores* (see Figure 4-68 and later discussion under Skin), or cutaneous habronemiasis/draschiasis.

Larvated eggs or larvae may be recovered on standard fecal flotation. The eggs of both genera are elongate and thin walled and measure 40 to 50 µm × 10 to 12 µm (Figure 4-57). These eggs (or hatched larvae) pass to the outside environment and are ingested by flies belonging to the family Muscidae. The larvae develop to the infective third stage within the fly, and if a horse accidentally ingests the fly, the larvae develop to the adult stage within the stomach of the horse. The prepatent period is approximately 60 days. Antemortem diagnosis of gastric habronemiasis is based on observation of eggs or larvae on fecal flotation. Symptoms for *H. microstoma, H. muscae,* and *D. megastoma* occur with heavy infections and include gastritis, colic, and diarrhea caused by inflammation of the stomach tissues.

> **TECHNICIAN'S NOTE** Larval infections of *Habronema* and *Draschia* cause "summer sores" in horses when the larvae parasitize skin lesions.

Benzimidazoles and ivermectin are the most common anthelmintics used for these species in horses. As with ruminants, equines are pasture animals, so pasture management plays an important role in treatment and prevention. In addition, a good fly control program will help reduce the infected flies in the horse's environment.

Parasite: 🅩 *Trichostrongylus axei*
Host: Horses, cattle, sheep, and pigs
Location of Adult: Stomach
Distribution: Worldwide
Derivation of Genus: Hair round
Transmission Route: Ingestion of infective larvae
Common Name: Stomach worms of horses and pigs
Zoonotic: Yes but not common (per CDC)

Trichostrongylus axei is another species of nematode that may reside in the stomach of horses, where they suck the host's blood. These unusual nematodes can cross species lines and can also infect cattle, sheep, and swine by ingesting the infective third-stage larvae. The egg of *T. axei* is classified as a strongyle or trichostrongyle type of egg and measures 79 to 92 μm × 31 to 41 μm (see following discussion on strongyles) when seen on standard fecal flotation.

> **TECHNICIAN'S NOTE** *Trichostrongylus axei* can cross species lines and infect cattle, sheep, and pigs.

Parasite: *Parascaris equorum*
Host: Horses
Location of Adult: Small intestine
Distribution: Worldwide
Derivation of Genus: Bearing worms
Transmission Route: Ingestion of ova
Common Name: Equine roundworm or equine ascarid
Zoonotic: No

Parascaris equorum is often called the *equine ascarid* or *equine roundworm*. These nematodes are found in the small intestine of young foals (Figure 4-58). These robust nematodes are the largest of the equine nematodes. Sometimes young foals pass these nematodes in their feces (Figure 4-59). The eggs are passed in the feces, which tend to be sticky, and the larvae grow and molt within the eggs. The egg containing an L2 larva is ingested by the young foal and hatches in the intestines. The larvae migrate to the liver through the hepatic portal vein, where they grow and molt to the next stage of larvae. The larvae are carried to the lungs through the circulatory system, where they are coughed up and swallowed. Once back in the intestines, the larvae mature into adults (Figure 4-60) that ingest blood.

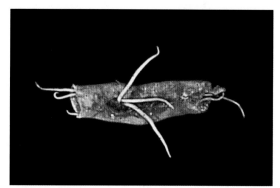

FIGURE 4-58 *Parascaris equorum* nematodes are often called *equine ascarids* or *equine roundworms*. These nematodes are found in the small intestine of young foals.

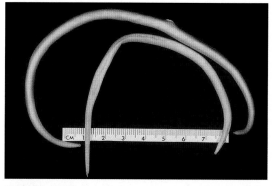

FIGURE 4-59 *Parascaris equorum* is the largest of the equine nematodes. Young foals may pass these large parasites in the feces.

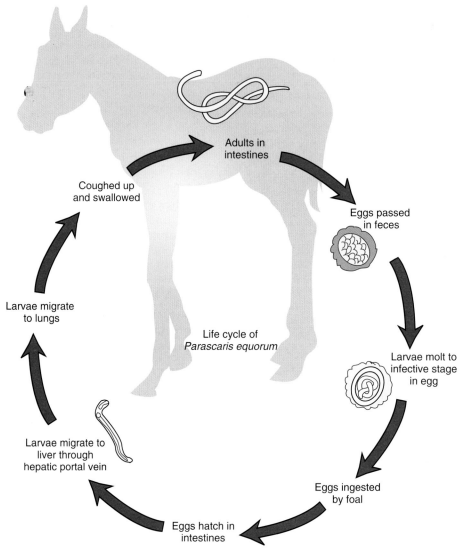

Coughed up
and swallowed

Adults in
intestines

Eggs passed
in feces

Larvae migrate
to lungs

Life cycle of
Parascaris equorum

Larvae molt to
infective stage
in egg

Larvae migrate to
liver through
hepatic portal vein

Eggs ingested
by foal

Eggs hatch in
intestines

FIGURE 4-60 Life cycle of *Parascaris equorum.*

The adult worms have large distinctive lips (Figure 4-61). The prepatent period for these ascarids is 75 to 80 days. The eggs are recovered from the feces of young horses and are round to oval and deeply pigmented. The shell is thickened, with a finely granular surface. These eggs measure 90 to 100 μm in diameter. The center of the egg contains one or two cells (Figure 4-62). Eggs can be easily recovered on standard fecal flotation.

The adult worms of *P. equorum* also may be passed in the feces of the young foal. This is one of the largest nematodes to infect horses and may grow to a length of 50 cm; however, such large specimens are the exception rather than the rule.

TECHNICIAN'S NOTE *Parascaris equorum* is the largest of the equine nematodes.

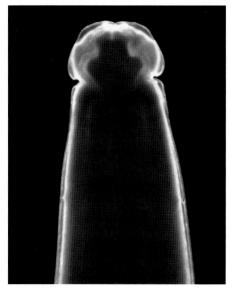

FIGURE 4-61 The distinctive lips of the adult *Parascaris equorum*. (From Bowman: *Georgis' Parasitology for Veterinarians*, ed 10, 2013, Elsevier.)

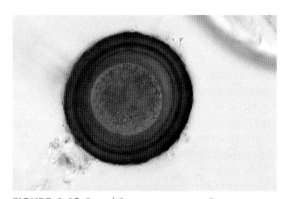

FIGURE 4-62 Egg of *Parascaris equorum*. Eggs are recovered from the feces of young horses and are round to oval and deeply pigmented. The shell is thickened, with a finely granular surface.

Mild infections of *P. equorum* are usually asymptomatic, but heavy infections can cause unthriftiness, depression, a potbellied appearance, anorexia, colic, and a cough with nasal discharge. Treatment involves pasture management to reduce chances of reinfection and a sound deworming program with benzimidazoles, ivermectin, piperazine, moxidectin, or

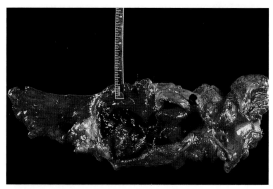

FIGURE 4-63 *Strongylus vulgaris* is often associated with thrombi in the anterior mesenteric artery of horses.

pyrantel. Prevention includes thoroughly washing the feeders and waterers to remove the contaminating eggs. In addition, pasture management involves rotating the pastures where the weanlings and foals graze.

Parasite: *Strongylus vulgaris, Strongylus edentatus,* and *Strongylus equinus*
Host: Horses
Location of Adult: Large intestines
Distribution: Worldwide
Derivation of Genus: Round and common
Transmission Route: Ingestion of infective larvae
Common Name: Strongyles of horses
Zoonotic: No

Strongyles are nematodes that parasitize the large intestine of horses and are typically divided into two types, large strongyles and small strongyles. The small strongyles comprise several genera that vary in pathogenicity. The large strongyles are the most pathogenic of the strongyles. *Strongylus vulgaris* is often associated with thrombi within the anterior mesenteric artery of horses (Figure 4-63). *S. vulgaris, Strongylus edentatus,* and *Strongylus equinus* are the large strongyles (Figure 4-64).

TECHNICIAN'S NOTE Although horses are infected with large and small strongyles, the large strongyles are the more pathogenic of the two types.

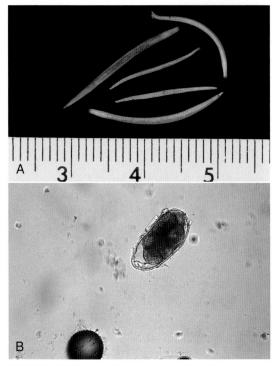

FIGURE 4-64 Strongyles are nematodes that parasitize the large intestine of horses and are typically divided into two types, large strongyles and small strongyles. **A,** Small strongyles comprise several genera that vary in pathogenicity. **B,** Large strongyles are the most pathogenic strongyles. Both large and small strongyles produce the typical strongyle type of egg.

Regardless of whether these endoparasites are a small strongyle or a large strongyle, their eggs are virtually identical. Identification to the species level is accomplished by fecal culture and identification of larvae. Strongyle eggs are most often observed during standard fecal flotation of horse feces. The eggs contain an 8- to 16-cell morula and measure approximately 70 to 90 μm × 40 to 50 μm. In addition, the life cycles of the strongyles are very similar. The eggs are passed in the feces and hatch in the environment. The infective-stage larvae migrate up and down blades of grass until the equine host ingests the larvae. The larvae are swallowed and migrate through the intestines to the mesenteric arteries and the liver where they grow and molt to the next larval stage. The larvae migrate back

toward the large intestine and grow and molt on their way. Once in the large intestine, the larvae enter the mucosa of the large intestine and mature to adults (Figure 4-65, large strongyles, and Figure 4-66, small strongyles). When these characteristic eggs are found on fecal flotation, the veterinary diagnostician should record their presence as a "strongyle type of egg" rather than trying to identify a particular species of large or small strongyles.

Clinical signs of a strongyle infection include colic, weight loss, lethargy, fever, and poor appetite. Most of the signs are related to the migration of the larvae through the mesenteric arteries and liver. The most common anthelmintics include fenbendazole, oxfendazole, thiabendazole, and ivermectin. Preventive measures include pasture management, a good deworming program, and routine fecal examinations.

> **TECHNICIAN'S NOTE** Most of the damage associated with strongyle infections is caused by the migration of larvae through the mesenteric arteries and liver.

Parasite: *Strongyloides westeri*
Host: Horses
Location of Adult: Small intestine
Distribution: Worldwide
Derivation of Genus: Roundlike shape
Transmission Route: Transmammary through colostrum and larval penetration through the skin
Common Name: Intestinal threadworm of horses
Zoonotic: No

Strongyloides westeri is the intestinal threadworm of horses, residing in the small intestine. These nematodes are unique in that only a parthenogenetic female is parasitic in the host. Parasitic males do not exist. The female parasitic worm has a near cylindric esophagus that is one quarter the length of the body (Figure 4-15). *S. westeri* produces larvated eggs measuring 40 to 52 μm × 32 to 40 μm. The mare can transmit the parasite to the foal through the colostrum. Larvae are able to enter the host through the skin or percutaneously. Eggs are usually

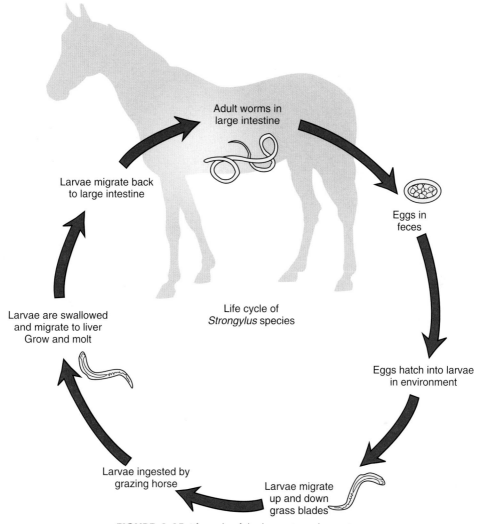

Adult worms in
large intestine

Eggs in
feces

Larvae migrate back
to large intestine

Larvae are swallowed
and migrate to liver
Grow and molt

Life cycle of
Strongylus species

Eggs hatch into larvae
in environment

Larvae ingested by
grazing horse

Larvae migrate
up and down
grass blades

FIGURE 4-65 Life cycle of the large strongyle species.

recovered on flotation of fresh feces. The prepatent period is 5 to 7 days (Figure 4-15). The clinical symptoms include diarrhea, weight loss, anemia, and poor appetite related to the adult feeding on the host's blood. A good deworming program for the mare and foal with oxibendazole, thiabendazole, or ivermectin helps control the parasite.

> 📎 *TECHNICIAN'S NOTE* The parthogenetic female is the only parasitic form of *Strongyloides westeri*. There are no parasitic males.

Parasite: *Oxyuris equi*
Host: Horses
Location of Adult: Cecum, colon, and rectum
Distribution: Worldwide
Derivation of Genus: Sharp tail
Transmission Route: Ingestion of infective ova
Common Name: Pinworm of horses
Zoonotic: No

Oxyuris equi is a pinworm of horses. The adult worms are found in the cecum, colon, and rectum. Adult worms are often observed protruding from

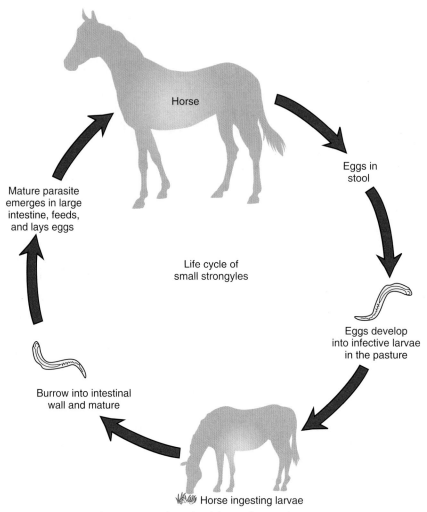

Horse

Eggs in stool

Life cycle of small strongyles

Eggs develop into infective larvae in the pasture

Mature parasite emerges in large intestine, feeds, and lays eggs

Burrow into intestinal wall and mature

Horse ingesting larvae

FIGURE 4-66 Life cycle of the small strongyle species.

the anus. Adult female worms attach their eggs to the exterior of the anus with a gelatinous, sticky material that produces inflammation and anal pruritus in infected horses. The eggs can be rubbed off the anus onto waterers, feeders, and fences, where the eggs can be ingested by the same host or a new host. Pinworm eggs can also be recovered from the feces; eggs are 90×40 μm and have a smooth, thick shell. They are operculate and slightly flattened on one side. Pinworm eggs may be larvated (Figure 4-67). The prepatent period is approximately 4 to 5 months.

Diagnosis of pinworms in horses is made by finding the characteristic eggs on microscopic examination of cellophane tape impressions or by scraping the surface of the anus. The pruritus produced often causes the horse to rub its rump against solid objects to relieve the itching. As a result, hairs in the region of the tail head are often broken. A good deworming program with oxibendazole, thiabendazole, or ivermectin and thoroughly washing the anus of infected horses will help control the spread of *O. equi*.

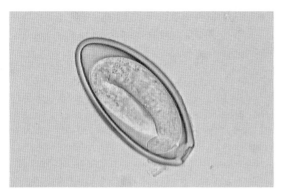

FIGURE 4-67 Egg of *Oxyuris equi*, the equine pinworm. Eggs are operculate and slightly flattened on one side. Pinworm eggs may be larvated.

> ❚*TECHNICIAN'S NOTE* The female *Oxyuris equi* attaches her eggs to the anus of the horse rather than laying them in the intestinal contents; thus it is rare to find ova on a fecal flotation test.

RESPIRATORY SYSTEM

Parasite: *Dictyocaulus arnfieldi*
Host: Horses, mules, and donkeys
Location of Adult: Bronchi and bronchioles
Distribution: Worldwide
Derivation of Genus: Netlike stalk
Transmission Route: Ingestion of larvae
Common Name: Equine lungworm
Zoonotic: No

Dictyocaulus arnfieldi, the equine lungworm, is found in the bronchi and bronchioles of horses, mules, and donkeys. The adults can cause obstruction of the bronchi and bronchioles. The eggs are ellipsoidal and embryonated and measure approximately 80 to 100 μm × 50 to 60 μm. Eggs can be recovered on fecal flotation of fresh feces (less than 24 hours old). Larvae hatch from the eggs within a few hours after feces are passed to the outside. The lungworm larvae become infective in the external environment; horses become infected by ingesting the larvae. The larvae migrate to the bronchi through lymphatic vessels. The prepatent period for the equine lungworm is 42 to 56 days. The ova or larvae can be found on standard fecal flotation. The common anthelmintics (thiabendazole, fenbendazole, ivermectin) used in a good deworming program will also treat *D. arnfieldi*.

> ❚*TECHNICIAN'S NOTE* The larvae of *Dictyocaulus arnfieldi* hatch from the ova within hours of being defecated.

SKIN

Parasite: *Habronema microstoma, Habronema muscae,* and *Draschia megastoma*
Host: Horses
Location of Adult: Stomach mucosa
Distribution: Worldwide
Intermediate Host: Muscidae flies
Derivation of Genus: Delicate thread (*Habronema*), worm named for Dr. Drasch
Transmission Route: Deposition of infected larvae into skin wounds by Muscid flies
Common Name: Cutaneous habronemiasis, cutaneous draschiasis, summer sores
Zoonotic: No

Adult *Habronema* species that occur in horses are gastrointestinal nematodes (see earlier discussion). The adults never parasitize the skin; however, the larval stages can be deposited by flies (*Musca domestica*) onto the skin wounds of horses. Here the larvae are aberrant, or "off course," and produce a condition known as cutaneous habronemiasis, cutaneous draschiasis, or summer sores. The lesions vary in size and have an uneven surface that consists of a soft, reddish-brown material and covers a mass of firmer granulation tissue. These lesions are seen on the parts of the body likely to be injured, such as the legs, withers, male genitalia, and medial canthus of the eye (Figure 4-68). These wounds tend to increase in size and do not respond to usual treatment until the following winter when they spontaneously heal.

Diagnosis of cutaneous habronemiasis is based on clinical signs and skin biopsies, which may reveal cross sections or longitudinal sections of these aberrant larvae.

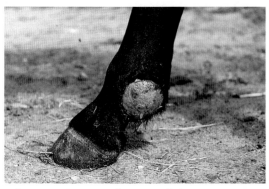

FIGURE 4-68 Lesions of cutaneous habronemiasis (cutaneous draschiasis, or summer sores) vary in size and have an uneven surface that consists of soft, reddish-brown material and covers a mass of firmer granulation tissue. Lesions are seen on body parts that are likely to be injured, such as the legs, withers, male genitalia, and medial canthus of the eye.

> **TECHNICIAN'S NOTE** Summer sores are caused by *Habronema* species and *Draschia* species becoming aberrant when the larvae are deposited in skin wounds by flies that carry the larval stage of the parasites.

Parasite: *Onchocerca cervicalis*
Host: Horses
Location of Adult: Ligamentum nuchae; microfilariae are found in the dermis
Intermediate Host: Biting midges of the *Culicoides* species
Distribution: Worldwide
Deriviation of Genus: Tumor tail
Transmission Route: Bite by infective *Culicoides* species, no-see-ums
Common Name: Equine filarial worm
Zoonotic: No

The microfilariae of *Onchocerca cervicalis,* the equine filarial parasite, produce recurrent dermatitis and periodic ophthalmia in horses. The adults live in the ligamentum nuchae of horses. The female worms produce microfilariae that migrate to the dermis through connective tissue. This parasite is spread by the biting midges of *Culicoides* species. The flies feed on host blood and ingest the microfilariae, which develop to the infective third stage within the fly. When the fly bites another horse,

larvae are injected into the connective tissue and develop to adults during migration to the ligamentum nuchae.

The microfilariae produce the characteristic lesions of cutaneous onchocerciasis as a result of the inflammation they cause: patchy alopecia and scaling on the head, neck, shoulders, and ventral midline that may be accompanied by intense pruritus.

Many infected horses are asymptomatic. Microfilariae of *Onchocerca* concentrate in certain areas, most often along the ventral midline. Because more than 90% of normal hosts are probably infected with *O. cervicalis*, detection of microfilariae in the skin of the ventral midline is not diagnostic for cutaneous onchocerciasis. However, the presence of microfilariae in diseased skin is highly indicative of, although not diagnostic of, cutaneous onchocerciasis.

> **TECHNICIAN'S NOTE** Cutaneous onchocerciasis is caused by the inflammation of the microfilariae within the skin. The inflammation causes patchy alopecia and scaling on the head, neck, shoulders, and ventral midline, which may be accompanied by intense pruritus.

Onchocerca microfilariae may be demonstrated by the following procedure. After clipping and a surgical scrub, a 6-mm punch biopsy specimen is obtained (see Chapter 17). With a single-edged razor blade or scalpel blade, half the tissue is minced in a small amount of preservative-free physiologic saline on a glass slide and allowed to stand for 5 to 10 minutes. Drying of the specimen is prevented by placing the slide in a covered chamber with a small amount of saline. The slide is then examined under a low-power (10×) objective on the microscope. Because the translucent microfilariae are difficult to observe, low-intensity light and high contrast (achieved by lowering the condenser) are essential. Live microfilariae are identified by the vigorous swimming activity at the edge of the tissue. *O. cervicalis* microfilariae are slender and 207 to 240 μm long. The other half of the biopsy should be submitted for routine histopathologic examination.

The unsheathed microfilariae of *O. cervicalis* have been incriminated in causing periodic ophthalmia and blindness in the eyes of horses. These may be detected by ophthalmic examination.

> **TECHNICIAN'S NOTE** *Onchocerca cervicalis* can be diagnosed by taking a biopsy of the infected skin lesion, mincing the biopsy tissue, and placing half of the sample in physiologic saline on a glass slide to identify the microfilariae.

EYE AND ADNEXA

Parasite: *Thelazia lacrymalis*
Host: Horse
Location of Adult: Conjunctival sac and lacrimal duct
Distribution: Worldwide
Indermediate Host: *Musca autumnalis*
Derivation of Genus: Nipple saliva
Transmission Route: Infective larvae deposited near the eyes when intermediate host, *M. autumnalis,* defecated after feeding on tears
Common Name: Eyeworm of the horse
Zoonotic: No

Thelazia lacrymalis is the eyeworm of horses throughout the world. Adult parasites can be recovered from the conjunctival sac and lacrimal duct where they can cause obstruction of the lacrimal ducts. Examination of the lacrimal secretions may reveal eggs or first-stage larvae.

ABDOMINAL CAVITY

Parasite: *Setaria equina*
Host: Horses
Location of Adult: Free within the peritoneal cavity
Distribution: Europe and North America
Intermediate Host: Mosquito
Derivation of Genus: Bristle
Transmission Route: Bite by infective mosquito
Common Name: Abdominal worm of horses
Zoonotic: No

Setaria equina is the abdominal worm of horses. Adults are large white worms and are found free within the peritoneal cavity. The sheathed microfilariae are 240 to 256 μm long. Antemortem diagnosis is by demonstration of microfilariae in peripheral blood smears. Adults may be observed freely within the peritoneal cavity during postmortem examination. The primary cause of pathology is migration of the larvae from the insertion point to the abdominal cavity.

> **TECHNICIAN'S NOTE** Adults of *Setaria equina* may be found free within the peritoneal cavity during abdominal surgery.

NEMATODES OF SWINE

GASTROINTESTINAL TRACT

Parasite: *Ascarops strongylina* and *Physocephalus sexalatus*
Host: Pigs
Location of Adult: Stomach
Distribution: Worldwide
Intermediate Host: Beetle
Derivation of Genus: *Ascarops*—Late worm; *Physocephalus*—Air head
Transmission Route: Ingestion of infective beetle
Common Name: Stomach worms of pigs
Zoonotic: No

Ascarops strongylina and *Physocephalus sexalatus* are the thick worms of the porcine stomach, where the adults suck the host's blood. Both nematodes produce thick-walled, larvated eggs that can be recovered on fecal flotation. The eggs of both species are similar in appearance. The egg of *A. strongylina* is 34 to 39 μm × 20 μm and has a thick shell surrounded by a thin membrane, producing an irregular outline (Figure 4-69). The egg of *P. sexalatus* is 34 to 39 μm × 15 to 17 μm. The larvated egg is ingested by a beetle and develops into an infective larva. The beetle is then ingested by the pig. The prepatent period for both species is approximately 42 days. Diagnosis is by observation of typical eggs on routine fecal flotation. Clinical signs include anemia, diarrhea, and weight loss. Anthelmintics used for treating *A. strongylina* and *P. sexalatus* are ivermectin, fenbendazole, thiabendazole, and oxfendazole.

> **TECHNICIAN'S NOTE** The stomach worms of the pig require a beetle intermediate host to harbor the infective larval stage.

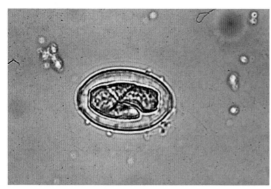

FIGURE 4-69 Egg of *Ascarops strongylina* is 34 to 39 μm × 20 μm and has a thick shell surrounded by a thin membrane that produces an irregular outline.

Parasite: *Hyostrongylus rubidus*
Host: Pigs
Location of Adult: Stomach
Distribution: Worldwide
Derivation of Genus: U-shaped and round
Transmission Route: Ingestion of infective ova
Common Name: Red stomach worm of pigs
Zoonotic: No

Hyostrongylus rubidus is the red stomach worm of swine. The egg is a trichostrongyle type of egg that is oval and thin shelled. It contains a morula with four or more cells and measures 71 to 78 μm × 35 to 42 μm. These eggs can be recovered on fecal flotation. As with the bovine trichostrongyles, definitive diagnosis can be made only by fecal culture and larval identification. The prepatent period is approximately 20 days. Clinical signs include dehydration, weight loss, diarrhea, and anemia related to the fact that the adult sucks the host's blood. Deworming with benzimidazoles (fenbendazole, thiabendazole, oxibendazole) and ivermectin controls the parasite.

> **TECHNICIAN'S NOTE** *Hyostrongylus rubidus,* or the red stomach worm of pigs, produces a trichostrongyle type of egg that contains a morula with four or more cells. It can be found on fecal flotation, but only a fecal culture and larval identification can provide a definitive diagnosis of specific genus and species.

Parasite: ⓩ *Trichostrongylus axei*
Host: Horses, sheep, cattle, and pigs
Location of Adult: Stomach
Distribution: Worldwide
Derivation of Genus: Hair round
Transmission Route: Ingestion of ova
Common Name: Stomach worm of horses, cattle, sheep, and pigs
Zoonotic: Yes but not common (per *CDC*)

T. axei is another species of nematode that may reside in the stomach of pigs and suck blood. It is important to remember that *T. axei* can cross species lines and also parasitize cattle, sheep, and horses. The eggs of *T. axei* are classified as the trichostrongyle type and measure 79 to 92 μm × 31 to 41 μm. As with bovine trichostrongyles, definitive diagnosis can be made only by fecal culture and larval identification. Benzimidazoles are the anthelmintics of choice. Diagnosis of trichostrongyle ova can be made with a standard fecal flotation technique.

Parasite: *Ascaris suum*
Host: Pigs
Location of Adult: Small intestine
Distribution: Worldwide
Derivation of Genus: Worm
Transmission Route: Ingestion of infective ova
Common Name: Swine ascarid or large intestinal roundworm of pigs
Zoonotic: No

Ascaris suum, the swine ascarid or large intestinal roundworm, is the largest nematode found in the small intestine of pigs (Figure 4-70). It may attain a length of 41 cm and can be as wide as 5 mm. Large numbers of these worms can cause intestinal obstruction. These large, robust nematodes may also be passed in feces. They produce eggs that are passed in the feces and hatch in the environment. The larvae grow to infective larvae within the eggs, which are ingested by the pig. The larvae hatch and migrate to the liver, where they grow to the next larval stage. The larvae migrate through the circulatory system to the lungs and the bronchial tree,

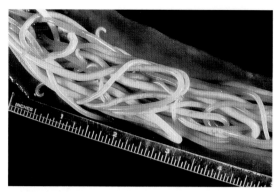

FIGURE 4-70 *Ascaris suum,* the swine ascarid or large intestinal roundworm, is the largest nematode found within the small intestine of pigs.

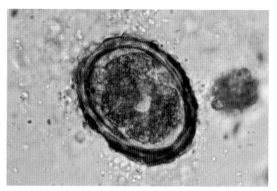

FIGURE 4-71 Eggs of *Ascaris suum* can be recovered on standard fecal flotation. Eggs are oval and golden brown with a thick, albuminous shell bearing prominent projections that give a lumpy, bumpy appearance.

where they are swallowed. Once in the intestines, the larvae mature into adults.

> **TECHNICIAN'S NOTE** *Ascaris suum* is the largest nematode found in the pig; the ova can be found on standard fecal flotation.

Eggs of *A. suum* can be recovered on standard fecal flotation. They are oval and golden brown with a thick, albuminous shell bearing prominent projections that give a lumpy, bumpy appearance. The eggs measure 70 to 89 µm × 37 to 40 µm (Figure 4-71). *A. suum* can cause a reduced growth rate, weight loss, unthriftiness, and respiratory symptoms (coughing, abdominal breathing, or thumps). Benzimidazoles, levamisole, ivermectin, pyrantel, piperazine, and hygromycin (a feed-additive dewormer) are the anthelmintics of choice.

Parasite: *Strongyloides ransomi*
Host: Pigs
Location of Adult: Small intestine
Distribution: Worldwide
Derivation of Genus: Roundlike
Transmission Route: Transmammary (through the colostrum), percutaneous
Common Name: Intestinal threadworm of pigs
Zoonotic: No

Strongyloides ransomi, the intestinal threadworm of pigs, is unique in that only a parthenogenetic female

is parasitic in the host. Parasitic males do not exist. These females produce larvated eggs measuring 45 to 55 µm × 26 to 35 µm. Eggs are usually recovered in the flotation of fresh feces. The life cycle of *S. ransomi* closely resembles that of *S. papillosus.* Transmission can occur through the colostrum. The prepatent period is 3 to 7 days (Figure 4-15). *S. ransomi* can produce diarrhea, anemia, and weight loss in the host as the parasite sucks its blood. Anthelmintics of choice are the benzimidazoles and ivermectin.

> **TECHNICIAN'S NOTE** *Strongyloides ransomi* is the intestinal threadworm of pigs; only the female is parasitic, and the larvae can enter a host through the skin or in the colostrum.

Parasite: *Oesophagostomum dentatum*
Host: Pigs
Location of Adult: Large intestine
Distribution: Worldwide
Derivation of Genus: Esophagus mouth; carry food mouth
Transmission Route: Ingestion of infective larvae
Common Name: Nodular worm of pigs
Zoonotic: No

Oesophagostomum dentatum, the nodular worm of swine, is found in the large intestine of swine (Figure 4-72). It is called the *nodular worm* because its larval stages induce the formation of large

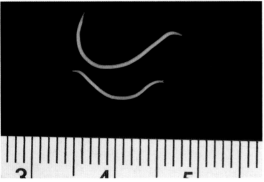

FIGURE 4-72 *Oesophagostomum dentatum,* the nodular worm of swine, is found in the large intestine of swine.

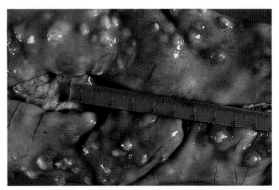

FIGURE 4-73 *Oesophagostomum dentatum* is called the *nodular worm* of swine because its larval stages induce the formation of large nodules within the wall of the large intestine.

nodules within the wall of the large intestine, which can cause intestinal disturbance and obstruction (Figure 4-73). The prepatent period is 50 days. The eggs of *O. dentatum* are of the trichostrongyle type, that is, oval thin-shelled eggs. They contain 4 to 16 cells and measure 40 × 70 μm. These eggs can be recovered on standard fecal flotation. As with the bovine trichostrongyles, definitive diagnosis can be made only by fecal culture and larval identification. The parasite can cause anorexia, diarrhea, weight loss, and gastrointestinal disturbances in the host. Benzimidazoles, ivermectin, levamisole, piperazine, and pyrantel are the anthelmintics of choice.

> **TECHNICIAN'S NOTE** The nodules formed by the third-stage larvae of *O. dentatum* in the large intestine cause intestinal disturbances and can cause a mechanical obstruction of the intestinal tract.

Parasite: *Trichuris suis*
Host: Pigs
Location of Adult: Cecum and colon
Distribution: Worldwide
Derivation of Genus: Hair tail
Transmission Route: Ingestion of infective ova
Common Name: Whipworm of pigs
Zoonotic: No

Trichuris suis, commonly called *whipworms,* infect the cecum and colon of swine. (See the previous discussion of nematodes of dogs and cats for gross morphology of adult worms and life cycle.) The egg of the whipworm is trichuroid or trichinelloid and has a thick, brown, barrel-shaped shell with polar plugs at both ends (Figure 4-17). The eggs are unembryonated (not larvated) when laid. Eggs of porcine whipworms measure 50 to 60 μm × 21 to 25 μm. The prepatent period is 42 to 49 days. Common symptoms seen in the host are anemia, bloody diarrhea, anorexia, and stunted growth related to the fact that the adult attaches to the intestinal wall and sucks the host's blood. Levamisole, dichlorvos, and fenbendazole are the anthelmintics of choice.

> **TECHNICIAN'S NOTE** The whipworm of the pig is similar in life cycle and appearance to dog and cat whipworms. The thin end of the adult was once thought to be the tail of the worm rather than the head.

Parasite: *Trichinella spiralis*
Host: Pigs can serve as both definitive and intermediate hosts.
Location of Adult: Small intestine
Distribution: Worldwide but does not occur in Australia or Denmark
Derivation of Name: Small hair
Transmission Route: Ingestion of contaminated raw and undercooked meat, usually pork
Common Name: Trichina worm
Zoonotic: Yes

The adult *Trichinella spiralis*, the "trichina worm," is found in the small intestine of the porcine definitive host. The adult worm is very fine and slender. The female is very tiny, only 4 mm in length; the male is even smaller. This stage is seldom recovered by the veterinarian. The egg is larvated and measures 30 × 40 μm. (See the discussion under musculoskeletal system for the larval stage in the porcine intermediate host.) *T. spiralis* is a very unusual parasite because the definitive host and the intermediate host may be the same animal. *T. spiralis* can be passed to humans in undercooked pork (see Chapter 16). Most animal hosts are asymptomatic (showing no symptoms); however, because larvae encyst in muscle tissue, they can cause damage to the muscle by their encysted presence.

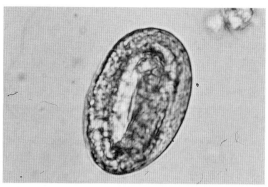

FIGURE 4-74 *Metastrongylus elongatus (apri)*, the swine lungworm, is found in the bronchi and bronchioles of pigs. Oval, thick-walled eggs measure 60 × 40 μm and contain larvae.

> **TECHNICIAN'S NOTE** Although *Trichinella spiralis* does not typically cause symptoms in the definitive host, it does cause problems in human muscles. The only test that can be used for diagnosis in the intermediate host is a biopsy of the muscle tissue for encysted larvae.

RESPIRATORY TRACT

Parasite: *Metastrongylus elongatus*
Host: Pigs
Location of Adult: Bronchi and bronchioles
Intermediate Host: Earthworm
Distribution: Worldwide
Derivation of Genus: After round
Transmission Route: Ingestion of infective earthworm
Common Name: Swine lungworm
Zoonotic: No

Metastrongylus elongatus, the swine lungworm, is found within the bronchi and bronchioles of pigs. The oval, thick-walled eggs measure 60 × 40 μm and contain larvae (Figure 4-74). Eggs can be recovered on fecal flotation using a flotation medium with a specific gravity greater than 1.25 or by using the fecal sedimentation technique. The prepatent period is approximately 24 days. *M. elongatus* uses the earthworm as an intermediate host. Therefore control of earthworms in the pig's environment will help eliminate this parasite. Control may include keeping pigs on concrete rather than pasture or dirt. Infected pigs may have a persistent cough, reduced growth rate, and unthriftiness as a result of partial obstructions in the airways. Infected pigs can be treated with fenbendazole, ivermectin, or levamisole.

> **TECHNICIAN'S NOTE** Fecal flotation with a solution having a specific gravity greater than 1.25 and the fecal sedimentation technique are the best ways to diagnose swine lungworm using feces.

URINARY TRACT

Parasite: *Stephanurus dentatus*
Host: Pigs
Location of Adult: Cystic spaces connected to the kidneys, ureters, and perirenal tissue
Intermediate Host: Earthworm
Distribution: Tropical and subtropical regions
Derivation of Genus: Encircling the urinary system
Transmission Route: Ingestion of infective intermediate host, earthworm, or percutaneous
Common Name: Swine kidney worm
Zoonotic: No

Stephanurus dentatus, the swine kidney worm, is found in cystic spaces that connect to the kidney, ureters, and perirenal tissues of pigs (Figure 4-75). The eggs are the oval, thin-shelled strongyle type containing 4 to 16 cells and measuring 90 to 120 μm × 43 to 70 μm. Eggs can be recovered from the urine using sedimentation (Figure 4-76). The prepatent period is extremely long, approximately 9 to 24 months. *S. dentatus* can use the earthworm as an intermediate host, or the infective larvae can enter the pig directly through the skin. Infected pigs may show signs of anorexia, decreased growth rate, and weight loss. Much of the damage caused by the parasite comes from the migration of larvae to the cystic spaces around the kidneys, ureters, and perirenal tissues. Anthelmintics of choice include fenbendazole, levamisole, and ivermectin.

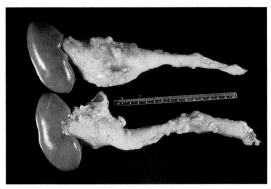

FIGURE 4-75 *Stephanurus dentatus,* the swine kidney worm, is found in cystic spaces that connect to the kidney, ureters, and perirenal tissues of pigs.

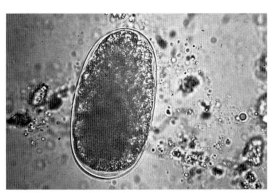

FIGURE 4-76 Eggs of *Stephanurus dentatus* are of the strongyle type, that is, oval, thin-shelled eggs. They contain 4 to 16 cells and measure 90 to 120 μm × 43 to 70 μm. Eggs can be recovered from urine using sedimentation.

> **TECHNICIAN'S NOTE** *Stephanurus dentatus* can have a direct life cycle by entering the host through the skin, or it can have an indirect life cycle by using an intermediate host, the earthworm.

MUSCULOSKELETAL SYSTEM

Parasite: *Trichinella spiralis*
Host: Pigs are the definitive host.
Location of Adult: Small intestine
Distribution: Worldwide but does not occur in Australia or Denmark
Derivation of Name: Small hairs
Transmission Route: Ingestion of contaminated raw and undercooked meat
Common Name: Trichina worm
Zoonotic: Yes

The larval form of *T. spiralis,* the trichina worm, is found in the musculature of the porcine intermediate host. The adult worm is very fine and slender and is found within the small intestine. The larval *T. spiralis* is found in striated muscle fibers. It measures approximately 1 mm in length and is found in cystic spaces within the musculature (Figures 4-77 and 4-78). The cyst measures 0.4 to 0.6 mm × 0.25 mm. In chronic cases the cyst may become calcified. (See the discussion under Gastrointestinal Tract for the adult stage of this parasite in the

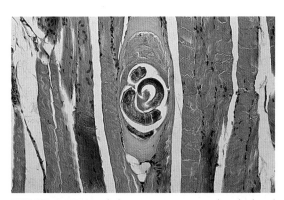

FIGURE 4-77 Muscle biopsy specimen revealing the larval form of *Trichinella spiralis,* the trichina worm, found in the musculature of the porcine intermediate host. Larvae measure approximately 1 mm in length and are found in cystic spaces in the musculature.

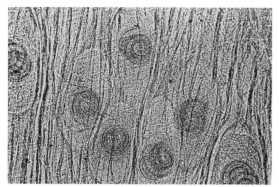

FIGURE 4-78 Histopathologic section revealing the larval form of *Trichinella spiralis*, the trichina worm, found in the musculature of the porcine intermediate host.

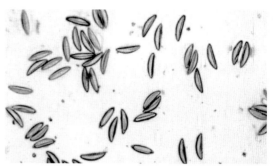

FIGURE 4-79 Eggs of *Syphacia obvelata*, the mouse cecal pinworm, as they appear on cellophane tape presentation.

definitive host.) Humans may become infected with *T. spiralis*.

Diagnosis of the larval stage of *T. spiralis* is made by performing a biopsy of muscle tissue and demonstrating encysted larvae within the skeletal musculature. As a result of the zoonotic potential for this parasite, pork should *always* be cooked thoroughly.

> 📎 *TECHNICIAN'S NOTE* *Trichinella spiralis* uses the pig as both the intermediate host and the definitive host. It can be passed to other hosts with the eating of raw or undercooked pork, thus using the pig as an intermediate host. However, it also uses the pig as the definitive host, reproducing within the pig to continue its life cycle.

NEMATODES OF MICE

GASTROINTESTINAL TRACT

Parasite: *Syphacia obvelata, Aspiculuris tetraptera,* and *Syphacia muris*
Host: Mice—*A. tetraptera;* mice, rats, hamsters, and gerbils—*Syphacia* species
Location of Adult: Cecum and rectum
Distribution: Worldwide
Derivation of Genus: *Syphacia*—love together; *Aspiculuris*—toward a small tail
Transmission Route: Ingestion of infective ova and retrograde infection
Common Name: Pinworms
Zoonotic: No

Oxyurids, or pinworms, of mice include *Syphacia obvelata, Aspiculuris tetraptera,* and to a lesser extent *Syphacia muris*, the common pinworm of rats. Patent *Syphacia* infections can be detected both antemortem and postmortem with the perianal cellophane test. The adults of *Syphacia* reside in the cecum of the mouse until the gravid female migrates the length of the colon to deposit a large batch of eggs in the perianal region, at which time the female dies.

Eggs of *A. tetraptera* cannot be detected with the perianal cellophane tape test. *A. tetraptera* adults reside mainly in the proximal loop of the colon of the mouse and do not migrate to deposit eggs on the perianal area, as do *Syphacia* species. Eggs of *A. tetraptera* can be detected antemortem by fecal flotation and occasionally by direct smear examination of feces.

The banana-shaped eggs of *S. obvelata* are elongated with pointed ends (Figure 4-79). They are flat on one side and convex on the other, measuring 118 to 153 μm × 33 to 55 μm. *S. muris* is found less frequently and in smaller numbers in mice than *S. obvelata*. The more symmetric, football-shaped eggs of *S. muris* are smaller than those of *S. obvelata*, measuring only 72 to 82 μm × 25 to 36 μm, and are blunted or rounded on the ends (Figure 4-80). When observed on fecal flotation, the eggs of *A. tetraptera* have a thinner shell than the eggs of the *Syphacia* species and do not have a flattened side. *A. tetraptera* eggs are 89 to 93 μm × 33 to 42 μm, symmetrically ellipsoid, and midway in size between eggs of the two *Syphacia* species.

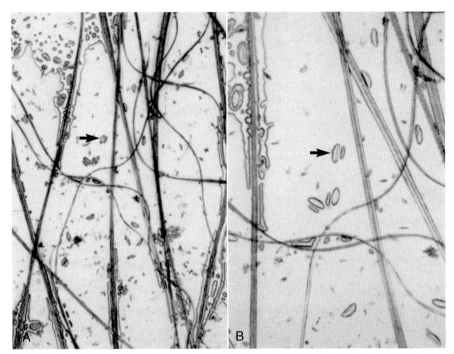

FIGURE 4-80 Cellophane tape presentation of *Syphacia muris* eggs viewed at **A**, low magnification, and **B**, medium magnification. The *arrow* points to the same egg at each magnification. The smaller object to the right of the egg is an artifact.

> **TECHNICIAN'S NOTE** *Aspiculurus tetraptera* females do not deposit ova on the perianal area as other pinworms do. Therefore the cellophane tape method cannot be used for diagnosis. Instead, standard fecal flotation or direct fecal smear is used to diagnose this species of pinworm.

On postmortem examination, pinworms of mice may be detected by placing a small piece of the cecum and proximal loop of the colon in a Petri dish with a small amount of normal saline. Within a few minutes, pinworms may be observed in the saline grossly or with the aid of a handheld magnifying lens or a dissecting microscope (Figure 4-81). The adult pinworms can be collected with a bulb and pipette, applied to a glass slide with a coverslip, and examined microscopically at low magnification (4× objective). *A. tetraptera* is usually recovered from the proximal colon and is easily distinguished from *Syphacia* species by its oval esophageal bulb and prominent cervical ala (Figure 4-82, *A*).

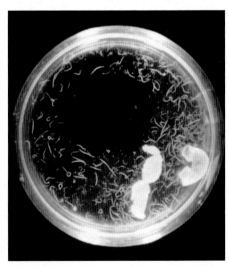

FIGURE 4-81 A 2-inch Petri dish containing saline and proximal loops of colon from three mice. White, hairlike objects are *Aspiculuris tetraptera* roundworms that have moved into the saline from colon sections.

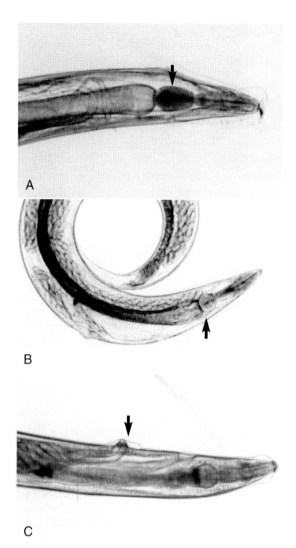

FIGURE 4-82 A, Cranial end of *Aspiculuris tetraptera* female, showing the oval esophageal bulb *(arrow)*. **B,** *Syphacia muris,* showing the round esophageal bulb *(arrow)*. **C,** Cranial end of *Syphacia obvelata* female *(arrow* indicates the vulva).

S. obvelata and *S. muris* are usually recovered from the cecum. *Syphacia* species have a rounded esophageal bulb and a small cervical ala (Figure 4-82, *B*). Additionally, the vulva is in the cranial one sixth of the body of *S. obvelata* females (Figure 4-82, *C*), whereas the vulva of *S. muris* is in the cranial one fourth of the body (Figure 4-82, *B*). Adult males of the two *Syphacia* species can be differentiated by the position of the three ventral mamelons. In

males of *S. obvelata,* the middle mamelon is located centrally on the length of the body (see Figure 4-86, *A*). The first mamelon is at the center of the male in *S. muris* (see Figure 4-86, *B*). Although differentiation of the adults of the two *Syphacia* species may be difficult and time-consuming for veterinary technicians, experienced diagnosticians can easily differentiate the eggs on cellophane tape preparations by size and shape (Figures 4-79 and 4-80).

In general, mice carry light to medium loads of pinworms without demonstrating clinical signs of infection. However, large numbers of pinworms may lead to rectal prolapse, enteritis, sticky stools, and pruritus, which result in biting at the base of the tail. Symptoms are caused by inflammation related to the female and eggs at the perianal region of the animal.

Pinworms are transmitted by the ingestion of the eggs. The eggs are hardy, resistant to environmental extremes, and light enough to aerosolize, making control difficult. Retrograde infection is also possible with *Syphacia* species. The multispecies owner should be instructed that *Syphacia* species can be easily transmitted among mice, rats, hamsters, and gerbils. *A. tetraptera* has also been diagnosed in rats. Rodent pinworms are not of zoonotic significance.

> *TECHNICIAN'S NOTE* Although pinworms are species specific, *Syphacia* species are able to survive and replicate in mice, rats, hamsters, and gerbils because they are all rodent species and are closely related.

NEMATODES OF RATS
GASTROINTESTINAL TRACT

The three oxyurids, or pinworms, discussed in the previous section (i.e., *S. muris, S. obvelata,* and *A. tetraptera*) may also infect rats. *S. muris* is by far the most common pinworm and is often referred to as the *rat pinworm.*

Parasite: *Trichosomoides crassicauda*
Host: Rats
Location of Adult: Urinary bladder
Distribution: Worldwide

Derivation of Genus: Body shaped like a hair
Transmission Route: Ingestion of ova from urine
   (urinary-oral route)
Common Name: Bladder worm of the rat
Zoonotic: No

Trichosomoides crassicauda is a nematode found in the urinary bladder of rats. The adult female *T. crassicauda* is approximately 10 mm long; it is a thin worm and is grossly visible in the wall of the urinary bladder. This parasite is unique in that the male is neotenic. This means that he is very small and resides in the vagina of the immature female and the uterus of the mature female *T. crassicauda*. The eggs are double operculate and approximately 65 × 33 μm and resemble whipworm eggs, especially those of *Trichuris* species. The main difference between them is that the eggs of *T. crassicauda* are lighter in color, are slightly smaller, and contain a single larva. This parasite has been associated with bladder tumors in rats; however, few clinical signs are associated with infection by *T. crassicauda*, most damage coming from the presence of the parasite in the bladder wall. Transmission is by the urinary-oral route. This parasite can be a significant problem in rat colonies but can be eliminated by cesarean delivery of neonates. This is a species-specific nematode and is not of zoonotic significance.

> **TECHNICIAN'S NOTE** The male urinary bladder worm of rats resides inside the vagina of the immature female or the uterus of the mature female.

Infections with *T. crassicauda* may be diagnosed in three ways: antemortem or postmortem observation of eggs in the urine, gross observation at postmortem of adult worms in the wall or lumen of the urinary bladder, and microscopic observation of the adult worms in histopathologic sections of the urinary bladder, ureters, or renal pelvis.

NEMATODES OF HAMSTERS

GASTROINTESTINAL TRACT

Hamsters are susceptible to infection with the mouse and rat pinworms *S. obvelata* and *S. muris*, although it is unlikely that hamsters will develop clinically apparent infections (see previous discussion of nematodes of mice).

NEMATODES OF GERBILS

GASTROINTESTINAL TRACT

Parasite: *Dentostomella translucida*
Host: Gerbil
Location of Adult: Stomach and proximal one third of the small intestine
Distribution: Worldwide
Derivation of Genus: Little tooth in mouth
Transmission Route: Ingestion of infective ova
Common Name: Pinworm of gerbils
Zoonotic: No

> **TECHNICIAN'S NOTE** Pinworms are not reported as commonly in gerbils as they are in other rodent species.

Dentostomella translucida, the gerbil pinworm, is not reported as frequently as other rodent pinworms (*Syphacia* species and *A. tetraptera*). This may be the result of a lack of information on its life cycle. Adult male and female nematodes have a short, muscular esophagus. The vulva of the female is located just cranial to the midbody (Figure 4-83). Males are distinguished by a cuticular inflation just cranial to the cloaca (Figure 4-84). Adults are 6 to 31 mm long, with the female generally larger than the male, as is true of other rodent pinworms. Eggs

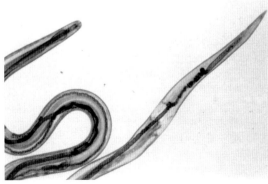

FIGURE 4-83 Adult female *Dentostomella translucida.*

of *D. translucida* are asymmetric and oval, measuring 120 to 140 μm × 30 to 60 μm (Figure 4-85). They resemble those of *A. tetraptera*, which are smaller, measuring 89 to 93 μm × 36 to 42 μm.

Fecal flotation may be used to detect eggs of *D. translucida*, but this method is unreliable because of the poorly understood life cycle (intermittent shedding of eggs). On postmortem examination, *D. translucida* may be found in the stomach and the proximal one third of the small intestine.

D. translucida has a direct life cycle and is transmitted by ingestion of infective eggs from feces of infected animals. The parasite has been found in the golden hamster and the gerbil. This parasite has no zoonotic significance.

As with hamsters, gerbils are susceptible to infection with the mouse and rat pinworms *S. obvelata* and *S. muris* (Figure 4-86; also Figures 4-79, 4-80, and 4-81 and previous discussion of nematodes of mice).

> **TECHNICIAN'S NOTE** As with other pinworm species, the damage done by *Dentostomella translucida* is most commonly caused by inflammation and irritation.

NEMATODES OF GUINEA PIGS

GASTROINTESTINAL TRACT

Parasite: *Paraspidodera uncinata*
Host: Guinea pig
Location of Adult: Cecum and colon

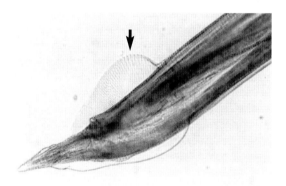

FIGURE 4-84 Cuticular inflation *(arrow)* on the tail of a male *Dentostomella translucida.*

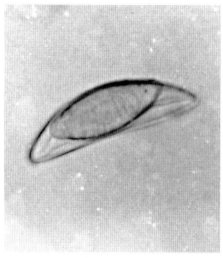

FIGURE 4-85 Egg of *Dentostomella translucida* in fecal flotation.

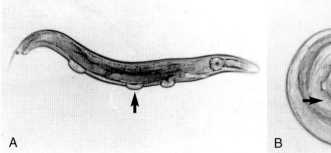
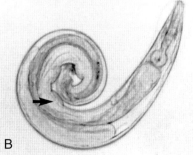

FIGURE 4-86 A, *Syphacia obvelata* male, showing the middle mamelon *(arrow)* at the center of the body. **B,** *S. muris* male, showing the first mamelon at midbody *(arrow).*

Distribution: Worldwide
Derivation of Genus: Bears a peculiar neck
Transmission Route: Ingestion of infective ova
Common Name: Ascarid of guinea pigs
Zoonotic: No

Paraspidodera uncinata is generally a nonpathogenic nematode of guinea pigs that can be found in cecal contents or in the mucosa of the cecum and colon. Adult worms are 11 to 28 mm × 0.3 to 0.4 mm. The male of *P. uncinata* has a sucker and two spicules of equal length immediately cranial to the anus. The eggs are oval and have a characteristic thick ascarid shell (Figure 4-87). Eggs are 40 to 50 μm × 30 to 40 μm. Antemortem, eggs may be detected by fecal flotation or direct fecal smear. Occasionally, extremely heavy infections may cause diarrhea and weight loss.

The life cycle of *P. uncinata* is direct, and transmission occurs through feed and water contaminated with infective eggs. *P. uncinata* has not been found in other species of animals and is not considered a public health hazard.

> **TECHNICIAN'S NOTE** The ascarid of guinea pigs is nonpathogenic but causes symptoms from intestinal disturbances with extremely heavy infections.

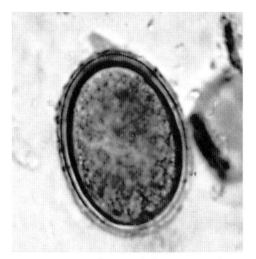

FIGURE 4-87 Egg of *Paraspidodera uncinata*, the cecal pinworm of guinea pigs.

NEMATODES OF RABBITS

GASTROINTESTINAL TRACT

Parasite: *Passalurus ambiguus*
Host: Rabbits
Location of Adult: Cecum and colon
Distribution: Worldwide
Derivation of Genus: Tailed worm named for a researcher named Passal
Transmission Route: Ingestion of infective ova
Common Name: Pinworm of rabbits
Zoonotic: No

Passalurus ambiguus is a nonpathogenic pinworm found in the cecum and colon of domestic and cottontail rabbits and hares. It is a pinworm that has an obvious round esophageal bulb. Adult females are approximately 10 mm long (Figure 4-88), and males are 4 to 5 mm long (Figure 4-89). Females have a long, finely pointed tail. Eggs are oval and slightly flattened on one side, measuring approximately 43 × 103 μm (Figure 4-90). Eggs are deposited in the feces and resemble the morulated hookworm eggs of dogs.

Infection with *P. ambiguus* can be detected antemortem by observing typical eggs in fecal flotation preparations. On postmortem examination the white, hairlike adult worms can be found in the cecum and proximal colon. Rabbits can tolerate heavy infections with no apparent clinical signs. It is believed that these pinworms feed on bacteria

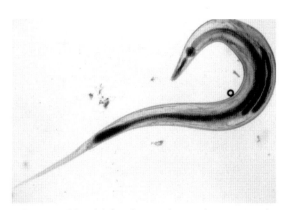

FIGURE 4-88 Adult female *Passalurus ambiguus*. Note the long, slender tail.

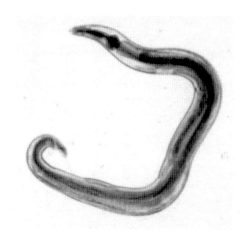

FIGURE 4-89 Adult male *Passalurus ambiguus.*

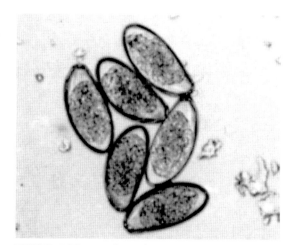

FIGURE 4-90 Ova of *Passalurus ambiguus* in fecal flotation.

in the intestinal contents without disturbing the mucosal lining of the cecum.

Eggs passed in the feces are immediately infective, so control of this parasite is quite difficult. Transmission is by ingestion of infective eggs. Clients should be advised to use feeders elevated off the floor of the rabbit hutch and to prevent wild hares and cottontail rabbits from having access to pet rabbits and their feed and bedding. *P. ambiguus* is species specific and has no zoonotic potential.

> **TECHNICIAN'S NOTE** The pinworm of rabbits is nonpathogenic and is believed to feed on the bacteria of the intestinal contents, thus not disturbing the intestinal mucosa.

Parasite: *Obeliscoides cuniculi* and *Trichostrongylus calcaratus*
Host: Rabbits
Location of Adult: Stomach (*O. cuniculi*) and small intestine (*T. calcaratus*)
Distribution: Worldwide
Derivation of Genus: Round hair (*T. calcaratus*); *Obeliscoides,* shaped like a pointed pillar
Transmission Route: Ingestion of infective larvae
Common Name: Trichostrongyles of rabbits
Zoonotic: No

Trichostrongyles are primarily parasites of ruminants and other large animals. However, these nematodes are also common in wild rabbits and uncommon in domestic rabbits. Diagnosticians must be aware of the possibility of infection with one or more rabbit trichostrongyles. Adult *Obeliscoides cuniculi* are found in the stomach of rabbits, and adult *Trichostrongylus calcaratus* are found in the small intestine where they feed on the host's blood. The males of these species are distinguished by the copulatory bursa on the posterior end. *O. cuniculi* females are 16 mm long and 0.5 mm wide, and males are 12 × 0.2 mm. Male and female adults may be found in the stomach on postmortem examination. Eggs are 80 × 45 μm and are thin shelled and oval. They may be easily observed with fecal flotation procedures. This nematode can produce hemorrhagic gastritis. Transmission is by ingestion of the larval form after eggs have been passed in the feces.

> **TECHNICIAN'S NOTE** The trichostrongyles of rabbits use a direct life cycle where a new host is infected by ingestion of infective larvae rather than using an intermediate host. The ova can be found on fecal flotation.

Adults of *T. calcaratus* are found in the small intestine and generally are smaller than those of *O. cuniculi.* Females of *T. calcaratus* are 6.4 mm × 100 μm, and males are 5.7 mm × 115 μm. The thin-shelled eggs are 65 × 33 μm and may be observed on fecal flotation. Rabbits infected with *T. calcaratus* may develop anemia. The life cycle of this trichostrongyle is direct, and transmission is by ingestion of infective larvae. As with other parasites that infect wild rabbits, prevention and control depend on keeping feed and bedding inaccessible to wild hares and cottontail rabbits.

> **TECHNICIAN'S NOTE** Rabbit trichostrongyles are typically found in wild rabbits rather than domestic rabbits.

NEMATODES OF PET AND AVIARY BIRDS

GASTROINTESTINAL TRACT

Parasite: *Ascaridia* species
Host: Lovebirds, cockatiels, macaws, parakeets, poultry, and waterfowl
Location of Adult: Small intestine
Distribution: Worldwide
Derivation of Genus: Intestinal worm
Transmission Route: Ingestion of infective ova
Common Name: Ascarids of birds
Zoonotic: No

Nematodes occur infrequently in pet and aviary birds. *Ascaridia* is occasionally seen in lovebirds, cockatiels, and macaws (Figures 4-91 and 4-92). Ascarids are very common in grass parakeets and can be demonstrated on both direct smear examination and fecal flotation. The eggs are thick-shelled roundworm type eggs (Figure 4-91). These roundworms are also common in backyard poultry and in waterfowl and can cause intestinal obstruction with large infections. In turkeys and peafowl, *Heterakis gallinarum* serves as an intermediate host for *Histomonas meleagridis,* the protozoan that produces infectious enterohepatitis.

> **TECHNICIAN'S NOTE** Although the ascarid of birds infects different bird species, it is most commonly seen in backyard poultry and waterfowl.

Parasite: *Spiroptera incesta, Dispharynx nasuta,* and *Tetrameres* species
Host: Australian finches—*S. incesta,* finches—*D. nasuta,* and pigeons—*Tetrameres* species
Location of Adult: Ventriculus, ventriculus, and proventriculus, respectively
Intermediate Host: Insect, insect, and sow bug, respectively
Distribution: Tropical and subtropical regions (*D. nasuta*)
Derivation of Genus: *Spiroptera:* coiled wing; *Dyspharynx:* abnormal throat; *Tetrameres:* made up of four parts

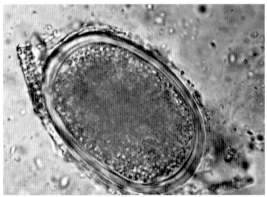

FIGURE 4-91 A roundworm (*Ascaridia*) egg in a fecal smear from a cockatiel.

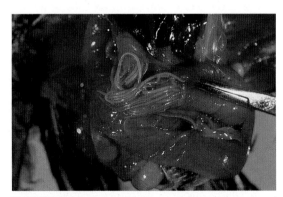

FIGURE 4-92 Nematodes occur infrequently in pet and aviary birds. *Ascaridia* is occasionally seen in the small intestine of lovebirds, cockatiels, and macaws.

Transmission Route: Ingestion of infective insect, ingestion of infective insect, and ingestion of infective sow bug, respectively
Common Name: Spirurids of birds
Zoonotic: No

Spirurids can infect a variety of avian species but are generally uncommon in pet birds. *Spiroptera incesta* can infect Australian finches; *Dispharynx nasuta* infects other finches. Infection by spirurids can be difficult to detect in finches. When spirurids are suspected, histologic examination of the ventriculus is recommended. The eggs of the spirurids are characterized by a thick wall and the presence of an embryonating larva within each egg. *Tetrameres,* a globose (spherical) spirurid, is typically found in the wall of the proventriculus of pigeons (Figure 4-4). Adults typically produce damage by living within the host.

> **TECHNICIAN'S NOTE** The spirurids of birds are not commonly found in pet birds.

Parasite: *Capillaria* species
Host: Pheasants, peafowl, and other poultry
Location of Adult: Crop and upper alimentary tract
Distribution: Worldwide

Derivation of Genus: Hairlike
Transmission Route: Ingestion of infective ova or paratenic host, earthworm
Common Name: Poultry capillarid
Zoonotic: No

Capillaria species may be found in the crop and upper alimentary tract of pheasants, peafowl, and other poultry. These hairlike nematodes have been reported in a variety of imported psittacine birds. The tiny adult worms can often be recovered from the wall of the esophagus or the crop, where they can cause inflammation and other disturbances. A direct smear of a sample from this area or a fecal flotation often reveals the characteristic thick-walled bipolar eggs, which are similar to those of whipworms, the *Trichuris* species. The eggs are shed in the feces and develop into infective ova. These infective ova can be ingested directly by a new host or by an earthworm as a paratenic host. The earthworm can then be ingested, and the parasite continues its life cycle in the bird.

> **TECHNICIAN'S NOTE** *Capillaria* species use a direct life cycle or a paratenic host, the earthworm, as a means of transmission from one host to another. The parasite does not undergo any life cycle stages in the earthworm. It is merely used to transport the parasite from one host to another.

CHAPTER FOUR TEST

MATCHING—Match the scientific name of each parasite with its common name, phrase, or term.

A. *Spirocerca lupi*

B. *Ollulanus tricuspis*

C. *Toxocara, Toxascaris* species

D. *Ancylostoma, Uncinaria* species

E. *Trichuris vulpis*

F. *Dirofilaria immitis*

G. *Dioctophyma renale*

H. *Aelurostrongylus abstrusus*

I. *Haemonchus, Ostertagia, Trichostrongylus,* and *Cooperia* species

J. *Thelazia rhodesii*

K. *Setaria cervi*

L. *Parascaris equorum*

M. *Strongylus vulgaris, S. edentatus,* and *S. equinus*

N. *Oxyuris equi*

O. *Strongyloides ransomi*

P. *Oesophagostomum dentatum*

Q. *Ascaris suum*

R. *Stephanurus dentatus*

S. *Trichinella spiralis*

T. *Syphacia obvelata*

U. *Passalurus ambiguus*

V. *Tetrameres* species

W. *Enterobius vermicularis*

X. *Pelodera strongyloides*

Y. *Physaloptera* species

Z. *Dracunculus insignis*

1. Hookworms of dogs and cats

2. Bovine trichostrongyles

3. Canine heartworm

4. Intestinal threadworm of swine

5. Swine kidney worm

6. Esophageal worm of dogs

7. Rabbit pinworm

8. Equine ascarid

9. Feline lungworm

10. Equine pinworm

11. Proventriculus worm of pigeons

12. Ascarids of dogs and cats

13. Abdominal worm of cattle

14. Feline trichostrongyle

15. Mouse pinworm

16. Free-living soil nematodes or facultative parasites

17. Large strongyles of horses

18. Whipworm of dogs

19. Swine ascarid

20. Guinea worm of dogs

21. Eyeworm of ruminants

22. Giant kidney worm

23. Human pinworm (pseudoparasite of dogs and cats)

24. Stomach worm of dogs and cats

25. Trichina worm

26. Nodular worm of swine

MATCHING—Match the parasite with the correct diagnostic technique or term.

A. *Spirocerca lupi*

B. *Dioctophyma renale*

C. *Trichuris vulpis*

D. *Oslerus osleri*

E. *Dirofilaria immitis*

F. *Stephanurus dentatus*

G. *Oesophagostomum dentatum*

H. *Oxyuris equi*

I. *Ollulanus tricuspis*

J. *Trichinella spiralis*

1. Observation of microfilariae using the modified Knott test in conjunction with commercially available ELISA

2. Observation of bipolar, football-shaped eggs in fecal flotation

3. Necropsy revealing large nodules within the wall of the large intestine

4. Observation of paper clip–shaped eggs on fecal flotation

5. Observation of infective first-stage larvae with an S-shaped appendage on the tail

6. Observation of large, rough, bipolar, barrel-shaped eggs on urine sedimentation

7. Flotation of feline vomitus revealing infective third-stage larvae

8. Microscopic examination of muscle biopsy specimen revealing encysted larvae in muscle tissue

9. Cellophane tape impressions of anus revealing larvated eggs

10. Observation of strongyle-type eggs in pig urine

MATCHING—Match the parasite with the pathology it produces.

A. *Physaloptera* species

B. *Toxocara canis*

C. *Trichuris vulpis*

D. *Oslerus osleri*

E. *Gongylonema pulchrum*

F. *Setaria equina*

G. *Ancylostoma caninum*

H. *Oxyuris equi*

I. *Spirocerca lupi*

J. *Dioctophyma renale*

1. Adult nematodes firmly attached to the mucosa of small intestine; voracious blood suckers

2. Blood suckers; tiny stylet in the tip of the whiplike anterior end that cannulates blood vessels

3. Ingestion of solid tissue; renal parenchyma

4. Physical blockage of the lumen of the small intestine

5. Parasite embedded in esophageal submucosa in a zigzag fashion

6. Adult nematodes firmly attached to the stomach mucosa; blood suckers

7. Formation of nodules in the esophagus

8. Formation of nodules at the bifurcation of the trachea

9. Pruritus in the anal region; hairs at the base of the tail broken off from attempts at scratching the anus

10. Nonpathogenic; solitary worms found free within the abdominal cavity

QUESTIONS FOR THOUGHT AND DISCUSSION

1. Why is it important to learn the life cycles of the nematode parasites of domesticated animals?

2. Why is it important to learn the scientific names, hosts, and locations of the nematode parasites of domesticated animals?

The Phylum Platyhelminthes, Class Cestoda

LEARNING OBJECTIVES

After studying this chapter, the reader should be able to do the following:

- Briefly discuss the external morphology of cestodes.
- Describe the important external morphologic features for differentiating both true tapeworms and pseudotapeworms.
- Describe the four types of cestode eggs.
- Compare the life cycle of a typical true tapeworm with that of a typical pseudotapeworm.
- Integrate vocabulary terms with the cestode parasites covered in Chapter 6.

KEY TERMS

Acetabula, suckers	Cysticercus	Neck	Rostellum
Armed tapeworm	Hermaphroditic	Plerocercoid	Scolex
Bothria	Hexacanth	Procercoid	Strobila
Cestodes	Hexacanth embryos	Proglottids	Tegument
Coenurus	Hydatid cyst	Pseudophyllidean egg	Tetrathyridium
Copepod	Immature proglottids	Pseudotapeworm	Trematodes
Coracidium	Mature proglottids	Pyriform apparatus	True tapeworm
Cysticercoid	Metacestode stage	type	Unarmed tapeworm

The phylum Platyhelminthes, the flatworms, includes the trematodes (or flukes) discussed in Chapters 7 and 8 and the cestodes (or tapeworms) detailed in this chapter and Chapter 6. Remember that the morphologic feature shared by these two classes is that they are both dorsoventrally flattened. However, whereas the flukes are flattened and leaf-shaped, the tapeworms are ribbonlike and segmented into identical compartments called proglottids (Figure 5-1).

> **TECHNICIAN'S NOTE** Cestodes are dorsoventrally flattened, ribbonlike, and segmented into identical compartments called *proglottids*.

Members of the phylum Platyhelminthes, class Cestoda, are often referred to as *cestodes* or *tapeworms*. Their bodies are usually long, segmented, and flattened, almost ribbonlike in appearance. Within the class Cestoda are two subclasses, Eucestoda (true

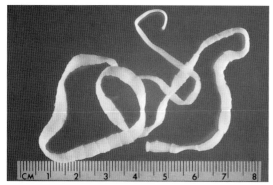

FIGURE 5-1 Example of a typical tapeworm with a dorso-ventrally flattened, ribbonlike appearance. Every tapeworm is segmented into identical compartments called *proglottids*.

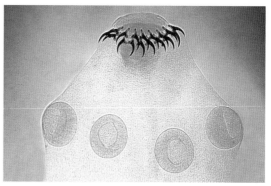

FIGURE 5-2 Located on the anterior end of the true tapeworm is the holdfast organelle, the scolex, or head. The scolex of the adult true tapeworm has four suckers, called *acetabula*, with which the tapeworm holds on to the lining of the small intestine, the predilection site of most adult tapeworms.

tapeworms) and Cotyloda (pseudotapeworms). Members of both of these classes are important parasites of domesticated and wild animals and of humans.

EUCESTODA (TRUE TAPEWORMS)

Phylum: Platyhelminthes
    Class: Cestoda

KEY MORPHOLOGIC FEATURES

As mentioned, tapeworms are long, segmented, flattened, almost ribbonlike parasites. On the extreme anterior end of the typical true tapeworm is the holdfast organelle, the scolex, or head (Figure 5-2). The scolex of the adult true tapeworm has four suckers called acetabula with which it holds on to the lining of the small intestine, the predilection site, or "home," of most adult tapeworms. Unlike the oral sucker of the digenetic trematode, the suckers of the true tapeworm are *not* associated with intake of food but rather serve as organs of attachment. True tapeworms do not have a mouth; instead they absorb the nutrients acquired from the host's intestine through their tegument, or body wall. In addition to the suckers, some true tapeworms may possess an anchorlike organelle called the rostellum (Figure 5-3). The rostellum usually has backward-facing hooks. With these hooks, the tapeworm further anchors itself in the mucosa of the small intestine. If the tapeworm has a rostellum, it is said to be an armed tapeworm; if the

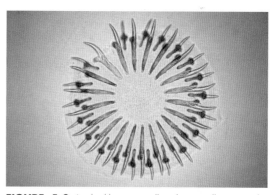

FIGURE 5-3 Anchorlike organelle, the rostellum, on the anterior end of the tapeworm. The rostellum usually has backward-facing hooks used to anchor the tapeworm farther into the mucosa of the small intestine. If the tapeworm has a rostellum, it is said to be an *armed* tapeworm; if the tapeworm lacks the rostellum, it is said to be an *unarmed* tapeworm.

tapeworm lacks the rostellum, it is said to be an unarmed tapeworm.

> **TECHNICIAN'S NOTE** The suckers on the cestode are not associated with food intake; instead the cestode absorbs nutrients from the host through its tegument.

Just posterior to the scolex of the true tapeworm is a germinal, or growth, region called the neck. It is from the neck that the rest of the true tapeworm's body, the strobila, arises. The strobila is composed of individual proglottids that are arranged much like the boxcars in a railroad train. The proglottids closest to the scolex and the neck of the true tapeworm are the **immature**, or youngest, proglottids (Figure 5-4); those that are intermediate in distance from the scolex and the neck are the mature proglottids (Figure 5-5), and those farthest from the scolex and the neck are the **gravid**, or oldest, proglottids (Figure 5-6).

As with the hermaphroditic digenetic trematodes, each proglottid of a true tapeworm contains complete sets of both male and female reproductive organs. As with the flukes, tapeworms are hermaphroditic. The sex organs of these tapeworms are usually located along the lateral aspects of the proglottid. Cross-fertilization and self-fertilization take place between and among individual proglottids. Immature proglottids contain male and female reproductive organs that are sexually immature; these are "prepuberty" proglottids. Mature proglottids contain male and female reproductive organs that are sexually mature and completely functional, or capable of reproduction. Gravid proglottids contain male and female reproductive organs that have grown old or are "spent," having

degenerated to the point that the only portion remaining is the uterus filled with tapeworm eggs. Tapeworm proglottids can usually be observed with the naked eye in the feces of the definitive host (Figure 5-7). Other organ systems (nervous,

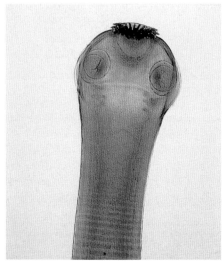

FIGURE 5-4 Proglottids closest to the scolex and neck of the true tapeworm are the immature, or youngest, proglottids. Immature proglottids contain immature, nonfunctional male and female reproductive organs.

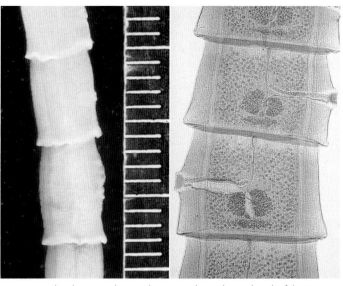

FIGURE 5-5 Tapeworm proglottids intermediate in distance to the scolex and neck of the true tapeworm are mature, or adolescent, proglottids. Mature proglottids contain mature, functional male and female reproductive organs.

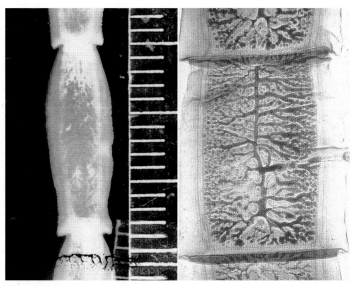

FIGURE 5-6 Tapeworm proglottids farthest from the scolex and neck of the true tapeworm are gravid, or aged, proglottids. Gravid proglottids contain male and female reproductive organs that have grown old and degenerated so that only the uterus filled with eggs remains.

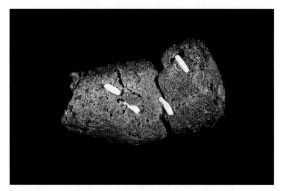

FIGURE 5-7 Tapeworm proglottids (*Dipylidium caninum*) observed in feces of the definitive host.

excretory) are represented; however, they are not as important as the reproductive system. As with the digenetic trematodes, or flukes, tapeworms are "designed" to reproduce and produce offspring.

> ◾ TECHNICIAN'S NOTE Each segment of the tapeworm contains male and female reproductive organs. Mature proglottids can self-fertilize or cross-fertilize with other segments. The gravid proglottids contain the eggs of the tapeworm.

The eggs found in the gravid proglottids contain the larval stage, or hexacanth, with six hooks. The hexacanths can be contained within one of four egg types: the pyriform apparatus type, *Dipylidium* type, *Taenia* type, and pseudophyllidean type. The pyriform apparatus type (Figure 5-8, *A*) is an egg with three coverings, the innermost of which is pear-shaped and is called the *pyriform apparatus*. The *Dipylidium* egg packet contains multiple hexacanths within one egg (Figure 5-8, *B*). The *Taenia* egg has a wide outer shell with a thicker outer covering and a six-hooked hexacanth within the egg (Figure 5-8, *C*). The oval pseudophyllidean egg has an operculum (Figure 5-8, *D*) at one end. The hexacanth within it contains six hooks.

> ◾ TECHNICIAN'S NOTE Tapeworms can produce one of four types of eggs: pseudophyllidean type, *Dipylidium* type, *Taenia* type, and pyriform apparatus type.

LIFE CYCLE OF THE TRUE TAPEWORM

The life cycle of a typical true tapeworm is more complicated than that of a digenetic

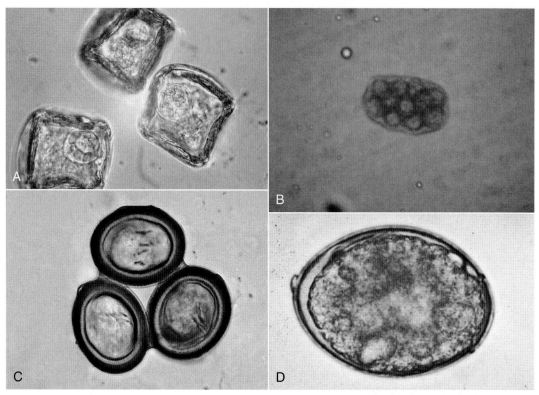

FIGURE 5-8 Tapeworm eggs can be seen in four basic types. **A,** Pyriform apparatus type egg. **B,** *Dipylidium* eggs, as seen in *Dipylidium caninum*. **C,** *Taenia* egg, as seen in *Taenia pisiformis*. **D,** Pseudophyllidean egg, as seen in *Diphyllobothrium latum*.

trematode. In most cases the gravid proglottids of the true tapeworm pass to the outside environment, sometimes singly and sometimes in chains, one behind the other. These proglottids rupture in the external environment and release thousands of hexacanth embryos, or eggs, to the outside environment (Figure 5-9). To continue the life cycle, the egg must be ingested by a suitable intermediate host, either an invertebrate or a vertebrate. Within this host, the egg develops into a metacestode stage, or larval tapeworm. The metacestode may take one of several forms: cysticercoid, cysticercus, coenurus, hydatid cyst, or tetrathyridium. These larval stages differ in their choice of host, their structure, their predilection site, and their pathogenicity to the intermediate host. Sometimes the metacestode, or larval stage of the tapeworm, is more pathogenic to the intermediate host than the adult or mature

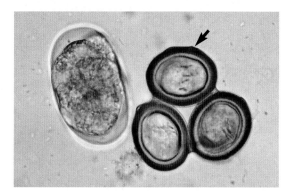

FIGURE 5-9 Tapeworm egg, or hexacanth embryo. Tapeworm eggs are released to the outside environment. Each tapeworm egg is infective for the intermediate host and produces one metacestode stage. The unmarked egg is an *Ancylostoma caninum*.

tapeworm is to the definitive host. The definitive host becomes infected by ingesting the intermediate host containing the metacestode stage. The "juvenile," or developing, tapeworm emerges from the metacestode stage, attaches to the lining of the small intestine, and begins to produce the strobila, which is composed of proglottids.

Tapeworm proglottids have muscles that enable them to move about. Owners of infected animals often observe these tapeworms as "little white worms" crawling on the animal's feces, hair coat, or bedding. Tapeworm proglottids often contain eggs when they are passed into the feces. These hexacanth embryos are eggs with embryos that have an internal structure and six hooks (Figure 5-9). The hexacanth embryos are ingested by the intermediate host in which the tapeworm develops.

> **TECHNICIAN'S NOTE** The owner of an animal infected with tapeworms often sees "little white worms" crawling in the animal's feces when the animal defecates. When the segment dries out, they often see "rice" in the stool.

The intermediate host may be an arthropod, such as a flea or a grain mite. In this host the hexacanth embryo develops into a microscopic larval stage known as a **cysticercoid** (Figure 5-10). The cysticercoid is tiny and contains a small, fluid-filled space. The definitive host becomes infected by ingesting the intermediate host containing the cysticercoid larval stage. Examples of tapeworms that develop into a cysticercoid stage in an intermediate host are the fringed tapeworm of cattle (*Thysanosoma actinoides*) and the double-pored tapeworm of dogs and cats (*Dipylidium caninum*).

Sometimes the intermediate host is a mammalian host such as a rabbit, in which the hexacanth embryo develops into a **cysticercus**, or "bladder worm," stage (Figure 5-11). The bladder worm is a fluid-filled larval stage within the tissues of the vertebrate intermediate host. The definitive host becomes infected by ingesting the intermediate host containing the bladder worm larval stage (Figure 5-12). Examples of tapeworms that have a bladder worm stage (or a variation of the bladder

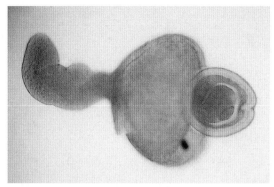

FIGURE 5-10 Microscopic larval (metacestode) stage known as a *cysticercoid*. The cysticercoid is tiny (microscopic) and contains a small, fluid-filled space; the cysticercoid develops within the intermediate host. The definitive host becomes infected by ingesting the intermediate host containing the cysticercoid larval stage. Examples of tapeworms that develop into the cysticercoid stage in the intermediate host are *Thysanosoma actinoides* of cattle, *Anoplocephala* species of horses, and *Dipylidium caninum* of dogs and cats.

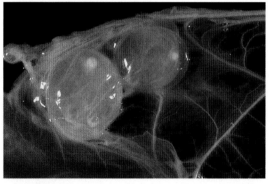

FIGURE 5-11 The hexacanth embryo of some tapeworms develops into the *cysticercus*, or bladder worm, stage. Bladder worm is a fluid-filled larval stage within tissues of a vertebrate intermediate host. The definitive host becomes infected by ingesting the intermediate host containing the bladder worm larval stage. Examples of tapeworms that develop into the cysticercus stage in an intermediate host are the *Taenia* species.

worm stage) in an intermediate host are the canine taeniid tapeworm (*Taenia pisiformis*) and the *Coenurus* tapeworm (*Multiceps multiceps*). Other tapeworms that use a variation of the bladder worm stage are *Echinococcus granulosus* and *Echinococcus multilocularis*, the hydatid cyst tapeworms. Chapter

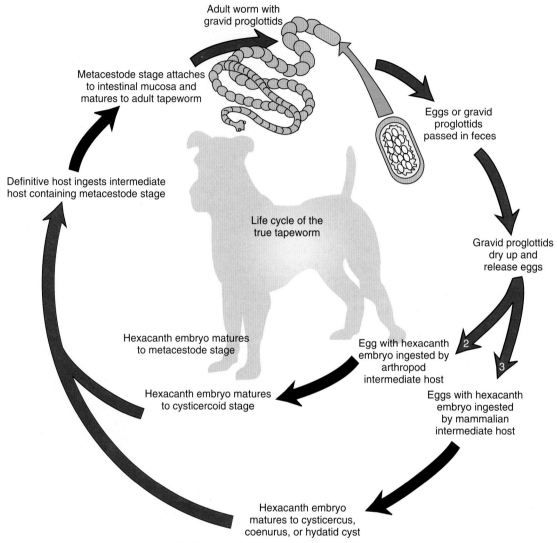

FIGURE 5-12 Life cycle of the true tapeworm.

6 covers these tapeworms and their larval stages in greater detail.

COTYLODA (PSEUDOTAPEWORMS)

Phylum: Platyhelminthes
    Class: Cestoda

KEY MORPHOLOGIC FEATURES

Members of the subclass Cotyloda, the pseudotapeworms, are tapeworms; they are long, segmented, flattened, almost ribbonlike parasites. These tapeworms resemble true tapeworms in that on the extreme anterior end of the typical pseudotapeworm is the holdfast organelle, the scolex, or head. Instead of possessing four holdfast suckers, or acetabula, the typical pseudotapeworm has two slitlike organelles called bothria (Figure 5-13). Bothria are longitudinal grooves along the length of the scolex. The pseudotapeworm attaches to the lining of the small intestine by means of the bothria. As with true tapeworms, pseudotapeworms do not have a

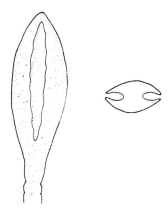

FIGURE 5-13 Slitlike bothria on the anterior end of the typical pseudotapeworm.

mouth; instead, they absorb the nutrients acquired from the host's intestine through their tegument, or body wall.

> **TECHNICIAN'S NOTE** Instead of using a scolex with suckers to attach to the host, the pseudotapeworm uses two slitlike organelles called *bothria* to attach to the host's intestines.

The strobila of the pseudotapeworm is similar to that of the true tapeworm. The neck, or growth region, is just posterior to the scolex, and the pseudotapeworm's body arises from this. The strobila of the pseudotapeworm also is composed of immature, mature, and gravid proglottids. As with true tapeworms, pseudotapeworms are hermaphroditic, and each proglottid of a pseudotapeworm contains complete sets of both male and female reproductive organs. The sex organs of these tapeworms are usually located along the central region of each proglottid. There is a centrally located uterine pore through which eggs are voided to the external environment. The eggs of the pseudotapeworm do not resemble those of the true tapeworm. Oddly, they resemble the eggs of a digenetic trematode—they are operculated. In most cases the spent proglottids of the pseudotapeworm pass to the outside environment in long chains.

> **TECHNICIAN'S NOTE** The body of the pseudotapeworm is composed of immature, mature, and gravid proglottids with male and female reproductive organs in each segment.

LIFE CYCLE OF THE PSEUDOTAPEWORM

The life cycle of the pseudotapeworm is slightly more complicated than that of a true tapeworm. The operculated eggs are passed singly to the external environment. If these eggs make contact with water, they hatch, releasing a ciliated hexacanth embryo out of the operculum. This ciliated hexacanth embryo is called a coracidium. The coracidium must be ingested by a suitable first intermediate host, an aquatic crustacean called a copepod. Within the copepod, the coracidium develops to a stage called a procercoid. If the copepod containing the procercoid is ingested by the second intermediate host, usually a fish of some type, the procercoid develops into the second stage, which is infective for the definitive host. This stage is called the plerocercoid stage. The definitive host becomes infected by ingesting the second intermediate host containing the plerocercoid stage. This plerocercoid stage is the juvenile, or developing, tapeworm; it possesses slitlike bothria. When the plerocercoid stage is ingested by the definitive host, it emerges from the metacestode stage, attaches to the lining of the small intestine, and begins to produce the strobila (Figure 5-14).

> **TECHNICIAN'S NOTE** The life cycle of the pseudotapeworm is more complex than that of the true tapeworm, using two intermediate hosts, the second of which is infective to the definitive host.

There are two important species of pseudotapeworms: *Diphyllobothrium latum*, the "broad fish tapeworm," and *Spirometra mansonoides*, the "zipper tapeworm."

Chapter 6 details the major true tapeworms and pseudotapeworms that infect domesticated animals.

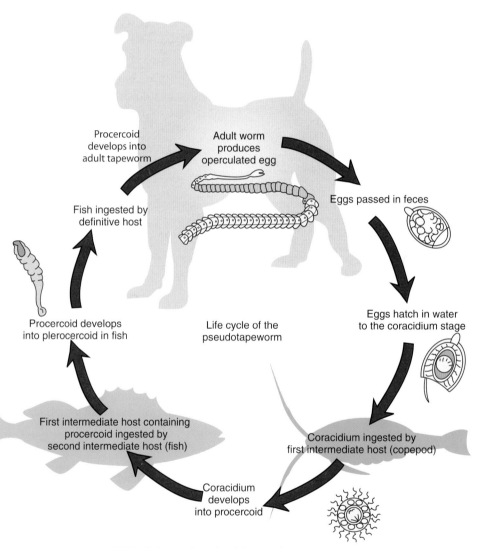

FIGURE 5-14 Life cycle of the pseudotapeworm.

CHAPTER FIVE TEST

MATCHING—Match the term with the correct phrase or term.

A. Eucestode

B. Armed scolex

C. Tegument

D. Hexacanth embryo

E. Coracidium

F. Hermaphroditic

G. Bothria

H. Metacestode

I. Strobila

J. Unarmed scolex

1. Slitlike structures on the scolex of the pseudotapeworm

2. Possessing both male and female reproductive organs

3. Lacking a rostellum

4. True tapeworm

5. Larval tapeworm

6. Ciliated stage emerging from an operculated pseudotapeworm egg

7. All of the connected proglottids (immature, mature, and gravid proglottids)

8. Tapeworm egg containing six hooks

9. Tapeworm's body wall

10. Possessing a rostellum

QUESTIONS FOR THOUGHT AND DISCUSSION

1. How can a gravid proglottid be used in making a definitive diagnosis of cestodiasis in any definitive host?

2. Compare and contrast the following types of cestode eggs. You may use drawings with labels to illustrate the differences. Give examples of cestodes that typify these egg types (see Chapter 6 for examples).
   • Egg packet
   • Egg with a pyriform apparatus
   • Hexacanth embryo
   • Pseudotapeworm egg

3. Compare and contrast the "typical cestode life cycle" of a true tapeworm versus the life cycle of a pseudotapeworm.

4. What are some external morphologic features used to identify intact adult cestodes, both true tapeworms and pseudotapeworms?

5. Define the following terms commonly used in a veterinary practice.
   • Gravid proglottid
   • Scolex
   • Hexacanth embryo
   • Egg packet
   • Cysticercoid

6 Tapeworms That Parasitize Domestic Animals and Humans

OUTLINE

LEARNING OBJECTIVES

After studying this chapter, the reader should be able to do the following:

- Identify the tapeworm parasites (both adult and larval forms) of the following domesticated animals: dog, cat, cattle, sheep, horse, and selected laboratory animals.
- Understand that many cestode parasites are associated with two scientific names, one scientific name for the adult form of the parasite and one scientific name for the larval (metacestode) stage of the parasite.
- Understand the correlation and integration between vertebrate or invertebrate hosts that

serve as intermediate hosts for larval (metacestode) stages of cestodes and the vertebrate hosts that serve as definitive hosts for the adult stages of their corresponding cestode parasites.
- Understand the concepts behind the following metacestode stages relative to their roles in the life cycles of both true tapeworms and pseudotapeworms.

KEY TERMS

Coenurus
Coracidium
Cysticercoid
Cysticercus or bladder
  worm
Egg packets
Embryophore
Hexacanth six-
  toothed embryo

Hydatid cyst
Lappets
Metacestode
Multilocular or
  alveolar hydatid
  cyst
Oncosphere

Operculated ovum
Oribatid grain mites
Plerocercoid
Procercoid
Pseudotapeworm
Psocids
Sparganum

Pyriform apparatus
Strobilocercus
Tetrathyridium
True tapeworm
Typical taeniid type
  of egg

EUCESTODA (TRUE TAPEWORMS)

Phylum: Platyhelminthes (flatworms)
  Class: Cestoda (tapeworms)
    Subclass: Eucestoda (true tapeworms)

MICE, RATS, GERBILS, AND HAMSTERS

Intestinal Tract

Parasite: ⬢ *Hymenolepis nana*
Parasite: *Hymenolepis diminuta*
Host: Mice, rats, gerbils, hamsters, dogs, and humans
Location of Adult: Small intestine
Distribution: Worldwide
Derivation of Genus: Membrane covering
Intermediate Host: None necessary (*H. nana*); fleas, flour beetles, and other arthropods (*H. diminuta*)
Transmission Route: Ingestion of infective fleas, grain beetle, or cockroach (*H. diminuta*); ingestion of infective egg or autoinfection (*H. nana*)
Common Name: Rodent tapeworm
Zoonotic: *H. nana:* Yes; *H. diminuta:* No

> **TECHNICIAN'S NOTE** Although *Hymenolepis nana* and *Hymenolepis diminuta* are mainly parasites of mice, rats, gerbils, and hamsters, they have been found in dogs and humans.

Hymenolepis nana and *Hymenolepis diminuta* parasitize mice, rats, gerbils, and hamsters. These tapeworms are small and slender. Adults of *H. nana* are 1 mm wide and 25 to 40 mm in length, and adults of *H. diminuta* are 3 to 4 mm wide and 20 to 60 mm in length. These true tapeworms reside in the small intestine of the rodent definitive host and are usually detected on postmortem examination of the small intestine. The scolex of *H. nana* has a ring of hooks on its anterior end; it has an armed rostellum (Figure 6-1). The scolex of *H. diminuta* has no hooks; it is unarmed (Figure 6-2).

H. nana has a direct life cycle, whereas *H. diminuta* requires an intermediate host for infection. The eggs of *H. nana* are passed in the feces and are swallowed by a host. The hexacanth enters the villus of the small intestine and matures into a

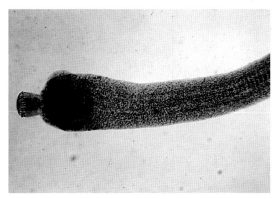

FIGURE 6-1 Scolex of *Hymenolepis nana*, showing armed rostellum on scolex.

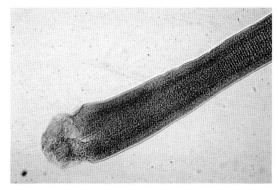

FIGURE 6-2 Scolex of *Hymenolepis diminuta*, showing unarmed scolex.

nontailed cysticercoid. The cysticercoid returns to the lumen of the small intestine, attaches to the lining, and matures to adulthood. *H. diminuta* also passes its eggs in the feces, which are ingested by an intermediate arthropod host. The hexacanth six-toothed embryo (embryo containing three pairs of hooks) matures into a tailed cysticercoid. The arthropod is ingested by a definitive host, and the cysticercoid attaches to the lining of the small intestine and matures into an adult.

> **TECHNICIAN'S NOTE** *Hymenolepis nana* is unique in that it is the only tapeworm that does not need an intermediate host for any developmental stage in its life cycle.

The eggs of *Hymenolepis* species may be detected on fecal flotation. Veterinary technicians should be

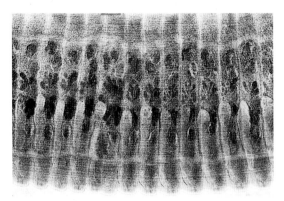

FIGURE 6-3 Stained proglottids of *Hymenolepis diminuta*.

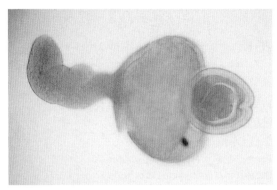

FIGURE 6-5 Cysticercoid (larval) stage has been dissected from the insect intermediate host.

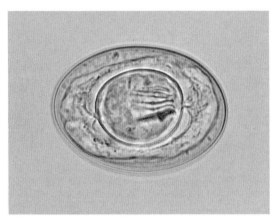

FIGURE 6-4 Oval egg of *Hymenolepis nana* measures 44 to 62 μm × 30 to 55 μm.

aware that the eggs of this tapeworm are shed intermittently in the feces. Sometimes individual proglottids are also recovered, but these do not float. Figure 6-3 shows stained proglottids of *H. diminuta*. The oval egg of *H. nana* measures 44 to 62 μm × 30 to 55 μm (Figure 6-4). The egg of *H. diminuta* is more spherical and measures 62 to 88 μm × 30 to 55 μm. The embryo within the egg of both species measures 24 to 30 μm × 16 to 25 μm and contains three pairs of hooks (hexacanth embryo). Infected animals may be treated with niclosamide or praziquantel.

Both of these tapeworms have zoonotic potential. *H. nana* is unique in that it does not require an intermediate host; therefore it is directly infective to other rodents and to humans. Autoinfection by

H. nana can occur when its eggs hatch in the small intestine of the host and subsequently infect that host. *H. diminuta* uses an insect (flea, grain beetle, or cockroach) as an intermediate host to complete its life cycle. The cysticercoid develops within the insect intermediate host (Figure 6-5).

> *TECHNICIAN'S NOTE* Both *Hymenolepis nana* and *Hymenolepis diminuta* can infect humans.

RUMINANTS
Intestinal Tract

Moniezia species and *Thysanosoma actinoides* are true tapeworms that infect the intestinal tract of ruminants.

Parasite: *Moniezia benedini* and *Moniezia expansa*
Host: Cattle (*M. benedini*); cattle, sheep, and goats (*M. expansa*)
Location of Adult: Small intestine
Intermediate Host: Grain mites
Distribution: Worldwide
Derivation of Genus: *Moniezia*—to be single
Transmission Route: Ingestion of infective grain mite
Common Name: Ruminant tapeworms
Zoonotic: No

Moniezia *Species*

Moniezia species are long (up to 6 m) tapeworms found in the small intestine of cattle, sheep, and goats. *Moniezia* species are large tapeworms and can be up to 1.6 cm at the widest margins (Figure 6-6). The scolex of *Moniezia* is unarmed; it lacks an armed rostellum (Figure 6-7). Individual proglottids are very short and wide—"squatty." Each proglottid contains two sets of laterally located genital organs and associated pores (Figure 6-8). These tapeworms produce eggs with a characteristic square or triangular shape. Both species will produce eggs with a three-layered egg shell; the innermost lining is a **pyriform** (pear-shaped) **apparatus.** Two species are common among ruminants: *Moniezia benedini* in cattle and *Moniezia expansa* in cattle, sheep, and goats. The eggs of both species can be easily differentiated using standard fecal flotation procedures.

The eggs of *M. expansa* are triangular or pyramidal and 56 to 67 μm in diameter. The eggs of *M. benedini* are square or cuboidal and approximately 75 μm in diameter (Figure 6-9). The prepatent period for these tapeworms is approximately 40 days.

> *TECHNICIAN'S NOTE* *Moniezia* species can be found with standard fecal flotation techniques. *Moniezia benedini* eggs have a square or cuboidal shape, whereas *Moniezia expansa* eggs are triangular or pyramidal.

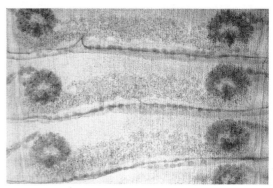

FIGURE 6-8 Each proglottid of the adult *Moniezia* species contains two sets of laterally located genital organs and genital pores.

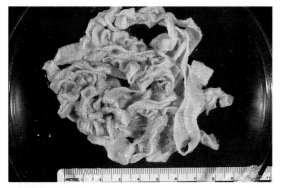

FIGURE 6-6 *Moniezia* species are large tapeworms. They can grow to 6 m long and up to 1.6 cm at the widest margins.

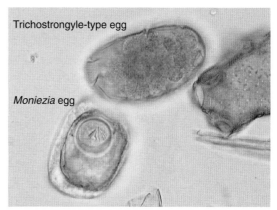

Trichostrongyle-type egg

Moniezia egg

FIGURE 6-9 *Moniezia* species produce eggs with a characteristic square or triangular shape. Two species are common among ruminants, *Moniezia benedini* in cattle and *Moniezia expansa* in cattle, sheep, and goats. Eggs of both species can be easily differentiated using standard fecal flotation procedures. Eggs of *M. expansa* are triangular or pyramidal and 56 to 67 μm in diameter. Eggs of *M. benedini* are square or cuboidal and approximately 75 μm in diameter. Both eggs contain a pyriform apparatus.

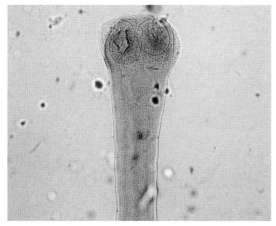

FIGURE 6-7 Scolex of *Moniezia* is unarmed; it lacks an armed rostellum.

The metacestode, or larval, stage of *Moniezia* is the cysticercoid stage, which may be found within the intermediate hosts, oribatid grain mites. Intact proglottids and eggs are found in the feces of the ruminant definitive host. Mites become infected by ingesting the hexacanth embryo, which develops into the cysticercoid stage within the body of the grain mite. Ruminants become infected by ingesting cysticercoid-infected mites that infest the grain. The cysticercoid is a tiny, microscopic stage and probably will not be observed by the veterinarian (Figure 6-5). For every cysticercoid that is ingested by the ruminant, one adult tapeworm will develop in the small intestine of that ruminant (Figure 6-10). Large numbers of adults can cause rupture of the gut or can obstruct the lumen of the intestines, especially in young animals. It is important that the veterinarian recognize the oribatid mite as the source of this tapeworm and understand the importance of effective tapeworm therapeusis (morantel, niclosamide, albendazole, fenbendazole, or oxfendazole) in cattle. Pasture rotation in addition to therapeusis is essential in greatly reducing the transmission of this parasite.

TECHNICIAN'S NOTE Pasture rotation is essential in reducing the transmission of ruminant tapeworms.

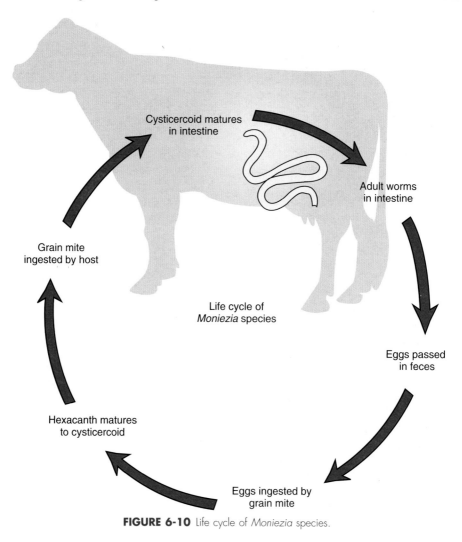

Cysticercoid matures in intestine

Adult worms in intestine

Grain mite ingested by host

Life cycle of *Moniezia* species

Eggs passed in feces

Hexacanth matures to cysticercoid

Eggs ingested by grain mite

FIGURE 6-10 Life cycle of *Moniezia* species.

Parasite: *Thysanosoma actinoides*
Host: Sheep, goats, and cattle
Location of Adult: Lumen of the bile duct, pancreatic ducts, and small intestine
Intermediate Host: Unknown, proposed hosts are psocids
Distribution: North and South America
Derivation of Genus: Fringed body
Transmission Route: Ingestion of unknown intermediate host
Common Name: Fringed tapeworm of sheep and goats
Zoonotic: No

Thysanosoma actinoides

T. actinoides is the fringed tapeworm found in the bile ducts (can cause bile duct obstruction), pancreatic ducts (can cause obstruction of the pancreatic duct), and small intestine of ruminants (Figure 6-11). The adult tapeworm measures 8 mm × 15 to 30 cm and possesses an unarmed scolex. As with *Moniezia* species, the proglottids are very short; however, these proglottids possess a unique feature: a very prominent fringe located on the posterior aspect of each proglottid. (Figure 6-12 shows the fringed adult *T. actinoides*.)

Eggs of this tapeworm occur in packets of 6 to 12 eggs, with individual eggs measuring 19 × 27 μm.

These eggs do not possess a pyriform apparatus. The eggs can be found on standard fecal flotation procedures. Adults can be identified at necropsy.

> **TECHNICIAN'S NOTE** These fringed tapeworms are unique among the adult tapeworms in that they possess a very prominent fringe along the posterior margin of each and every proglottid. The adults are also found in an unusual location for tapeworms, the lumen of the bile duct.

The metacestode (larval) stage of *T. actinoides* is the cysticercoid stage, which may be found within the proposed intermediate hosts, psocids. Psocids are primitive insects often associated with vegetation. These insects become infected by ingesting the hexacanth embryo, which develops into the cysticercoid stage within the body of the psocid. Ruminants may become infected by accidentally ingesting cysticercoid-infected psocids that infest vegetation. The cysticercoid is a microscopic stage and probably will not be observed by the veterinarian. For every cysticercoid that is ingested by a ruminant, one adult tapeworm will develop in the small intestine of that ruminant. It is important that the veterinarian recognize psocids as the source of this tapeworm and understand the importance of

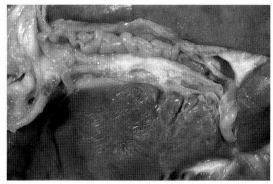

FIGURE 6-11 *Thysanosoma actinoides*, the fringed tapeworm, is unusual in that it is not found in the intestine (as are most adult tapeworms). Instead it resides in the bile duct of sheep.

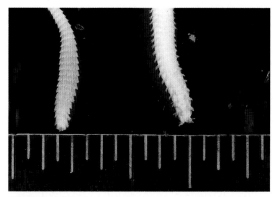

FIGURE 6-12 The adult *Thysanosoma actinoides* measures 8 mm × 15 to 30 cm. Note that proglottids are very short. They demonstrate a unique morphologic feature, a conspicuous fringe located on the posterior aspect of each proglottid, thus the common name *fringed tapeworm*.

effective tapeworm therapeusis (niclosamide or praziquantel, as well as pasture rotation) in cattle.

METACESTODE (LARVAL) STAGES FOUND IN THE MUSCULATURE OF FOOD ANIMALS

Parasite: 🅩 *Taenia saginata* (adult tapeworm)/ *Cysticercus bovis* (metacestode [larval] stage)

Host: Humans

Location of Adult: Small intestine

Intermediate Host: Cattle

Distribution: Worldwide

Derivation of Genus: Flat band, bandage, or tape/ bladder tail

Transmission Route: Ingestion of raw or under- cooked infective beef

Common Name: Beef tapeworm of humans, beef measles, measly beef of cattle

Zoonotic: Yes

Cattle may serve as intermediate hosts for a tape- worm of humans, *Taenia saginata*. The adult tape- worm is unusual among the *Taenia* species in that it does not have an armed rostellum like the rest of the species. Adults possess 14 to 32 lateral branches of the uterus within the gravid proglottid. The eggs are typical taeniid-type ova with a striated embryophore (shell) surrounding an oncosphere with six hooklets inside. The adults can cause obstruction of the intestinal tract if present in suf- ficient numbers.

> 📖 TECHNICIAN'S NOTE *Taenia saginata* is unusual in that it has an unarmed rostellum, whereas all other *Taenia* species possess an armed rostellum.

The larval stage for this tapeworm is a cysticercus, or bladder worm, called *Cysticercus bovis*. A cysti- cercus is a single invaginated scolex in a large fluid- filled cyst, cavity, or vesicle. This condition in cattle is often referred to as *beef measles* or *measly beef*. These infective metacestodes are found in the mus- culature (skeletal and cardiac muscles) of cattle. If enough cysticerci are present in the muscle tissue, they can interfere with muscle function and produce

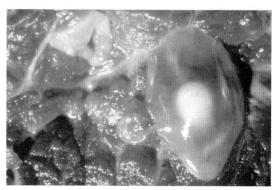

FIGURE 6-13 Gross view of the cysticercus of the larval form of the beef tapeworm, *Taenia saginata* (*Cysticercus bovis*), within the muscle of a beef cow.

pain and myositis. Humans become infected with this zoonotic tapeworm by ingesting poorly cooked beef. (Figure 6-13 shows the cysticercus of *C. bovis* within beef muscle.)

Parasite: 🅩 *Taenia solium* (adult tapeworm)/ *Cysticercus cellulosae* (metacestode [larval] stage)

Host: Human

Location of Adult: Small intestine

Intermediate Host: Pigs

Distribution: Underdeveloped countries including Latin America, India, Africa, and the Far East

Derivation of Genus: Flat band, bandage, or tape/ bladder tail

Transmission Route: Ingestion of infective under- cooked or raw pork

Common Name: Pork tapeworm of humans, measly pork, pork measles of swine

Zoonotic: Yes

Pigs may serve as the intermediate host for a similar tapeworm of humans, *Taenia solium*. The adult possesses an armed rostellum with a double row of hooks. It is best identified by its 7 to 16 lateral branches of the uterus within each gravid proglot- tid. The eggs are typical taeniid-type ova with a striated embryophore surrounding an oncosphere with six hooklets inside. In large numbers the adult worms can cause intestinal obstruction. The ova can be found on standard fecal flotation. The adults can be identified by their characteristic lateral branches of the uterus.

The larval stage for this tapeworm is a cysticercus, or bladder worm, known as *Cysticercus cellulosae*. This metacestode stage in pigs is often referred to as *pork measles* or *measly pork*. These metacestodes are found in the musculature (skeletal and cardiac muscles) of pigs. Humans become infected with this zoonotic tapeworm by ingesting poorly cooked pork. It is also important to note that if humans ingest the eggs of *T. solium*, the cysticercus can develop within their muscles (Figure 6-14) and within nervous tissue such as the brain, eye, and spinal cord.

The adult stages of the metacestode stages (*C. bovis* and *C. cellulosae*) are found in the small intestine of humans. Because humans may become infected by ingesting poorly cooked beef or pork, these are important zoonotic tapeworms.

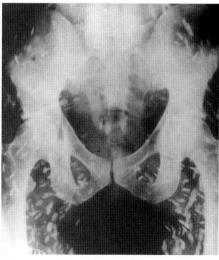

FIGURE 6-14 Radiographic view of cysticerci of the larval form of pork tapeworm, *Taenia solium* (*Cysticercus cellulosae*), within human muscle.

METACESTODE (LARVAL) STAGES FOUND IN THE ABDOMINAL CAVITY OF FOOD ANIMALS

Parasite: *Taenia hydatigena* (adult tapeworm)/*Cysticercus tenuicollis* (metacestode [larval] stage)
Host: Dogs
Location of Adult: Small intestine
Intermediate Host: Cattle, sheep, goats
Distribution: Worldwide
Derivation of Genus: Flat band, bandage, or tape/bladder tail
Transmission Route: Ingestion of infective abdominal omentum of ruminants
Common Name: Canine taeniid/bovine bladder worm
Zoonotic: No

For *Taenia hydatigena*, an adult tapeworm found in the small intestine of dogs, the larval stage is a ping-pong ball–sized, fluid-filled bladder called *Cysticercus tenuicollis*, which is usually attached to the greater omentum or other abdominal organs of the ruminant intermediate host (Figure 6-15) and is considered nonpathogenic to the intermediate host. The adult worm has an armed rostellum. The proglottids have a single lateral genital pore. The eggs are typical taeniid-type ova with a striated embryophore surrounding an oncosphere with six hooklets inside. In large numbers the adults can cause obstruction of the intestinal tract. To acquire this

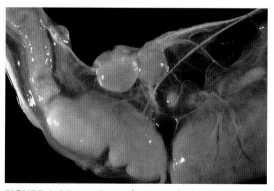

FIGURE 6-15 Larval stage for *Taenia hydatigena* is a ping-pong ball–sized, fluid-filled bladder (*Cysticercus tenuicollis*) that is usually attached to the greater omentum or other abdominal organs of the ruminant intermediate host.

tapeworm, dogs become infected by ingesting the abdominal viscera of cysticercus-infected ruminants. For every cysticercus that is ingested by the dog, one adult tapeworm will develop in the small intestine of that dog. Diagnosis is made by finding the taeniid ova on standard fecal flotation. It is important that the veterinarian recognize the ruminant as the source of this tapeworm and understand the importance of preventing predation or ingestion of ruminant offal by the dog. Necropsy of the intermediate host reveals the cysticercus stage in the abdominal cavity of the ruminant intermediate host.

> **TECHNICIAN'S NOTE** **Typical-taeniid type** eggs can be found on standard fecal flotation.

HORSES

Intestinal Tract

Parasite: *Anoplocephala perfoliata, Anoplocephala magna,* and *Paranoplocephala mamillana*

Host: Horses

Location of Adult: Small intestine, large intestine, and cecum (*A. perfoliata*); small intestine and occasionally stomach (*A. magna* and *P. mamillana*)

Intermediate Host: Grain mites

Distribution: Worldwide

Derivation of Genus: Unarmed head/Bearing an unarmed head

Transmission Route: Ingestion of infective grain mites

Common Name: Lappeted equine tapeworm (*A. perfoliata*) and equine tapeworm with large scolex (*A. magna*); dwarf tapeworm (*P. mamillana*); collectively, equine tapeworms

Zoonotic: No

> **TECHNICIAN'S NOTE** *Anoplocephala perfoliata* adults are easily identified by their morphologic features (lappets just posterior to the scolex) and characteristic ovum with its pyriform apparatus.

Anoplocephala perfoliata, Anoplocephala magna, and *Paranoplocephala mamillana* are the equine tapeworms. *A. perfoliata* is found in the small and large intestine and cecum; *A. magna* and *P. mamillana* are found in the small intestine and occasionally the stomach. *A. perfoliata* can measure from 5 to 8 cm in length and up to 1.2 cm in width. The scolex is oblong, 2 to 3 mm in diameter, unarmed, with very prominent **lappets** (two round protuberances) behind each of the four suckers. The proglottids are wider than long, and each proglottid has only one set of male and female reproductive organs (Figure 6-16). *A. magna* can measure up to 80 cm in length and 2.5 cm in width. The scolex is large and oblong, 4 to 6 mm in diameter, unarmed but lacking the lappets of *A. perfoliata* (Figure 6-17). *P. mamillana,* also known as the *dwarf*

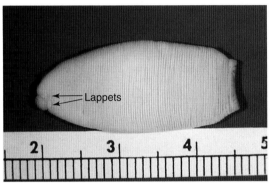

FIGURE 6-16 Adult specimen of *Anoplocephala perfoliata,* an equine tapeworm. The scolex is oblong, 2 to 3 mm in diameter, and has very prominent lappets behind each of four suckers. Proglottids are wider than long, and each has only one set of male and female reproductive organs.

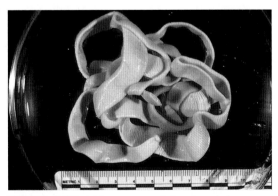

FIGURE 6-17 Adult specimen of *Anoplocephala magna,* an equine tapeworm. The scolex is quite large, 4 to 6 mm in diameter, and lacks prominent lappets.

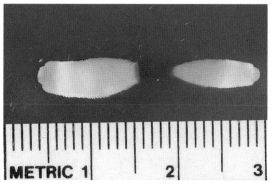

FIGURE 6-18 Adult specimens of *Paranoplocephala mamillana*, the dwarf equine tapeworm. The scolex is quite narrow and lacks prominent lappets. Note: These specimens are entire specimens and not individual proglottids.

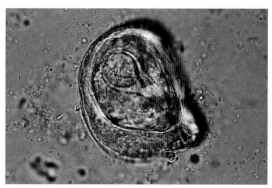

FIGURE 6-19 Fecal flotation revealing the egg of *Anoplocephala perfoliata*. The egg is thick-walled, with one or more flattened sides measuring 65 to 80 μm in diameter; those of *Anoplocephala magna* are similar but slightly smaller, measuring 50 to 60 μm. Eggs have an innermost lining called the *pyriform* (pear-shaped) *apparatus*.

tapeworm, is only 6 to 50 mm in length and 4 to 6 mm in width (Figure 6-18). The scolex is quite narrow. The adults of all three species can cause granulation tissue at the site of attachment in the intestinal wall.

The eggs of *A. perfoliata* are thick walled, with one or more flattened sides measuring 65 to 80 μm in diameter; those of *A. magna* are similar but slightly smaller, measuring 50 to 60 μm. The eggs of *P. mamillana* are oval and thin walled, measuring 51 × 37 μm. Eggs of all three species have a three-layered eggshell; the innermost lining is a pyriform (pear-shaped) apparatus. The hexacanth embryo can be visualized just inside the pyriform apparatus (Figure 6-19). Eggs of all equine tapeworms can be recovered using standard fecal flotation. The prepatent period for all three species ranges from 28 to 42 days.

> *TECHNICIAN'S NOTE* All three species of equine tapeworms can be identified on standard fecal flotation by observing their triangular, three-layered–shell ova with the pyriform apparatus.

As in *Moniezia* species in ruminants, the metacestode (larval) stage of equine tapeworms is the cysticercoid stage, which may be found within the intermediate hosts, oribatid grain mites. Intact proglottids and eggs are found in the feces of the equine definitive host. Mites become infected by ingesting the hexacanth embryo, which develops

into the cysticercoid stage within the body of the grain mites. Horses become infected by ingesting cysticercoid-infected mites infesting the grain. The cysticercoid is a microscopic stage and probably will not be observed by the veterinarian. For every cysticercoid that is ingested by the ruminant, one adult tapeworm will develop in the small intestine of that ruminant (Figure 6-10). It is important that the veterinarian recognize the oribatid mite as the source of this tapeworm and understand the importance of pasture rotation and effective tapeworm therapeusis (pyrantel pamoate and pyrantel tartrate; praziquantel has been used with success but is not approved by the Food and Drug Administration [FDA]) in horses.

> *TECHNICIAN'S NOTE* Pasture rotation and deworming protocols are effective in reducing these equine tapeworms in horses.

TRUE TAPEWORMS OF DOGS AND CATS

Tapeworms that infect dogs and cats are *Dipylidium caninum, Taenia pisiformis, Taenia hydatigena, Taenia ovis, Taenia taeniaeformis, Multiceps multiceps, Multiceps serialis, Echinococcus granulosus, Echinococcus multilocularis,* and *Mesocestoides* species.

Dipylidium caninum

Parasite: 🅉 *Dipylidium caninum*
Host: Dogs and cats
Location of Adult: Small intestine
Intermediate Host: Adult fleas
Distribution: Worldwide
Derivation of Genus: Having two entrances
Transmission Route: Ingestion of infective adult flea
Common Name: Double-pored tapeworm or cucumber seed tapeworm
Zoonotic: Yes

Dipylidium caninum is often called the *double-pored* or *cucumber seed tapeworm*. This is the most common tapeworm found in the small intestine of the dog and cat because the dog or cat becomes infected by ingesting the flea intermediate host. Fleas often contain this parasite's infective cysticercoid stage. The adult tapeworm can grow to a length of 50 cm (Figure 6-20). The scolex of this tapeworm is armed and consists of a prominent proboscis covered with rearward-facing, rose thorn–like hooks (Figure 6-21). This tapeworm usually demonstrates its presence by the release of and the appearance of its motile, terminal, gravid proglottids, which are usually found on the feces

(Figure 6-22). They may also be found on the pet's hair coat or in the bedding of the host. In the fresh state, these proglottids resemble cucumber seeds (cucumber seed tapeworm). These proglottids have a lateral pore located along the midpoint of each of their long edges (double-pored tapeworm) (Figure 6-23). Gravid proglottids contain thousands of unique egg packets, each containing 20 to 30 hexacanth embryos (Figure 6-24). (Figure 6-25 shows an individual egg packet of *D. caninum* containing hexacanth embryos.) The proglottids of *D. caninum* often dry out in the external environment. As they lose moisture they shrivel up, resembling uncooked grains of rice (Figure 6-26). If reconstituted with water, the dried proglottids usually assume their former cucumber seed appearance. The prepatent period for *D. caninum* is 14 to 21 days.

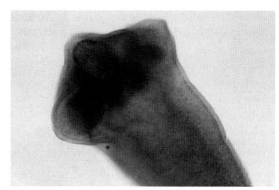

FIGURE 6-21 Scolex of *Dipylidium caninum* is armed and consists of a prominent proboscis covered with rearward-facing, rose thorn–like hooks.

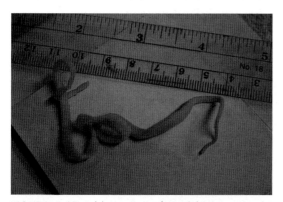

FIGURE 6-20 Adult specimen of *Dipylidium caninum*, the double-pored or cucumber seed tapeworm of dogs and cats. Adult tapeworms can grow to 50 cm long. This tapeworm usually demonstrates its presence by the release of and appearance of motile, terminal, gravid proglottids, which are usually found on feces, the hair coat, or bedding. In the fresh state, proglottids resemble cucumber seeds, thus the common name *cucumber seed tapeworm*.

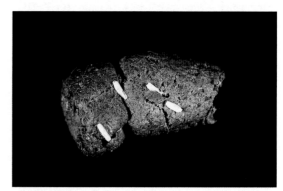

FIGURE 6-22 *Dipylidium caninum* usually demonstrates its presence by the release of and appearance of motile, terminal, gravid proglottids, which are usually found on feces.

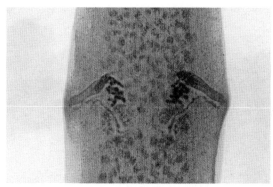

FIGURE 6-23 These proglottids of *Dipylidium caninum* have a lateral pore along the midpoint of each long edge, thus the second common name *double-pored tapeworm*.

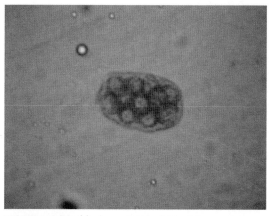

FIGURE 6-25 If fresh proglottids of *Dipylidium caninum* are teased or broken open, they may reveal thousands of egg packets, each containing 20 to 30 hexacanth embryos.

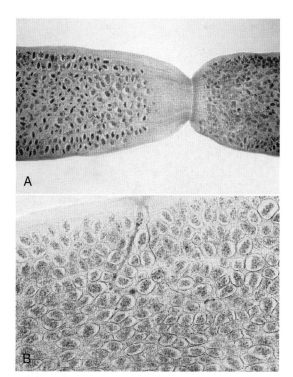

A

B

FIGURE 6-24 Gravid proglottids of *Dipylidium caninum* are filled with thousands of egg packets. **A,** Gravid proglottid showing egg packets. **B,** Close-up of gravid proglottid showing egg packets containing hexacanth embryos.

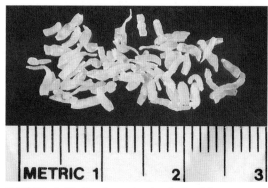

FIGURE 6-26 Dried proglottids of *Dipylidium caninum* resemble uncooked grains of rice. When water is added, they assume their natural state.

The metacestode (larval) stage of this tapeworm is the cysticercoid stage, which may be found within the flea intermediate host. Larval fleas become infected by ingesting the hexacanth embryo, which develops into the cysticercoid stage within the body of the adult flea. Dogs and cats become infected by ingesting cysticercoid-infected adult fleas (Figure 6-27). The cysticercoid is a microscopic stage and probably will not be observed by the veterinarian. For every cysticercoid that is ingested by the dog or cat, one adult tapeworm will develop in the small intestine of that dog or cat. If a human (e.g., child) ingests a flea containing the cysticercoid stage, this tapeworm will develop to the adult stage within the small intestine. It is a zoonotic parasite.

> **⬛ TECHNICIAN'S NOTE** In sufficient numbers, adult *Dipylidium caninum* tapeworms can cause intestinal obstruction in the host.

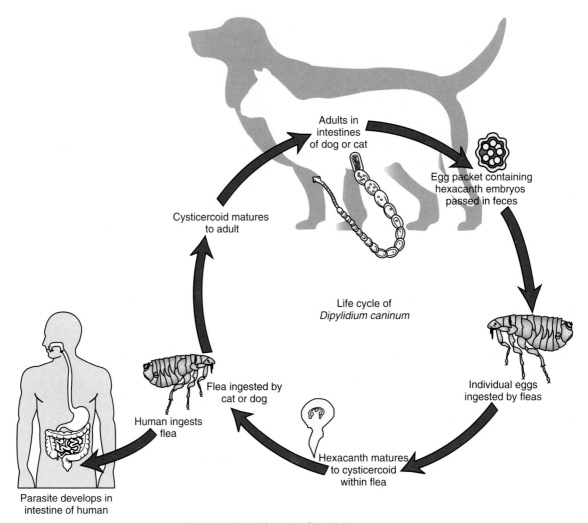

FIGURE 6-27 Life cycle of *Dipylidium caninum*.

This tapeworm is typically diagnosed in one of two ways. The egg packets can be found on fecal flotation (Figure 6-24) if the gravid proglottids dry up and release the egg packets. The gravid proglottids may also be seen by the client in the feces, on bedding, or in the hair coat. It is important that the veterinarian recognize the flea as the source of this tapeworm and understand the importance of flea control in effective tapeworm therapeusis. *D. caninum* is typically treated with a single dose of praziquantel or epsiprantel. All pets in the household must be treated for both fleas and tapeworms.

TECHNICIAN'S NOTE *Dipylidium caninum* can be diagnosed by finding the characteristic egg packets on standard fecal flotation (this tends to be rare) or by observing the gravid proglottids in the feces.

Taenia pisiformis, Taenia hydatigena, and *Taenia ovis/Cysticercus pisiformis, Cysticercus tenuicollis,* and *Cysticercus ovis* (Metacestode [larval] tapeworm)

Parasite: *Taenia pisiformis, Taenia hydatigena,* and *Taenia ovis*

CASE PRESENTATION 6-1

Setting up the Scenario

Mr. Michelson presented Pixie, a 3-year-old spayed Persian cat, for her annual physical examination and routine vaccinations. During the history-taking session, Mr. Michelson revealed to you that Pixie had what appeared to be tapeworm proglottids, moving "creatures" resembling grains of cooked white rice, in her fresh stool sample and on the living room couch where she often naps. A fecal sample was performed, and one of the tapeworm proglottids was torn open to release the characteristic egg packets of *Dipylidium caninum.* Dr. James will administer a cestocide to remove this very common problem tapeworm but has asked you as the veterinary technician to educate Mr. Michelson regarding the details of *D. caninum*'s life cycle and zoonotic importance.

What Information Must the Veterinary Technician Convey to Mr. Michelson?

The veterinary technician enters the examination room and begins the explanation. "Mr. Michelson, Pixie has been diagnosed with *D. caninum,* a helminth parasite often referred to as the *cucumber seed tapeworm* or the *double-pored tapeworm.* To complete its life cycle, this tapeworm uses the flea as an intermediate host. The flea is the means by which this tapeworm is transmitted from an infected dog or cat to an uninfected dog or cat. Because Pixie is not subjected to any routine flea control programs, she has become infested with fleas. If Pixie is infested with fleas within her hair coat, I am sorry to inform

you that your home will also be infested with fleas; in fact there are several developmental life cycle stages of fleas that may be found throughout Pixie's environment (your home or your yard). It is the flea that makes the transmission of *D. caninum* possible. Pixie was infected by ingesting at least one adult flea containing the infective stage of the tapeworm. Dr. James has prescribed medication to remove the tapeworms, but you must use additional flea control programs to reduce the flea population in/on Pixie, your other pets, your home, and your yard. Removing fleas from the environment will prevent reinfection with the tapeworms and infection in your other pets if they happen to ingest infected fleas. Because fleas can be found year-round, we recommend treating all of your pets with an established year-round flea control program to prevent reinfestation with fleas and the accompanying reinfection with tapeworms.

It is also important to understand that humans, especially children, can become infected with *D. caninum* if these infective fleas are ingested. Therefore flea treatment on your pets and in your house and yard will protect you and your family from infection with this tapeworm. Do you have any questions?"

The veterinary technician noted in Pixie's medical record that these discussions regarding flea control and prevention, especially the portion regarding the zoonotic potential of *D. caninum,* had taken place with Mr. Michelson.

Host: Dogs
Location of Adult: Small intestine
Intermediate Host: Rabbits and hares (*T. pisiformis*); ruminants (*T. hydatigena*); sheep (*T. ovis*)
Distribution: Worldwide
Derivation of Genus: Flat band, bandage, or tape
Transmission Route: Ingestion of infective intermediate host
Common Name: Canine taeniid (*T. pisiformis* and *T. hydatigena*); mutton tapeworm of dogs (*T. ovis*)
Zoonotic: No

Taenia pisiformis, T. hydatigena, and *T. ovis* are the canine taeniids. The canine taeniids measure from 1 to 2 cm (*T. ovis*) to 200 cm (*T. pisiformis*) and up to 75 to 500 cm (*T. hydatigena*) in length. These adult taeniids are found within the small intestine of the canine definitive host (Figure 6-28) where, in sufficient numbers, they can cause intestinal obstruction. The scolex of all these tapeworms is armed, consisting of two rows of rostellar hooks (Figure 6-29). As with *D. caninum,* the *Taenia* species manifest by the appearance of motile, terminal, gravid proglottids on the feces, on the pet's hair

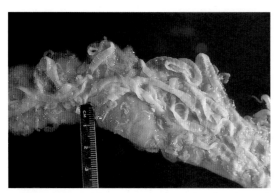

FIGURE 6-28 Adult canine taeniids are found in the small intestine of the canine definitive host.

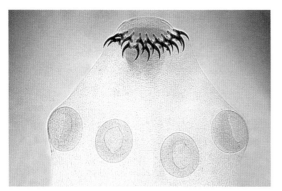

FIGURE 6-29 Details of the scolex of the canine taeniid. Note the four suckers and armed rostellum.

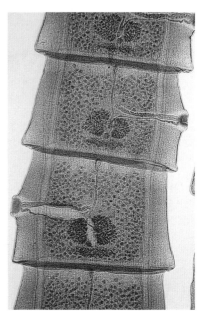

FIGURE 6-30 Mature proglottids of *Taenia* species demonstrating a single lateral pore located along the midpoint of long edges (as opposed to the double-pored tapeworm).

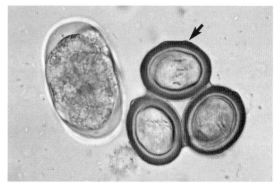

FIGURE 6-31 Tapeworm egg, or hexacanth embryo. Tapeworm eggs are released to the outside environment. Each tapeworm egg is infective for the intermediate host and produces one metacestode stage. The unmarked egg is an *Ancylostoma caninum*.

coat, or in the bedding of the host. In the fresh state, these proglottids have a single lateral pore located along the midpoint of either of their long edges (unlike the double-pored tapeworm) (Figure 6-30).

> **TECHNICIAN'S NOTE** Gravid proglottids found in the feces can be teased open and the ova identified as *Dipylidium* or taeniid-type ova to speciate the genus of the tapeworm represented by the gravid proglottids.

As with *D. caninum,* if the fresh proglottids are teased or broken open, they may reveal typical hexacanth embryos (Figure 6-31). These hexacanth embryos have a striated eggshell (called the **embryophore**) and contain six hooks (or teeth) within the interior of the egg. This egg is referred to as a **typical taeniid type of egg**. The proglottids of

Taenia species also dry out in the external environment and resemble uncooked grains of rice. If reconstituted with water, they usually assume their former single-pored appearance. If gravid proglottids of *Taenia* species are recovered from a dog's or cat's feces, the proglottid should be torn open or macerated in a drop of saline solution on a glass slide to reveal the characteristic eggs under the compound microscope.

The eggs of the taeniid tapeworms are slightly oval and are 43 to 53 µm × 43 to 49 µm in diameter (*T. pisiformis*), 36 to 39 µm × 31 to 35 µm in diameter (*T. hydatigena*), and 19 to 31 µm × 24 to 26 µm in diameter (*T. ovis*). Eggs of *Taenia* species contain a single oncosphere (literally a "growth ball") with three pairs (6) of hooks. The oncosphere is often called a *hexacanth embryo*. The eggs of the taeniids are very similar to those of *Echinococcus* and *Multiceps* species.

The metacestode (larval) stage for *T. pisiformis*, *T. hydatigena*, and *T. ovis* is the cysticercus, or bladder worm stage, which may be found within the respective rabbit, ruminant, or ovine intermediate hosts.

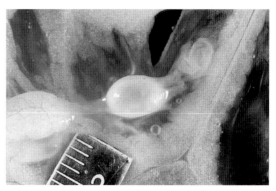

FIGURE 6-32 Larval stage for *Taenia pisiformis* is a pea-sized, fluid-filled bladder (*Cysticercus pisiformis*). The larval stage is usually attached to the greater omentum or other abdominal organs of the rabbit intermediate host.

> **TECHNICIAN'S NOTE** The intermediate hosts of the canine taeniid tapeworms ingest the ova from the feces of the canine host. The ova then develop into a cysticercus stage in the intermediate host.

For *T. pisiformis* and *T. hydatigena*, the rabbit and the ruminant become infected by ingesting the taeniid eggs or hexacanth embryos, often found close to canine feces. These embryos hatch and develop into the cysticercus stage within the peritoneal cavity of the intermediate hosts. For *T. pisiformis* the larval stage is a pea-sized, fluid-filled bladder (called *Cysticercus pisiformis*), usually attached to the greater omentum or other abdominal organs of the rabbit (Figure 6-32). Dogs become infected by killing and ingesting cysticercus-infected rabbits. For every cysticercus that is ingested by the dog, one adult tapeworm develops in the small intestine of that dog (Figure 6-33). It is important that the veterinarian recognize the rabbit as the source of this tapeworm and understand the importance of preventing predation or the ingestion of rabbit carrion by the dog. *T. pisiformis* can be treated with praziquantel or epsiprantel.

For *T. hydatigena* the tenuicollis stage is a ping-pong ball–sized, fluid-filled bladder (called *Cysticercus tenuicollis*), usually attached to the greater omentum or other abdominal organs of the

ruminant intermediate host (Figure 6-34; see also Figure 6-15). To acquire this tapeworm, dogs become infected by ingesting the abdominal viscera of cysticercus-infected ruminants (Figure 6-33). For every cysticercus that is ingested by the dog, one adult tapeworm will develop in the small intestine of that dog. It is important that the veterinarian recognize the ruminant as the source of this tapeworm and understand the importance of preventing predation or ingestion of ruminant offal by the dog.

For *T. ovis* the larval stage is a fluid-filled bladder (called *Cysticercus ovis*) found within the musculature of the ovine intermediate host (very similar to the cysticerci of *C. bovis* and *C. cellulosae* described earlier) (see Figure 6-13). To acquire this tapeworm, dogs become infected by ingesting the musculature of cysticercus-infected sheep (Figure 6-33). For every cysticercus that is ingested by the dog, one adult tapeworm will develop in the small intestine of that dog. It is important that the veterinarian recognize sheep muscle (uncooked mutton) as the source of this tapeworm and understand the importance of preventing predation and ingestion of sheep muscle by dogs.

> **TECHNICIAN'S NOTE** The dog is infected with the canine taeniid by eating the intermediate host containing the cysticercus stage of the tapeworm. Preventing predation of the intermediate host will stop the life cycle of the tapeworm.

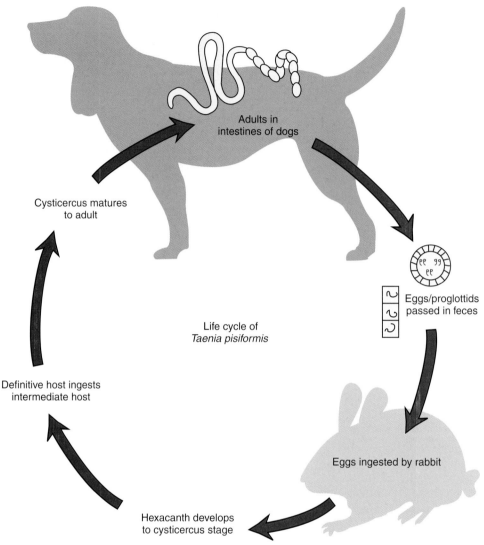

Adults in
intestines of dogs

Cysticercus matures
to adult

Life cycle of
Taenia pisiformis

Eggs/proglottids
passed in feces

Definitive host ingests
intermediate host

Eggs ingested by rabbit

Hexacanth develops
to cysticercus stage

FIGURE 6-33 Life cycle of *Taenia pisiformis*.

Taenia taeniaeformis (*Hydatigera taeniaeformis*)

Parasite: *Taenia taeniaeformis/Cysticercus fasciolaris* (Metacestode [larval] stage)

Host: Cats

Location of Adult: Small intestines

Intermediate Host: Rats and mice

Distribution: Worldwide

Derivation of Genus: Flat band, bandage, or tape

Transmission Route: Ingestion of infective rats or mice

Common Name: Feline taeniid or feline tapeworm

Zoonotic: No

Taenia taeniaeformis, or *Hydatigera taeniaeformis,* is called the feline tapeworm or the feline taeniid. This tapeworm, which may be up to 60 cm in length, is observed infrequently in cats that are

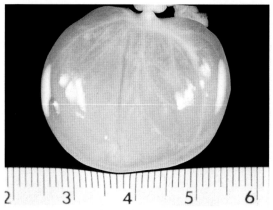

FIGURE 6-34 Larval stage for *Taenia hydatigena* is a ping-pong ball–sized, fluid-filled bladder (*Cysticercus tenuicollis*), usually attached to the greater omentum or other abdominal organs of the ruminant intermediate host.

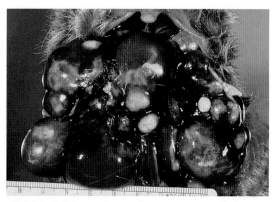

FIGURE 6-35 Larval stage for *Taenia taeniaeformis* is a strobilocercus (*Cysticercus fasciolaris*). The strobilocercus is a scolex attached to a long neck, which connects to a bladder.

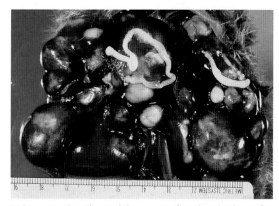

FIGURE 6-36 The strobilocercus is found in the liver of a rodent intermediate host.

allowed to roam and prey on rabbits and rodents. The armed scolex is similar to that of the canine taeniids, as are the proglottids; however, in the fresh or intact state the terminal proglottids of *T. taeniaeformis* are said to be bell-shaped. The egg of this tapeworm is 31 to 36 μm in diameter and contains a single oncosphere with three pairs of hooks. For this reason the oncosphere is often called a *hexacanth* (or six-toothed) *embryo*. As with the eggs of the canine taeniids, the egg is very similar to that of the *Echinococcus* species. (See Figure 6-31 for unique features of this taeniid type of tapeworm egg.)

> **TECHNICIAN'S NOTE** *Taenia taeniaeformis* produces a taeniid-type ovum and appears similar to that of the canine taeniids except the terminal proglottids are bell-shaped.

The metacestode (larval) stage for *T. taeniaeformis* is the strobilocercus, a morphologic variation of the cysticercus (bladder worm) stage. For *T. taeniaeformis* to develop, the rodent intermediate host becomes infected by ingesting the taeniid eggs, or hexacanth embryos, often found in proximity to feline feces. The embryo hatches and develops into the cysticercus stage within the liver of the intermediate host. For the first 42 days in this location, it

develops as a cysticercus. On day 42, however, the cysticercus changes its form into that of a strobilocercus. For *T. taeniaeformis,* the strobilocercus is a scolex attached to a long neck, which connects to a bladder; this stage has the scientific name *Cysticercus fasciolaris* (Figures 6-35, 6-36, and 6-37). The cat becomes infected by killing the rat and ingesting the strobilocercus from the liver. The neck and its connected bladder are digested, the scolex attaches, and the tapeworm begins to grow in the cat's intestine (Figure 6-33). For every strobilocercus that is ingested by the cat, one adult tapeworm will develop in the small intestine of that cat. It is important that the veterinarian recognize the rat as the source of

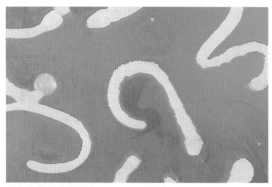

FIGURE 6-37 Detail of an individual strobilocercus, *Cysticercus fasciolaris.*

this tapeworm and understand the importance of preventing predation or the ingestion of rat or mouse carrion by the cat. The cat can be treated with praziquantel.

> **TECHNICIAN'S NOTE**   *Taenia taeniaeformis* uses a strobilocercus as its metacestode stage. The strobilocercus is a fluid-filled bladder that connects to a long strobila that connects to a scolex. This life cycle is unique because it is like no other taeniid tapeworm life cycle.

Multiceps multiceps and Multiceps serialis

Parasite: *Multiceps multiceps* and *Multiceps serialis/ Coenurus cerebralis, Coenurus serialis* (Metacestode [larval] tapeworm)

Host: Dogs

Location of Adult: Small intestines

Intermediate Host: Sheep (*M. multiceps*) and rabbits (*M. serialis*)

Distribution: Worldwide (*M. multiceps*)

Derivation of Genus: Many heads

Transmission Route: Ingestion of infected intermediate host

Common Name: Coenurus-producing tapeworm

Zoonotic: No

Multiceps multiceps and *Multiceps serialis* are also taeniid tapeworms of the small intestine of canids. The adults of *M. multiceps* are 40 to 100 cm in length; those of *M. serialis* can grow up to 72 cm. Both possess a scolex with a double row of rostellar hooks. In sufficient numbers, the adult tapeworms can obstruct the intestinal tract.

The eggs of *M. multiceps* are 29 to 37 µm in diameter, and those of *M. serialis* are elliptic and measure 31 to 34 µm × 29 to 30 µm. Both contain a single oncosphere with three pairs of hooks. As with the eggs of the canine and feline taeniids, the eggs of *Multiceps* species are very similar to those of *Taenia* and *Echinococcus* species. (See Figure 6-31 for unique features of this taeniid type of tapeworm.)

> **TECHNICIAN'S NOTE**   The taeniid-type ova of *Multiceps* species can be found on standard fecal flotation.

The metacestode (larval) stage for *M. multiceps* and *M. serialis* is the coenurus stage, which may be found within the respective ovine or rabbit intermediate host. This coenurus also has a scientific name: *Coenurus cerebralis* for *M. multiceps* and *Coenurus serialis* for *M. serialis*. It is essentially a single large bladder with several invaginated scolices attached to its inner wall. The coenurus is found within the tissues of the respective intermediate host. For each coenurus that is ingested by the dog, several adult tapeworms develop, one for each invaginated scolex ingested.

For *M. multiceps*, the sheep intermediate host becomes infected by ingesting taeniid eggs, or hexacanth embryos, which are often found close to canine feces. These embryos hatch and migrate to neurologic tissue (either brain or spinal cord tissue), where they develop into the coenurus stage within the tissue hosts. Naturally, the presence of these large space-occupying lesions within the brain and spinal cord can produce neurologic signs in the infected sheep. The larval stage of *M. multiceps* may be up to 5 cm in diameter and is a fluid-filled bladder (called *C. cerebralis*) with many individual scolices lining the walls of the bladder. Dogs become infected either by killing the sheep and ingesting coenurus-infected neural tissue or by being fed such tissues by their sheepherder owners. For every coenurus that is ingested by the dog, many adult tapeworms will develop in the small intestine of that dog. It is important that the veterinarian recognize the sheep as the source of this tapeworm and understand the importance of preventing predation or the ingestion of sheep carrion or offal by the dog.

> TECHNICIAN'S NOTE   *Multiceps multiceps* is associated with the formation of a coenurus in the brain or nervous tissue of the ovine intermediate host.

For *M. serialis*, the rabbit intermediate host becomes infected by ingesting the taeniid eggs or hexacanth embryos often found in proximity to canine feces. These embryos hatch and migrate to the rabbit's subcutaneous tissues, where they develop into the coenurus stage. The presence of these large bladder-like cysts within the subcutaneous tissues of the rabbit can interfere with movement and speed, making the rabbit easy prey. For *M. serialis*, the larval stage may be up to 4 cm in diameter and is a fluid-filled bladder called *C. serialis* (Figure 6-38), with many individual invaginated scolices lining the walls of the bladder. Dogs become infected either by killing the slow-moving rabbit and ingesting coenurus-infected subcutaneous tissues or by being fed such tissues by their rabbit-hunting owners. For every coenurus that is ingested by the dog, many adult tapeworms will develop in the small intestine of that dog. It is important that the

veterinarian recognize the rabbit as the source of this tapeworm and understand the importance of preventing predation or the ingestion of rabbit carrion or offal by the dog.

> TECHNICIAN'S NOTE   *Multiceps serialis* is associated with the formation of a coenurus in the subcutaneous or intermuscular connective tissue of the rabbit intermediate host.

Echinococcus granulosus and *Echinococcus multilocularis*

Parasite: 🅩 *Echinococcus granulosus* and *Echinococcus multilocularis*

Host: Dogs (*E. granulosus*); cats (*E. multilocularis*)

Location of Adult: Small intestine

Intermediate Host: Sheep, cattle, and other herbivores (*E. granulosus*); rats, mice, and voles (*E. multilocularis*); humans (both)

Distribution: Worldwide (*E. granulosus*); countries in the Northern Hemisphere (*E. multilocularis*)

Derivation of Genus: Spiny berry

Transmission Route: Ingestion of infective intermediate host

Common Name: Unilocular hydatid tapeworm (*E. granulosus*); multilocular hydatid tapeworm (*E. multilocularis*)

Zoonotic: Yes

Echinococcus granulosus and *Echinococcus multilocularis* are the hydatid disease tapeworms associated

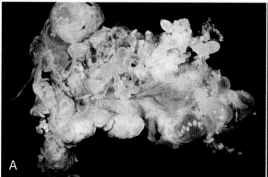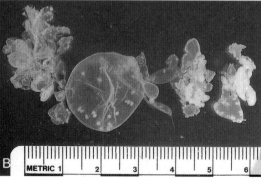

FIGURE 6-38 **A,** *Coenurus serialis* from subcutaneous connective tissues of a rabbit. **B,** Note the individual invaginated scolices lining the walls of the bladder.

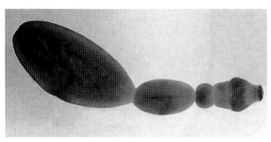

FIGURE 6-39 Adult *Echinococcus* species is a tiny tapeworm, only 1.2 to 7 mm in length. The entire tapeworm has only three proglottids: immature, mature, and gravid.

with **unilocular** and **multilocular** hydatid disease. *E. granulosus* is the hydatid cyst tapeworm of dogs, and *E. multilocularis* is the hydatid cyst tapeworm of cats. These are important parasites because of their extreme zoonotic potential.

The adult *Echinococcus* is a tiny tapeworm, only 1.2 to 7 mm in length. The entire tapeworm has a scolex followed by only three proglottids: immature, mature, and gravid (Figure 6-39). When passed, the tiny gravid proglottids likely will be overlooked by the client, the veterinary technician, and the veterinarian. Definitive diagnosis of *Echinococcus* species infection is best achieved by identifying adult tapeworms taken from the host's intestinal tract. In the rare instance in which *Echinococcus* species infection is suspected, antemortem diagnosis is accomplished by purging the dog or cat using arecoline hydrobromide, 3.5 mg/kg body weight, and collecting its feces.

> **TECHNICIAN'S NOTE** The adult *Echinococcus* tapeworms cannot accumulate in sufficient numbers to cause intestinal blockage. Their pathogenicity lies in the fact that their eggs can develop into unilocular or multilocular (depending on species) hydatid cysts in the liver, lungs, or brain of the intermediate hosts.

Purging the infected dog or cat is usually performed only when infection is strongly suspected. Entire worms or their proglottids may be collected from the final clear mucus. Because of serious zoonotic potential, all evacuated material should be handled with caution. After the feces have been examined,

the evacuate should be incinerated. Rubber gloves should be worn when handling suspect feces.

Diagnosis of *Echinococcus* species in either a definitive or an intermediate host warrants reporting to state and federal authorities.

The egg of *E. granulosus* is ovoid, 32 to 36 μm × 25 to 30 μm, and contains a single oncosphere with three pairs of hooks. The egg of *E. multilocularis* is ovoid, 30 to 40 μm, and contains a single oncosphere with three pairs of hooks. Because of serious zoonotic potential (see Chapter 16), any "suspect" eggs of *Echinococcus* species should be handled with extreme caution. These eggs are very similar in appearance to those of *Taenia* and *Multiceps* species. (See Figure 6-31 for unique features of this taeniid type of tapeworm.)

The metacestode (larval) stage for *E. granulosus* and *E. multilocularis* is the **hydatid cyst** stage, which may be found within the respective ruminant or rodent intermediate host. The hydatid cyst for *E. granulosus* is a unilocular hydatid cyst found within the liver, lung, and other organs of the ruminant intermediate host. The hydatid cyst for *E. multilocularis* is a multilocular or alveolar hydatid cyst found within the liver or lungs of the rodent intermediate host. Humans may also serve as an intermediate host for both of these tapeworms. Humans become infected by ingesting eggs of these tapeworm species.

The unilocular (single-compartment) hydatid cyst of *E. granulosus* has a thick cyst wall with a thin germinal membrane located just inside it. Brood capsules containing protoscolices "bud" from this germinal membrane. When a dog ingests the hydatid cyst containing the brood capsules and protoscolices, each protoscolex develops into an adult tapeworm (Figure 6-40).

> **TECHNICIAN'S NOTE** Humans can serve as an intermediate host for both species of *Echinococcus* tapeworms.

The multilocular (multicompartment) hydatid cyst of *E. multilocularis* lacks the thick cyst wall of the unilocular hydatid cyst. It is often described as *alveolar* or similar to a "bunch of grapes." Lacking the thick cyst wall of the unilocular cyst, the

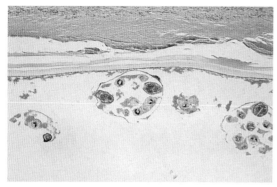

FIGURE 6-40 Photomicrograph of a unilocular hydatid cyst of *Echinococcus granulosus* showing a thick multilayered wall and a thin granular germinal membrane. Spherical brood capsules containing protoscolices arise from the germinal membrane.

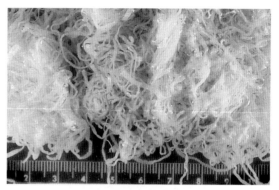

FIGURE 6-41 Adult *Mesocestoides* species are medium-sized tapeworms, ranging from 12 cm to more than 2 m long.

multilocular cyst is very invasive, often replacing normal tissue, similar to a malignant cancer. It also possesses a thin germinal membrane. Brood capsules containing protoscolices bud from the germinal membrane. When a cat ingests the hydatid cyst containing the brood capsules and protoscolices, each protoscolex will develop into an adult tapeworm in the intestine of the cat.

Praziquantel can be used to treat adult *Echinococcus* worms but will not affect the hydatid cyst stage. The best treatment for the hydatid cyst stage of the parasites is preventing ingestion of the eggs.

> **TECHNICIAN'S NOTE** *Echinococcus* species are the tiniest tapeworms of veterinary parasitology, but "dynamite comes in little packages." As zoonotic diseases go, these tapeworms pack a BIG PUNCH! If diagnosed, this parasite must be reported to state and federal authorities.

Mesocestoides Species

Parasite: *Mesocestoides* species
Host: Dogs, cats, and other carnivores
Location of Adult: Small intestine
Intermediate Host: First intermediate host, oribatid mite; second intermediate host, rats and mice
Distribution: North America, Asia, Europe, and Africa
Derivation of Genus: The form of a middle girdle

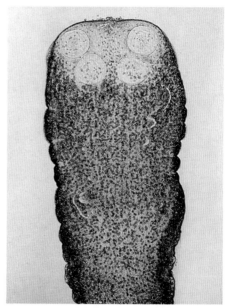

FIGURE 6-42 Scolex of *Mesocestoides* species is oblong, has four suckers, and is unarmed.

Transmission Route: Ingestion of infective intermediate host
Common Name: Tetrathyridium tapeworm
Zoonotic: No

Mesocestoides species may parasitize the small intestine of carnivores, including the dog and the cat. These are small- to medium-sized true tapeworms, ranging from 12 cm to more than 2 m in length (Figure 6-41). The scolex of this tapeworm is oblong with four suckers, is unarmed (Figure 6-42), and

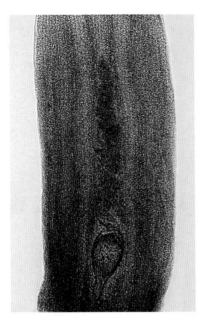

FIGURE 6-43 Gravid proglottids of *Mesocestoides* have a unique appearance.

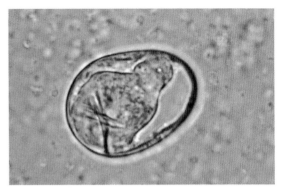

FIGURE 6-44 Eggs of *Mesocestoides* species contain a single oncosphere with three pairs of hooks. The oncosphere is often called a *hexacanth embryo*.

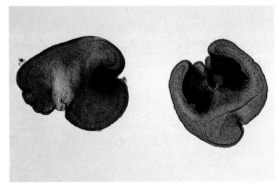

FIGURE 6-45 Metacestode stage for *Mesocestoides* species is a tetrathyridium, a solid-bodied metacestode stage with a deeply invaginated, acetabular scolex.

has a centrally located uterine pore. In sufficient numbers the adult tapeworms can cause intestinal obstruction. Gravid proglottids of *Mesocestoides* have a unique appearance (Figure 6-43). The eggs of *Mesocestoides* species contain a single oncosphere (hexacanth embryo) with three pairs of hooks. (See Figure 6-44 for features of this egg.) The striated embryophore (shell) is lacking.

> **TECHNICIAN'S NOTE** *Mesocestoides* species of tapeworms are unusual true tapeworms in that they use two intermediate hosts instead of one intermediate host.

Mesocestoides is an unusual genus among the true tapeworms in that it is the only one that uses two intermediate hosts. (The pseudotapeworms described in the next section use two intermediate hosts.) The egg is a hexacanth embryo. If it is ingested by an oribatid mite, it develops into a cysticercoid within that mite (much like the cysticercoids of *Dipylidium, Moniezia, Thysanosoma,* and *Anoplocephala* species). If this cysticercoid-containing mite is ingested by a mouse or reptile, the cysticercoid develops into a tetrathyridium, a solid-bodied metacestode stage with a deeply invaginated, acetabular scolex (Figure 6-45). This tetrathyridium is approximately 1 cm in diameter and is capable of multiplying exponentially; that is, one tetrathyridium becomes two, two become four, four become eight, and so on (Figures 6-46 and 6-47). This type of asexual reproduction produces large numbers of tetrathyridia that are infective to the canine or feline definitive host. The tetrathyridia multiply in the body of the second intermediate host and are often confined to the serous cavities, particularly the peritoneal cavity (Figure 6-48), and other internal organs such as the liver (Figures 6-49 and 6-50). Tetrathyridia often multiply so much within the abdominal cavity that they greatly

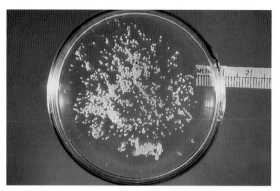

FIGURE 6-46 Tetrathyridium is about 1 cm in diameter and is capable of multiplying exponentially (i.e., one tetrathyridium becomes two, two become four, four become eight).

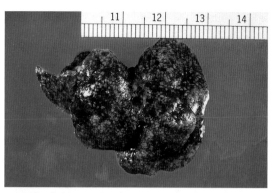

FIGURE 6-49 Tetrathyridia multiply in internal organs such as the liver.

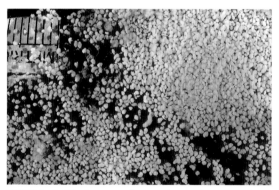

FIGURE 6-47 This type of asexual reproduction produces large numbers of tetrathyridia that are infective to the canine or feline definitive host.

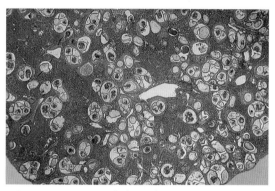

FIGURE 6-50 Histopathology of the liver of a rat infected with tetrathyridia.

expand the girth of the intermediate host. When ingested by the definitive host, each tetrathyridium becomes an adult tapeworm within the intestine of that definitive host.

> **TECHNICIAN'S NOTE** The ova of the tetrathyridium tapeworms can be found with standard fecal flotation procedures.

COTYLODA (PSEUDOTAPEWORMS)

Phylum: Platyhelminthes
   Class: Cestoda
      Subclass: Cotyloda

Members of the subclass Cotyloda, or pseudotapeworms, grossly resemble the members of the

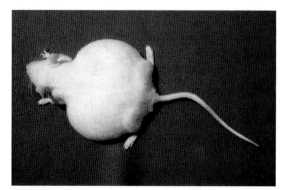

FIGURE 6-48 Tetrathyridia multiply in the body of a second intermediate host and are often confined to serous cavities, particularly the peritoneal cavity.

subclass Eucestoda. These flatworms are ribbonlike and divided into a long chain of proglottids. These are hermaphroditic tapeworms, but instead of possessing laterally located reproductive organs and genital pores, they have centrally located reproductive organs and genital pores (Figure 6-51). The egg for members of this subclass is operculated (Figure 6-52) and almost identical to the egg of the digenetic trematodes. Most pseudotapeworms release their operculated eggs directly from the uterus; the eggs then pass out to the external environment in the feces of the definitive host. The adult tapeworms occasionally release chains of gravid proglottids when these terminal proglottids have become aged or spent. Instead of possessing four suckers and (possibly) a rostellum, the pseudotapeworm has two slitlike organs of attachment (known as **bothria**) on the lateral aspects of the scolex. Figure 6-53 shows the scolex of *Diphyllobothrium latum*.

During its life cycle, the pseudotapeworm uses two intermediate hosts. The pseudophyllidean-type operculated egg makes contact with water and releases a ciliated hexacanth embryo. This stage is called a coracidium. The coracidium is a motile hexacanth embryo that is covered with tiny hairs (cilia). It emerges through the operculum of a pseudotapeworm egg. Following emergence, it swims in the water. The coracidium is ingested by a microscopic aquatic crustacean and, within that crustacean, develops into a stage called a procercoid. The crustacean with the procercoid is later ingested by a fish or an amphibian and, within the musculature of that host, develops into a solid-bodied metacestode stage called a plerocercoid, or sparganum. The definitive host becomes infected by ingesting the second intermediate host with this plerocercoid (sparganum) stage. The scolex attaches in the small intestine and begins to "grow" a new tapeworm.

The important pseudotapeworms of animals are the *Spirometra* species and *Diphyllobothrium* species.

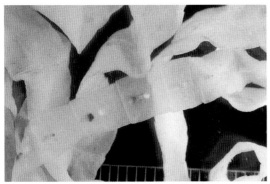

FIGURE 6-51 Representative pseudotapeworm (*Diphyllobothrium latum*), with centrally located reproductive organs and genital pores.

TECHNICIAN'S NOTE   The pseudotapeworms use two intermediate hosts in their life cycle.

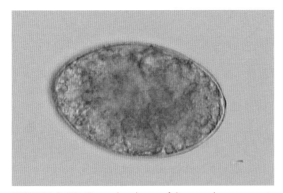

FIGURE 6-52 Operculated egg of the pseudotapeworm is almost identical to the egg of digenetic trematodes. Most pseudotapeworms release eggs directly from the uterus; eggs then pass out to the external environment in the feces of the definitive host.

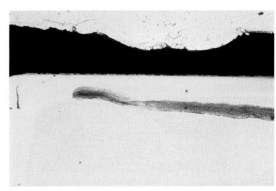

FIGURE 6-53 Anterior end (scolex) of *Diphyllobothrium latum*.

SPIROMETRA SPECIES

Parasite: 🇿 *Spirometra* species
Host: Dogs and cats
Location of Adult: Small intestine
Intermediate Hosts: First intermediate host, aquatic crustacean; second intermediate host, fish or frogs
Distribution: North and South America, Far East, and Australia
Derivation of Genus: Coiled or spiral uterus
Transmission Route: Ingestion of infective fish or frog
Common Name: Zipper tapeworm or sparganosis tapeworm
Zoonotic: Yes

Spirometra species are often referred to as *zipper* or *sparganosis tapeworms*. These medium-sized tapeworms are often found in the small intestine of both the dog and the cat and are often found in pets residing in Florida and along the Gulf Coast of North America. The adult pseudotapeworm possesses four suckers on its anterior end. This pseudotapeworm has two slitlike holdfast organs called *bothria*. In sufficient numbers, the adults can cause intestinal obstruction. This tapeworm is a clinical oddity because it produces an operculated egg. Each proglottid of *Spirometra* species possesses a centrally located, spiraled uterus and an associated uterine pore through which eggs are released. These tapeworms characteristically release eggs until they exhaust their uterine contents. Gravid segments are usually not discharged into the pet's feces. The tapeworm is unique because while it is attached to the host's jejunum, the mature proglottids often separate along the longitudinal axis for a short distance. The tapeworm appears to "unzip," thus its common name, the *zipper tapeworm*. Spent "zipped" and "unzipped" proglottids often appear in the feces of the pet. (See Figure 6-54 for unique features of this pseudotapeworm.)

> 📎 *TECHNICIAN'S NOTE* Dogs and humans are capable of serving as second intermediate hosts—becoming infected by ingesting copepods with procercoid-stage larvae.

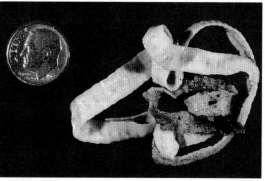

FIGURE 6-54 Adult *Spirometra* species with centrally located, spiraled uterus and uterine pore through which eggs are released. Gravid segments usually are not discharged into the feces. This tapeworm is unique because while attached to the host's jejunum, mature proglottids often separate along the longitudinal axis for a short distance. The tapeworm appears to unzip, thus its common name, *zipper tapeworm*.

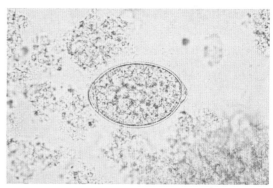

FIGURE 6-55 Egg of *Spirometra mansonoides* is operculated, resembling the egg of a fluke (digenetic trematode).

The egg of *Spirometra* species resembles that of a fluke (digenetic trematode). The egg has a distinct operculum at one end of the pole of the shell (**operculated ovum**). The eggs are oval and yellowish-brown. They average 60 × 36 μm, have an asymmetric appearance, and tend to be rather pointed at one end (Figure 6-55). When the eggs rupture, a distinct operculum is visible. The eggs are unembryonated when passed in the feces.

The metacestode (larval) stage for *Spirometra* species is the sparganum, a solid-bodied stage with slitlike mouthparts. This stage is found in the musculature of its intermediate hosts, fish and amphibians such as frogs. Dogs and cats can become infected with both the tetrathyridial and adult

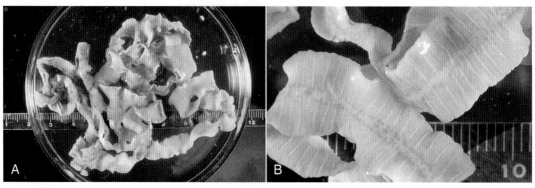

FIGURE 6-56 A, Adult *Diphyllobothrium* species can measure 2 to 12 m long, although this tapeworm probably does not attain maximum length in dogs and cats. B, Each proglottid has a centrally located, rosette-shaped uterus and an associated uterine pore through which eggs are released.

stages of the parasites by ingesting the fish and amphibian intermediate hosts. It is important that the veterinarian recognize the fish and the amphibian as the sources of this tapeworm and understand the importance of preventing predation or the ingestion of carrion or offal by the dog and cat.

> **TECHNICIAN'S NOTE** The eggs of the zipper tapeworm can be found with standard fecal flotation procedures.

DIPHYLLOBOTHRIUM SPECIES

Parasite: 🅩 *Diphyllobothrium latum*
Host: Dogs, cats, and humans
Location of Adult: Small intestine
Intermediate Hosts: First intermediate host, aquatic crustacean; second intermediate host, fish
Distribution: Scandinavian countries, Ukraine, and North America
Derivation of Genus: Double leaf
Transmission Route: Ingestion of infective fish
Common Name: Broad fish tapeworm
Zoonotic: Yes

Diphyllobothrium species are often referred to as *broad fish tapeworms*. This tapeworm can be 2 to 12 m in length; however, it probably does not attain this maximum length in dogs and cats. Instead of possessing four suckers on its anterior end, this pseudotapeworm has two slitlike holdfast organs called *bothria*. The adults absorb vitamin B$_{12}$ to the point that the tapeworm can produce pernicious

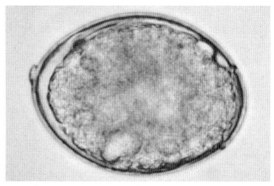

FIGURE 6-57 Egg of *Diphyllobothrium* species also resembles that of a fluke (digenetic trematode). The egg is oval, with a distinct operculum at the opposite end of the pole of the shell. Eggs are light brown and average 67 to 71 µm × 40 to 51 µm. Eggs tend to be rounded on one end, with an operculum on the opposite end. Eggs are unembryonated when passed in the feces.

anemia in the host as well as causing intestinal obstruction. Each proglottid of this tapeworm has a centrally located, rosette-shaped uterus and an associated uterine pore through which the eggs are released (Figure 6-56). These tapeworms continually release eggs until they exhaust their uterine contents. The terminal proglottids become senile rather than gravid and detach in chains rather than individually. The egg of *Diphyllobothrium* species also resembles that of a fluke (digenetic trematode). The egg is oval and possesses a distinct operculum at one end of the pole of the shell. The eggs are light brown, averaging 67 to 71 µm × 40 to 51 µm, and tend to be rounded on one end (Figure 6-57). The operculum is present on the end opposite the rounded pole. The eggs are unembryonated when passed in the feces.

> **TECHNICIAN'S NOTE** The eggs of *D. latum* are unembryonated with an operculum opposite the rounded pole. The eggs can be found with standard fecal flotation procedures.

The metacestode (larval) stage for *Diphyllobothrium* species is the plerocercoid, a solid-bodied stage with slitlike mouthparts. This stage is found in the musculature of the fish intermediate host. Dogs and cats become infected by ingesting the fish intermediate host. It is important that the veterinarian recognize the fish as the source of this tapeworm and understand the importance of preventing predation or the ingestion of raw fish by the dog and cat.

CHAPTER SIX TEST

MATCHING—Match the term with the correct phrase or term.

A. *Coenurus cerebralis*

B. *Cysticercus fasciolaris*

C. *Echinococcus granulosus*

D. *Anoplocephala perfoliata*

E. *Dipylidium caninum*

F. *Paranoplocephala mamillana*

G. *Cysticercus bovis*

H. *Cysticercus cellulosae*

I. Typical taeniid-type ova

J. *Moniezia* species

K. Egg packet

L. Hexacanth embryo

M. Pyriform apparatus

N. *Hymenolepis nana*

O. Cysticercoid

P. *Taenia hydatigena*

Q. *Thysanosoma actinoides*

R. *Mesocestoides* species

S. *Spirometra mansonoides*

T. Ovum of pseudotapeworm

U. *Diphyllobothrium latum*

V. Plerocercoid

W. Procercoid

X. *Echinococcus multilocularis*

Y. Praziquantel

Z. Metacestode stage

1. Noninvaginated scolex in a small cavity or vesicle or bladder found in invertebrates

2. Zipper tapeworm

3. Double-pored tapeworm or the cucumber seed tapeworm

4. Ruminant tapeworm

5. Neurologic signs in infected sheep

6. Embryo containing three pairs of hooks

7. Sparganum

8. Lappets behind scolex

9. Strobilocercus in rats

10. Rat tapeworm

11. Broad fish tapeworm

12. *Dipylidium caninum*

13. *Taenia saginata*

14. *Taenia* or *Multiceps* or *Echinococcus* species

15. Found in *Cyclops* species—aquatic crustacean

16. Fringed tapeworm

17. Larval tapeworm

18. Innermost lining of eggs of *Moniezia* species, *Anoplocephala* species

19. Dwarf equine tapeworm

20. Unilocular hydatid cyst

21. *Cysticercus tenuicollis* in bovine omentum

22. Measly pork, pork measles

23. Effective cestocide; kills tapeworms

24. Tetrathyridium

25. Alveolar hydatid disease in rodents

26. Operculated on one end

QUESTIONS FOR THOUGHT AND DISCUSSION

1. How might *Coenurus cerebralis* and *Coenurus serialis* affect the behavior of the intermediate host, thus facilitating transmission to the definitive host?

2. Compare and contrast the following types of metacestode stages. You may use drawings with labels to illustrate differences. Give examples of cestodes that typify these metacestode stages (see this chapter for examples).
   - Cysticercoid and cysticercus
   - Cysticercus and coenurus
   - Unilocular and multilocular hydatid cysts

3. Why is a single gravid proglottid of *Dipylidium caninum* so important in facilitating the transmission of the parasite to the flea intermediate host?

4. What feature makes the tetrathyridia of *Mesocestoides* species so pathogenic to the second intermediate host?

5. Three genera of taeniid tapeworms (*Taenia, Multiceps,* and *Echinococcus* species) produce similar ova (typical taeniid-type ova) in a canine fecal flotation. Why is it important to wear disposable gloves when performing fecal examinations? HINT: The ovum of one of these three genera is capable of infecting humans; that is, one is a very serious zoonotic parasite. What might happen if a human ingested this pathology-producing ovum?

6. Why are the following terms or phrases so important in a veterinary clinical practice, either small animal or large animal?
   - Identifying the gravid proglottid of *Dipylidium caninum*
   - *Cysticercus bovis* and *Cysticercus cellulosae*
   - Unilocular and multilocular hydatid cysts

7 The Phylum Platyhelminthes, Class Trematoda

OUTLINE

LEARNING OBJECTIVES

After studying this chapter, the reader should be able to do the following:
- Identify the external and internal morphologic features of the digenetic fluke.
- Identify the developmental stages in the life cycle of a typical digenetic fluke.
- Compare and contrast monogenetic trematodes and digenetic trematodes.

KEY TERMS

Acetabulum (ventral
  sucker)
Adult fluke
Cercaria

Digenetic fluke
Hermaphroditic
Metacercaria

Miracidium
Monogenetic fluke
Operculum

Oral sucker
Redia
Sporocyst

The phylum Platyhelminthes, the flatworms, includes two of the strangest classes in the animal kingdom, the trematodes (or flukes) and the cestodes (or tapeworms). The morphologic feature common to these two classes is that the worms are dorsoventrally flattened.

Members of the phylum Platyhelminthes, class Trematoda, are often referred to as *trematodes* or *flukes*. Their bodies are often flattened, unsegmented, and leaflike. An example of a typical fluke is *Fasciola hepatica* (Figure 7-1). Within this class are two subclasses, the subclass Monogenea (the monogenetic trematodes) and the subclass Digenea (the digenetic trematodes). Monogenetic trematodes usually parasitize fish, amphibians, and

reptiles, whereas digenetic trematodes are usually associated with wild and domestic animals and humans.

> **TECHNICIAN'S NOTE** Trematodes are dorsoventrally flattened, unsegmented, and leaflike.

SUBCLASS MONOGENEA

Phylum: Platyhelminthes
  Class: Trematoda
    Subclass: Monogenea

Monogenetic flukes or trematodes are usually ectoparasites of fish, amphibians, and reptiles. They

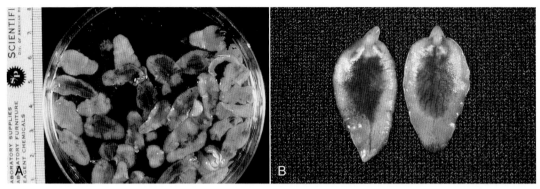

FIGURE 7-1 A, Representative flukes. B, *Fasciola hepatica* with flattened, unsegmented, leaflike bodies.

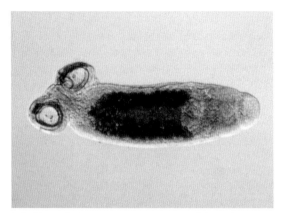

FIGURE 7-2 Representative monogenetic fluke with a posterior adhesive organ that may have suckers, hooks, or clamps.

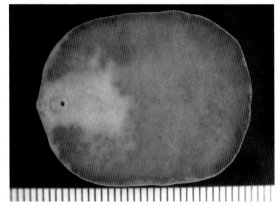

FIGURE 7-3 Digenetic flukes are usually broad, leaf-shaped, and flattened (Figure 7-1), although a few are thick and fleshy.

attach to the exterior surfaces, such as the gills, skin, fins, and mouth. These trematodes attach to the host with a posterior adhesive organ that may have suckers, hooks, or clamps (Figure 7-2). These parasites are usually diagnosed in veterinary practices that specialize in treating saltwater or freshwater aquarium fish or in aquacultural environments (e.g., fish farming). Because monogenetic trematodes are diagnosed so infrequently in veterinary practice, the emphasis in this chapter (and the next) is on the digenetic trematodes.

> **TECHNICIAN'S NOTE** Monogenetic trematodes are seen in aquatic fish, amphibians, and reptiles.

SUBCLASS DIGENEA

Phylum: Platyhelminthes
 Class: Trematoda
  Subclass: Digenea

Digenetic trematodes, or flukes, are usually endoparasites of both domestic and wild animals and occasionally humans. Digenetic flukes are generally broad, leaf-shaped, and flattened, although a few, such as *Fascioloides magna,* are thick and fleshy (Figure 7-3). One group of trematodes (the schistosomes) are long, thin, and wormlike, resembling the nematodes or roundworms.

KEY MORPHOLOGIC FEATURES

Figure 7-4 details the internal morphology of a representative digenetic fluke. On or near the anterior end is the fluke's mouth, which is surrounded by a muscular oral sucker. This mouth connects to a muscular pharynx, which in turn leads to an esophagus, which bifurcates into two blind ceca. Flukes do not possess an anus; to release digested food, they regurgitate their cecal contents back into the tissues or organs they infect. These contents are often observed in the tissues on histopathologic section and are colloquially referred to as *fluke puke*. Flukes also possess a muscular organ of attachment called an acetabulum, or ventral sucker. This organ is used as a "holdfast organ" and is not associated with feeding.

With the exception of the schistosomes, or blood flukes, all flukes are hermaphroditic; that is, each fluke possesses complete sets of both male and female reproductive organs. The male reproductive organs consist of two testes, the vas efferens, the vas deferens, the seminal vesicle, and the cirrus (the fluke's version of a penis). The female reproductive organs consist of an ovary, an oviduct, a seminal receptacle, the yolk glands, the ootype, the Mehlis gland, vitelline glands, and the uterus. Self-fertilization usually takes place; however, cross-fertilization between two adult flukes also occurs.

LIFE CYCLE OF THE FLUKE

The female portion of the fluke's reproductive tract produces operculated eggs that have been stored in the uterus (Figure 7-5). Eggs pass out of the uterus through the genital pore and are usually passed out to the external environment within the host's feces. The operculated eggs embryonate in the external environment. If the egg makes contact with water, it will hatch and produce a motile stage called a miracidium (Figure 7-6). The miracidium is

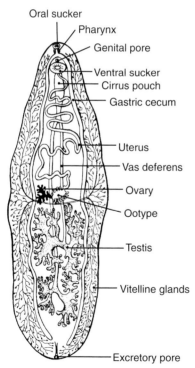

Oral sucker
Pharynx
Genital pore
Ventral sucker
Cirrus pouch
Gastric cecum
Uterus
Vas deferens
Ovary
Ootype
Testis
Vitelline glands
Excretory pore

FIGURE 7-4 Internal morphology of representative digenetic fluke. Note that digenetic flukes are hermaphroditic; that is, they contain both male and female reproductive organs.

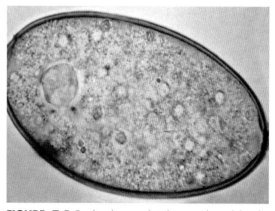

FIGURE 7-5 Fertilized operculated egg released by the female portion of the reproductive system of the hermaphroditic fluke. The operculum is a tiny "trapdoor" through which the miracidium emerges.

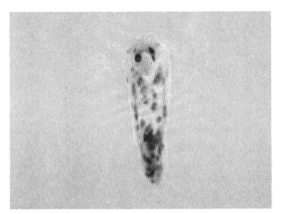

FIGURE 7-6 The miracidium is the motile, ciliated stage that emerges through the operculum and eventually penetrates the snail, the first intermediate host.

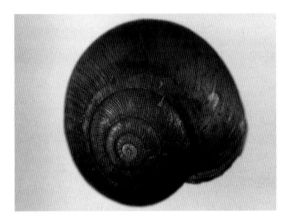

FIGURE 7-7 For most digenetic flukes, a snail is the first intermediate host.

covered with tiny hairs called *cilia.* The movement of the cilia allows the miracidium to swim in the water. The miracidium seeks out an aquatic snail (Figure 7-7), the first intermediate host, then penetrates the skin of the snail and develops to the next stage, the sporocyst. The sporocyst is merely a sack in which the next stage, the redia, develops. Many rediae develop within the sporocyst. Within each redia, many cercariae develop (Figure 7-8). The cercarial stage often has a tail and emerges from the snail and swims in the water (Figure 7-9). Depending on the species of fluke, at this point the cercaria will take one of the following three paths:

1. The cercaria may directly penetrate the skin of the definitive host.

2. The cercaria may attach to vegetation, lose its tail, secrete a thick cyst wall around itself, and thus develop into a metacercaria (Figure 7-10). The vegetation with the attached encysted metacercaria will be ingested by the definitive host.

3. The cercaria may lose its tail, penetrate the second intermediate host, secrete a thick cyst wall around itself, and develop into a metacercaria within the second intermediate host. The second intermediate host with the encysted metacercaria will be ingested by the definitive host.

> **TECHNICIAN'S NOTE** The cercarial stage of the trematode life cycle can use one of three ways to enter a definitive host: penetrate the skin directly, attach to vegetation and await ingestion, or penetrate the skin of a second intermediate host and await ingestion.

If the fluke takes the first option, the cercaria migrates to its predilection site (the site of infection) and develops into the adult fluke. If the fluke takes the second option, the thick cyst wall is digested by the host and the juvenile fluke is released. The juvenile fluke then migrates to the predilection site and develops into an adult fluke. If the fluke takes the third option, the second intermediate host and the thick cyst wall are digested and the juvenile fluke is released. The juvenile fluke then migrates to the predilection site and develops into an adult fluke. Most of the predilection sites of the flukes are associated with the digestive system. The exceptions are *Paragonimus kellicotti*, the lung fluke of dogs and cats, and the schistosomes, or blood flukes, which reside in the blood vessels. Once the adult stage of the fluke is reached, self-fertilization and cross-fertilization occur and the life cycle begins again, with operculated eggs being released to the outside environment.

> **TECHNICIAN'S NOTE** With two exceptions, flukes may be found within the digestive system.

Chapter 8 details some of the important flukes of domestic animals (and in some cases, wild animals) in North America. As individual species, adult

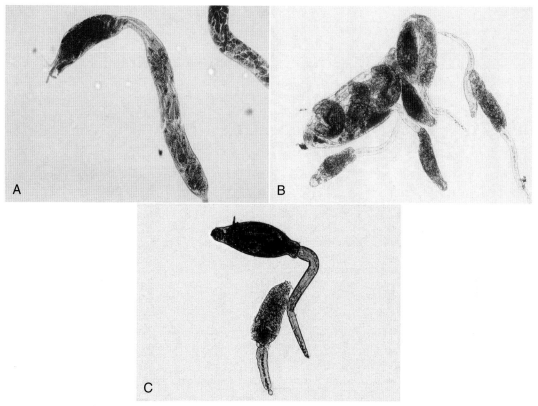

FIGURE 7-8 After the snail intermediate host has been penetrated, the next developmental stage, **A,** the sporocyst, is formed by the miracidium. **B,** The sporocyst stage forms many internal redial stages. **C,** Each redial stage forms many internal cercarial stages.

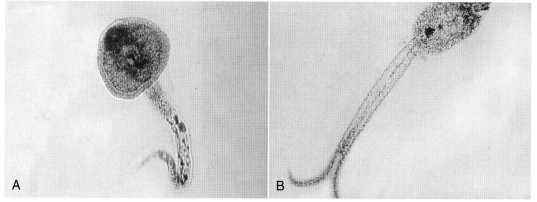

FIGURE 7-9 The cercarial stage is released from the redial stage. This stage often has a tail and emerges from the snail to swim in the water. Rarely, the cercarial stage penetrates the skin of the definitive host.

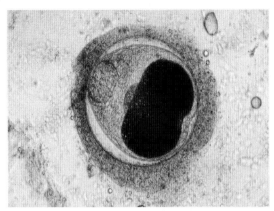

FIGURE 7-10 Metacercarial stage dissected from the muscles of salmonid fish. The cercarial stage may swim to vegetation, drop its tail, secrete a thick cyst wall, and develop into the metacercarial stage, or the cercarial stage may drop its tail, penetrate or be eaten by a second intermediate host, secrete a thick cyst wall around itself, and develop to a metacercaria within the second intermediate host.

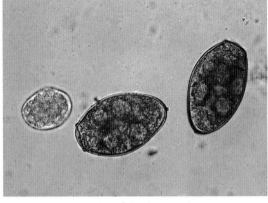

FIGURE 7-11 Digenetic flukes have a characteristic ovum, the operculated egg, which is almost unique to this subclass. Most of these flukes possess this oval egg with a distinct operculum, or door, on one end of the egg. The egg of *Paragonimus kellicotti* has an operculum that is easily observed.

flukes can be quite distinctive in appearance. Flukes tend to be found in certain predilection tissue or organ sites within the host's body. Although some may "wander" off course in the developmental life cycle, adult flukes are usually associated with certain tissue or organ sites. It is important for the diagnostician to associate certain flukes with their predilection sites.

Finally, digenetic flukes have a characteristic ovum that is almost unique to this subclass—the operculated egg (Figure 7-11). Most of these flukes possess an oval egg with a distinct operculum, or door, on one pole (either end) of the egg. There are a few exceptions, and they are noted when these flukes are discussed.

TECHNICIAN'S NOTE Digenetic trematodes have a characteristic operculated egg.

CHAPTER SEVEN TEST

MATCHING—Match the term with the correct phrase or term.

A. Monogenetic trematodes

B. Acetabulum

C. Miracidium

D. Sporocyst

E. Redia

F. Cercaria

G. Operculum

H. Hermaphroditic

I. Metacercaria

J. Digenetic trematodes

1. Developmental stage after penetration of the miracidium into a snail (first intermediate host)

2. Door or cap at one end, or pole, of the trematode egg

3. Ectoparasites of fish, amphibians, and reptiles

4. Encysted stage in the life cycle of the trematode usually found on vegetation or within the second intermediate host

5. Endoparasitic flukes of both domestic and wild animals

6. Stage that follows the redia; stage that emerges from the second intermediate host

7. Motile stage emerging from the operculated fluke egg

8. Ventral sucker that is used as a holdfast organ of attachment for digenetic flukes

9. Simultaneously possessing both male and female reproductive organs

10. Stage that develops on the inside of the sporocyst

QUESTIONS FOR THOUGHT AND DISCUSSION

1. How are monogenetic trematodes different from digenetic trematodes?

2. Describe the developmental stages in the life cycle of a typical digenetic fluke.

Trematodes (Flukes) of Animals and Humans

LEARNING OBJECTIVES

After studying this chapter, the reader should be able to do the following:
- Identify digenetic flukes to genus and/or species when given a trematode specimen and the host and location where the specimen was found within that host.

KEY TERMS

Amphistomes
Black spot

Operculum
Schistosomes

Schistosome cercarial dermatitis

The following organisms are flukes that may parasitize domesticated and wild animals. A few species are known to parasitize humans.

FLUKES OF RUMINANTS (CATTLE, SHEEP, AND GOATS)

Parasite: ⓩ *Dicrocoelium dendriticum*
Host: Sheep, goats, and cattle
Location of Adult: Bile duct
Intermediate Hosts: First intermediate host, *Cionella lubrica*, land snail; second intermediate host, *Formica fusca*, ant
Distribution: Worldwide
Derivation of Genus: Forked bowel
Transmission Route: Ingestion of infected ants
Common Name: Lancet fluke
Zoonotic: Yes (per *The Merck Veterinary Manual*)

> **TECHNICIAN'S NOTE** The lancet fluke is an unusual trematode in that it uses intermediate hosts from dry habitats rather than a first intermediate host from an aquatic habitat.

Dicrocoelium dendriticum is commonly referred to as the *lancet fluke* of sheep, goats, and cattle. This tiny, flattened, leaflike fluke is only 6 to 10 mm long and 1.5 to 2.5 mm wide (Figure 8-1) and has an oral sucker, a ventral sucker, tandem testes, and lateral **vitellaria** (accessory genital glands that secrete the yolk and shell for the fertilized ovum). These flukes are found in the fine branches of the bile duct and can produce hyperplasia of the bile duct's glandular epithelial lining resulting in bile duct obstruction. This fluke produces brown embryonated eggs that are 36 to 46 μm × 10 to

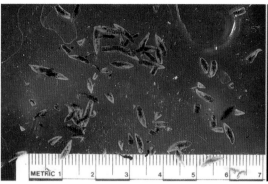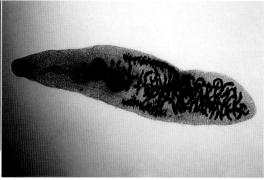

FIGURE 8-1 Adult *Dicrocoelium dendriticum* is commonly referred to as the *lancet fluke* of sheep, goats, and cattle. This tiny, flattened, leaflike fluke (6-10 mm long and 1.5-2.5 mm wide) is found in fine branches of the bile duct.

20 μm. The egg possesses an operculum (similar to a hinged hatch) on one pole (end) of the egg. This operculum is said to be indistinct. The first intermediate host is the land snail, *Cionella lubrica*, whereas the second intermediate host is the ant, *Formica fusca*. The eggs can be found on standard fecal flotation and fecal sedimentation procedures.

> **TECHNICIAN'S NOTE** *Dicrocoelium dendriticum* alters the behavior pattern of both the land snail and the ant.

Parasite: *Paramphistomum* species and *Cotylophoron* species
Host: Cattle, sheep, goats, and other ruminants
Location of Adult: Rumen and reticulum
Intermediate Hosts: First intermediate host, aquatic snail; second intermediate host, none; cercariae encyst on aquatic vegetation
Distribution: Worldwide (*Paramphistomum* sp.)
Derivation of Genus: Beyond a mouth on both sides (*Paramphistomum* sp.); ridge cup (*Cotylophoron* sp.), bears a cup shape
Transmission Route: Ingestion of aquatic vegetation with metacercariae
Common Name: Rumen flukes
Zoonotic: No

Rumen flukes comprise two genera of veterinary importance, *Paramphistomum* and *Cotylophoron*

(Figure 8-2). Rumen flukes belong to a group of flukes called amphistomes (*amphi* means "on both sides" or "double," and *stome* means "mouth"); these flukes appear to possess a "mouth" at both ends of their body. Amphistomes have an oral sucker (the feeding organelle, or "true mouth") on the anterior end and a large ventral sucker (an organ of attachment) on the posterior end. The adult flukes closely resemble Kellogg's Rice Krispies. In the fresh state, amphistomes are light-colored to bright red and pear-shaped, approximately 5 to 13 mm × 2 to 5 mm. They attach with the oral sucker to the lining of the rumen and reticulum of cattle, sheep, goats, and many other ruminants and expose the ventral suckers (Figure 8-3). The adult flukes are nonpathogenic; the pathogenicity of these flukes lies in the migration of the juvenile forms in the small intestine. These juvenile forms are known for the ability to ingest large plugs of intestinal lining. The eggs of *Paramphistomum* species measure 114 to 176 μm × 73 to 100 μm; the eggs of *Cotylophoron* species measure 125 to 135 μm by 61 × 68 μm. The prepatent period for *Paramphistomum* species is 80 to 95 days.

> **TECHNICIAN'S NOTE** The oral sucker of the rumen fluke is on one end of the fluke, and the ventral sucker is on the other end.

Parasite: 🅩 *Fasciola hepatica*
Host: Cattle, sheep, and other ruminants
Location of Adult: Bile duct

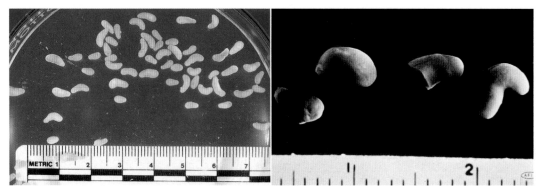

FIGURE 8-2 Rumen flukes, or amphistomes (*Paramphistomum* and *Cotylophoron* species), have an oral sucker (feeding organelle) on the anterior end and a large ventral sucker (organ of attachment) on the posterior end.

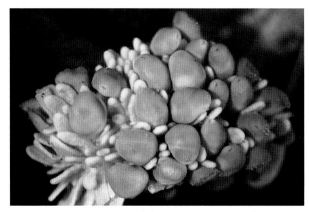

FIGURE 8-3 Rumen flukes among rumen papillae.

Intermediate Hosts: First intermediate host, aquatic snail; second intermediate host, none; cercariae encyst on aquatic vegetation

Distribution: Worldwide

Derivation of Genus: Small band

Transmission Route: Ingestion of aquatic vegetation with metacercariae

Common Name: Liver fluke

Zoonotic: Yes (per *The Merck Veterinary Manual*)

Fasciola hepatica is the liver fluke of cattle, sheep, and other ruminants. It is perhaps the most economically important fluke in veterinary medicine because it causes "liver rot," clay pipe–stem fibrosis or liver condemnation, at slaughter as a result of obstruction of the bile ducts. This fluke is the best-known fluke among those parasitizing food animals; parasitologists have studied *F. hepatica* more than any other fluke. Adult flukes are found in the bile ducts of the liver and possess a unique appearance. They are flattened and leaflike, measuring 30 × 13 mm (Figure 8-4). These liver flukes are broader in the anterior region than in the posterior region and possess an anterior cone-shaped projection that is followed by a pair of prominent, laterally directed shoulders. The internal morphology is not easily discernible because of the superimposition of the highly branched ceca over highly branched testes, ova, and vitellaria. These flukes are tan to reddish brown in the fresh state; preserved specimens take on a grayish appearance. Their eggs are oval and yellow brown and measure 130 to

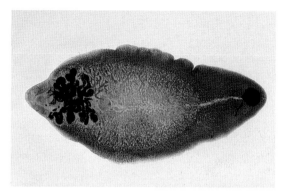

FIGURE 8-4 Adult liver flukes (*Fasciola hepatica*) are broader in the anterior region and have a prominent anterior cone-shaped projection followed by prominent shoulders. In the fresh state, these flukes are grayish brown and measure 30 × 13 mm.

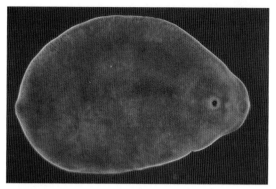

FIGURE 8-6 Adult *Fascioloides magna* are large, flattened, flesh-colored, oval flukes measuring up to 10 cm in length, 2.5 cm in width, and 4.5 mm in thickness. These flukes lack the anterior conelike projection of adult *Fasciola hepatica*.

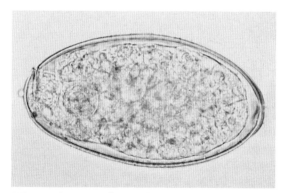

FIGURE 8-5 Egg of *Fasciola hepatica*. Eggs are oval, operculated, and yellow brown and measure 130 to 150 μm × 60 to 90 μm.

150 μm × 60 to 90 μm. Each egg possesses a distinct operculum (Figure 8-5). The eggs can be found on fecal sedimentation.

> **TECHNICIAN'S NOTE** *Fasciola hepatica* is the most studied fluke affecting domestic livestock, and it is a very important fluke in terms of economic effects on the hosts.

Parasite: *Fascioloides magna*
Host: White-tailed deer
Location of Adult: Liver parenchyma
Intermediate Host: Aquatic snail; the cercariae encyst on aquatic vegetation

Distribution: North America, Central and Southwestern Europe
Derivation of Genus: Band shape
Transmission Route: Ingestion of vegetation with metacercariae
Common Name: Liver fluke of wild ruminants (deer)
Zoonotic: No

Fascioloides magna is also a liver fluke; however, this fluke has the white-tailed deer as its true definitive host. It may also use cattle, sheep, and pigs as incidental hosts. The adult flukes are found in the liver parenchyma and possess a unique appearance. They are large, flattened, flesh-colored, oval flukes measuring up to 10 cm in length, 2.5 cm in width, and 4.5 mm in thickness, approximately the size of a U.S. gold dollar (Figure 8-6). These flukes lack the anterior conelike projection of *F. hepatica*. The egg is operculated, up to 170 μm in length and 100 μm in width. *F. magna* flukes produce open cysts in the liver parenchyma of white-tailed deer. These cysts communicate with the bile ducts, allowing eggs to be passed to the external environment. Thus eggs are often found during fecal sedimentation procedures of these infected hosts. In incidental hosts such as cattle and sheep, however, these flukes produce closed cysts in the liver parenchyma. These cysts do not communicate with the bile ducts, so the egg of *F. magna* cannot pass to the external environment. Incidental hosts act as "dead-end" hosts; that is, they are not capable of transmitting this parasite to other animals.

Eggs of the flukes just mentioned may be recovered from feces using either the fecal sedimentation procedure or a commercially available fluke egg recovery test.

> **TECHNICIAN'S NOTE** The eggs of *F. magna* can be found on fecal sedimentation technique from feces of the white-tailed deer. Necropsy is necessary to find the adult flukes in the incidental hosts.

FLUKES OF SMALL ANIMALS (DOGS AND CATS)

Parasite: *Platynosomum fastosum*
Host: Cats
Location of Adult: Bile ducts
Intermediate Host: First intermediate host, land snail; second intermediate host, lizard
Distribution: South America, southern United States, West Africa, Pacific Islands, Malaysia, and the Caribbean
Derivation of Genus: Flat disease-causing
Transmission Route: Ingestion of infected lizards
Common Name: Lizard-poisoning fluke of cats
Zoonotic: No

Platynosomum fastosum is the "lizard-poisoning fluke" of cats. This fluke received this common name because cats become infected by ingesting the lizard second intermediate host that contains the infective metacercarial stages of the fluke. These adult flukes are found in the liver, gallbladder, and bile ducts and less often in the small intestine of cats, producing signs such as diarrhea, vomiting, icterus, and even death from the obstruction of the bile duct. *P. fastosum* is a tiny, flattened, leaflike fluke that is only 4 to 8 mm long and 1.5 to 2.5 mm wide, with an oral sucker, ventral sucker, parallel (side-by-side) testes, and lateral vitellaria found in the fine branches of the bile duct of cats; it can produce desquamation (stripping) of the bile duct's glandular epithelial lining (Figure 8-7). The fluke's brownish operculated eggs are oval, measuring 34 to 50 μm × 20 to 35 μm (Figure 8-8). The eggs can be found on standard fecal flotation. Adults can be found in the bile ducts on necropsy.

> **TECHNICIAN'S NOTE** *Platynosomum fastosum* is associated with "lizard poisoning" in cats.

Parasite: ⓩ *Nanophyetus salmincola*
Host: Dogs
Location of Adult: Small intestine
Intermediate Host: First intermediate host, freshwater snail; second intermediate host, salmon

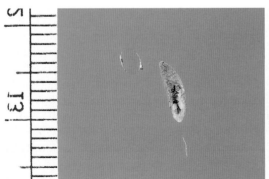 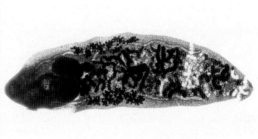

FIGURE 8-7 Adult *Platynosomum fastosum*, the lizard-poisoning fluke of cats, is a tiny, flattened, leaflike fluke (only 4-8 mm long and 1.5-1.2 mm wide) found in the fine branches of the bile duct of cats.

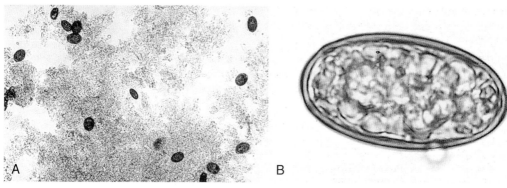

FIGURE 8-8 **A,** Eggs of *Platynosomum fastosum*. **B,** These oval, brown, operculated eggs measure 34 to 50 μm by 20 to 35 μm.

Distribution: Pacific Northwest region of North America

Derivation of Genus: Dwarf form

Transmission Route: Ingestion of infected salmon

Common Name: Salmon-poisoning fluke of dogs

Zoonotic: Yes (per Companion Animal Parasite Council)

Nanophyetus salmincola is the "salmon-poisoning fluke" of dogs in the Pacific Northwest region of North America. This fluke received its common name because dogs become infected by ingesting the salmon (fish) second intermediate host that contains the infective metacercarial stage of this fluke. The adult fluke inhabits the small intestine and serves as a vector for rickettsial agents that produce "salmon poisoning" and "Elokomin fluke fever" in dogs. Whereas *F. magna* is the largest fluke of our domesticated animals, *N. salmincola* is the smallest, measuring only 0.5 to 1.1 mm in length (Figure 8-9). The color of adult flukes is white to cream. The eggs are yellowish brown, with an indistinct operculum and a small, blunt point at the end opposite to the operculum. Eggs are 52 to 82 μm × 32 to 56 μm (Figure 8-10).

> **TECHNICIAN'S NOTE** The salmon-poisoning fluke causes pathology to the host by harboring the rickettsial agents that produce salmon poisoning and Elokomin fluke fever.

Parasite: *Alaria* species
Host: Dogs and cats

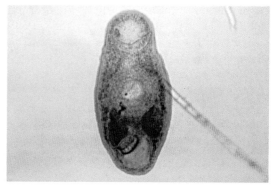

FIGURE 8-9 Adult *Nanophyetus salmincola*, the salmon-poisoning fluke of the Pacific Northwest. This fluke measures only 0.5 to 1.1 mm in length. The color of adult flukes is white to cream.

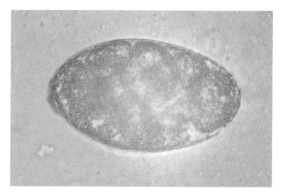

FIGURE 8-10 Egg of *Nanophyetus salmincola* is yellowish brown, with an indistinct operculum and a small, blunt point at the end opposite the operculum. Eggs are 52 to 82 μm × 32 to 56 μm.

Location of Adult: Small intestine
Intermediate Host: First intermediate host, snail; second intermediate host, frog, snake, or mouse
Distribution: Northern United States and Canada
Derivation of Genus: Winged
Transmission Route: Ingestion of infected frog, snake, or mouse
Common Name: Intestinal flukes of dogs and cats
Zoonotic: No

Alaria species are intestinal flukes of dogs and cats and are found throughout the northern half of the North American continent. This fluke is 2 to 6 mm in length. It has a unique appearance among the flukes in that its anterior half is flattened and expanded and its posterior half is rounded and globose. The eggs are large, golden brown, and operculated. They measure 98 to 134 μm × 62 to 68 μm (Figure 8-11).

> **TECHNICIAN'S NOTE**   The adult *Alaria* does not seem to cause any apparent effect in the host. It is the migration of the larvae that seems to cause pathologic findings/conditions in the host.

All the flukes covered in this chapter so far (in both ruminants and small animals) are parasites of portions of the digestive system, either the intestine or the ducts within the liver. The following flukes, however, are found in sites other than those associated with the digestive system. *Paragonimus kellicotti* is the lung fluke of dogs and cats found in cystic spaces in the lung parenchyma. *Heterobilharzia americana*, the canine schistosome, is a blood fluke that parasitizes the mesenteric veins of the small and large intestines and the portal veins of the dog.

Parasite: 🅩 *Paragonimus kellicotti*
Host: Dogs and cats
Location of Adult: Lung parenchyma
Intermediate Host: First intermediate host, operculated snail; second intermediate host, crayfish
Distribution: North America
Derivation of Genus: Alongside gonads
Transmission Route: Ingestion of infective crayfish
Common Name: Lung fluke of dogs and cats
Zoonotic: Yes but rare and only if raw crayfish are ingested (per *The Merck Veterinary Manual*)

Adult *P. kellicotti* flukes are found in cystic spaces within the lung parenchyma of both dogs and cats (Figure 8-12). These cystic spaces connect to the terminal bronchioles. The eggs are found in sputum or feces. Adults are thick, brownish-red flukes measuring up to 16 mm long × 8 mm wide (Figure 8-13). Eggs are yellowish brown, with a rather distinct operculum. The eggs are 75 to 118 μm × 42 to 67 μm; the shell at the pole opposite the operculum

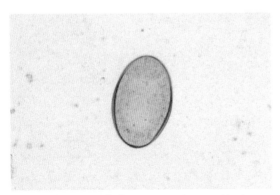

FIGURE 8-11 Egg of *Alaria* species is large, golden brown, and operculated, measuring 98 to 134 μm × 62 to 68 μm.

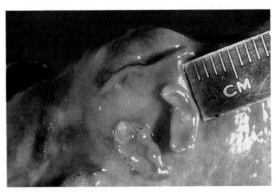

FIGURE 8-12 Adult *Paragonimus kellicotti* flukes are unusual in that they are found in the lung parenchyma, not the gastrointestinal tract.

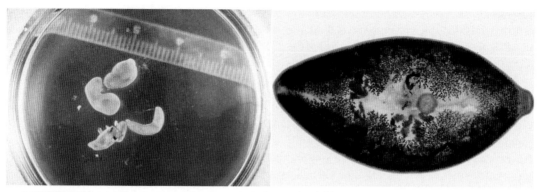

FIGURE 8-13 Adult *Paragonimus kellicotti* are thick, brownish-red flukes measuring up to 16 mm long × 8 mm wide. Adult flukes are found within the lung parenchyma.

is somewhat thickened (Figure 8-14). These fluke eggs can be recovered using fecal sedimentation techniques; however, the eggs of *P. kellicotti* are usually recovered using standard fecal flotation solutions. These eggs can also be recovered in the sputum by tracheal washing. The adult flukes within the cystic spaces in the lung parenchyma can be observed with thoracic radiography.

> **TECHNICIAN'S NOTE** Eggs of the lung fluke can be found on fecal sedimentation of feces or sputum. The adults may be seen in cystic spaces in the lung parenchyma on thoracic radiographs.

Parasite: ⬡**Z** *Heterobilharzia americana*
Host: Dogs
Location of Adult: Mesenteric veins of the small and large intestines and the portal veins
Intermediate Host: Freshwater snail
Distribution: North America, particularly the gulf states of the United States
Derivation: Another fluke named after Theodor Bilharz, German physician
Transmission Route: Metacercariae enter through the skin of the dog
Common Name: Schistosome of the dog
Zoonotic: Yes (per Companion Animal Parasite Council)

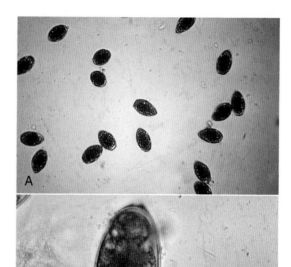

FIGURE 8-14 The distinctly operculated eggs of *Paragonimus kellicotti* are yellowish brown and 75 to 118 μm × 42 to 67 μm. The shell at the pole opposite the operculum is somewhat thickened.

H. americana, the canine schistosome, is a blood fluke that parasitizes the mesenteric veins of the small and large intestines and the portal veins of the dog (Figures 8-15 and 8-16). *Schistosome* means "split body." The blood flukes, or schistosomes, are unique flukes in that they are not hermaphroditic. Separate sexes exist, so there are male schistosomes and female schistosomes. Because these flukes reside in the fine branches of the mesenteric veins where they can obstruct the veins, they are long and slender. Females may be as long as 9 mm, and males are about 6.5 mm in length (Figure 8-17). This fluke is enzootic in the mudflats of the Mississippi delta and the coastal swampland of Louisiana. Although *H. americana* inhabits the blood vasculature, it manifests its presence by a bloody diarrhea. Infected dogs also exhibit emaciation and anorexia. Diagnosis is by identification of the thin-shelled egg, about 80 × 50 μm, which contains a miracidium on fecal sedimentation. (See Figure 8-18 for morphologic features of the egg of *H. americana.*)

> **TECHNICIAN'S NOTE** The canine schistosome does not use a second intermediate host. Instead the cercariae leave the freshwater snail and enter the dog by penetration of the skin.

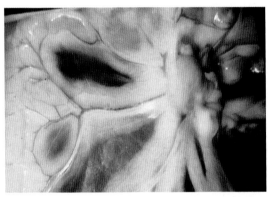

FIGURE 8-15 Gross necropsy revealing adult *Heterobilharzia americana* in the mesenteric veins of a dog.

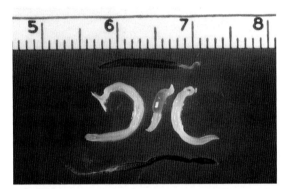

FIGURE 8-17 Adult male and female *Heterobilharzia americana* recovered from the mesenteric veins of a dog.

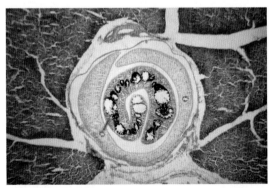

FIGURE 8-16 Histopathology of adult *Heterobilharzia americana* in the mesenteric veins of a dog.

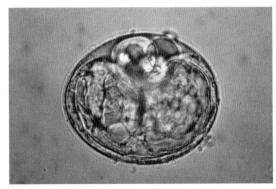

FIGURE 8-18 Thin-shelled egg of *Heterobilharzia americana,* approximately 80 × 50 μm. Miracidium sometimes are observed within the egg.

BOX 8-1 | A Few Words About Flukes of Humans

Parasite: *Schistosoma (Bilharzia)* species
Host: Humans
Location of Adult: Mesenteric veins of the small and large intestines and the urinary bladder
Intermediate Host: Freshwater snails
Distribution: Africa, the Middle East, the Caribbean
Derivation of Genus: Split body
Transmission Route: Cercariae enter through skin penetration
Common Name: Blood flukes of humans

Humans serve as definitive hosts for an important group of flukes called the *schistosomes*, or the *blood flukes*. These flukes are similar to *Heterobilharzia americana* and inhabit the blood vasculature of the mesenteric veins and the blood vasculature associated with major organs (large and small intestines and urinary bladder) of the abdominal cavity of humans. These flukes are members of the genus *Schistosoma* (also known as *Bilharzia*) and are important parasites of humans in Africa, the Middle East, the Caribbean, and other areas of the world. These parasites are important in human medicine; however, other than this mention, they are beyond the scope of this textbook. The cercarial stage of this important fluke infects the definitive host by direct penetration of the skin of humans as they are wading or bathing in water. Some members of the genus *Schistosoma* infect the blood vasculature of the mesenteric and portal veins of cattle; however, these schistosomes occur in Africa, the Mediterranean, and the Middle East and are not usually associated with domesticated animals in North America. Schistosomes are species specific; that is, human schistosomes infect humans, and bovine schistosomes infect cattle. Schistosomes of domestic animals are not zoonotic. The veterinary technician who has interest in the schistosomes of humans should consult a textbook on the parasitology of humans.

BOX 8-2 | A Few Words About Flukes of Wild Birds

Parasite: *Schistosoma (Trichobilharzia, Gigantobilharzia species)* and assorted other species found in birds
Host: Birds
Location of Adult: Blood vasculature
Intermediate Host: Freshwater snails
Distribution: North America
Derivation of Genus: Split body
Transmission Route: Cercariae enter through skin penetration
Common Name: Avian schistosomes

Avian schistosomes occur in the blood vasculature of many wild birds (particularly aquatic birds) that migrate across the North American continent along seasonal flyways. Migrating aquatic birds frequently rest in rivers and lakes of North America along their seasonal journeys. These birds are frequently infected with avian schistosomes in their blood vessels. The schistosomes produce eggs that pass to the external environment in the birds' feces. The eggs often make contact with water, hatch, and release the miracidia, the stage infective for the snail intermediate host. The miracidia penetrate aquatic snails and, within the snails, develop into the cercarial stage. The cercariae emerge from the snail and usually complete the life cycle by penetrating the skin of the appropriate avian definitive host. However, if the cercariae penetrate the skin of a human (who is swimming or playing in the lake, river, or ocean), with repeated exposure the cercariae can produce a severe papular or pustular dermatitis called **swimmer's itch** or **schistosome cercarial dermatitis** (Figure 8-19). This pruritic dermatitis is one of the few zoonotic parasitic conditions/diseases found among the digenetic trematodes. The dermatitis is quite pruritic and can ruin a vacation at the lake or the seashore.

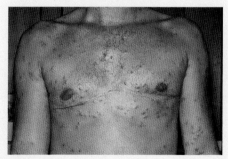

FIGURE 8-19 Severe papular or pustular dermatitis (swimmer's itch, or schistosome cercarial dermatitis) in a human. This pruritic dermatitis is the only zoonotic digenetic trematode. Courtesy of: James W, Berger T, Elston D: Andrews' Diseases of the Skin, 12th edition. St. Louis, Elsevier, 2015.

BOX 8-3 | A Few Words About Flukes of Game Fish

Birds near a lake or seashore may have flukes that reside in the gastrointestinal tract. As with the avian schistosomes described in Box 8-2, these flukes produce eggs that pass to the external environment and often make contact with water. The eggs hatch, releasing the miracidia. The miracidia penetrate aquatic snails and, within the snails, develop into the cercarial stage. The cercariae emerge from the snails and normally penetrate the skin of fish. When the cercariae penetrate the skin of fish, they produce a metacercarial stage. The metacercaria is actually a juvenile fluke. Fish often react to the presence of metacercariae by depositing melanin (black) pigment around the organism, producing a condition called **black spot** (Figure 8-20). Aquatic birds become infected with the fluke by ingesting the fish containing the metacercarial stage. Sometimes fishermen catch these fish and during the cleaning process may notice these conspicuous black metacercarial stages in the skin or in the muscles of the fish. If the fish is properly cooked, it is safe for human consumption. Humans

are not harmed when they ingest these stages; humans cannot become infected with this avian fluke. Therefore this is not a zoonotic condition; however, it may not be aesthetically pleasing! The unsightly appearance of these metacercarial spots in the fish's tissues may prevail over the hungry fisherman's appetite.

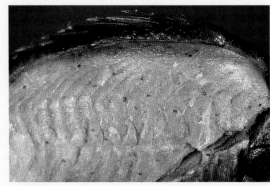

FIGURE 8-20 Fish exhibiting black spot, deposition of melanin pigment in response to the presence of metacercariae.

CHAPTER EIGHT TEST

MATCHING—Match the term with the correct phrase or term.

A. *Dicrocoelium dendriticum*

B. *Paramphistomum* and *Cotylophoron*

C. *Fasciola hepatica*

D. *Fascioloides magna*

E. *Platynosomum fastosum*

F. *Nanophyetus salmincola*

G. *Paragonimus kellicotti*

H. *Heterobilharzia americana*

I. Swimmer's itch

J. Black spot

1. Salmon-poisoning fluke of dogs

2. Canine schistosomes (blood flukes)

3. Liver fluke of cattle

4. The lancet fluke of ruminants

5. Rumen flukes

6. Melanin deposition in response to the presence of metacercariae

7. Schistosome cercarial dermatitis

8. Liver fluke of white-tailed deer

9. Lizard-poisoning fluke of cats

10. Lung fluke of dogs and cats

QUESTIONS FOR THOUGHT AND DISCUSSION

1. Discuss the zoonotic potential for the digenetic trematodes. In what way are trematodes zoonotic?

2. Trematodes are usually associated with the gastrointestinal tract or with some duct associated with the gastrointestinal tract. Which digenetic trematode is the exception to this rule?

3. Explain how schistosomes are different from other digenetic flukes.

The Phylum Acanthocephala

LEARNING OBJECTIVES

After studying this chapter, the reader should be able to do the following:

- Identify acanthocephalans relative to their morphology and egg type.
- Correctly spell *Macracanthorhynchus hirudinaceus,* the swine acanthocephalan. This

parasite has the longest scientific name among all the parasites of wild and domesticated animals.

KEY TERMS

Acanthella
Acanthocephalan

Acanthor
Cystacanth

Tegument

The phylum Acanthocephala consists of the "thorny-headed worms," or "spiny-headed worms." With regard to the number of acanthocephalan parasites that infect domesticated animals, the phylum Acanthocephala is very small.

COMMON ACANTHOCEPHALANS

Most acanthocephalans are parasites of marine and freshwater fish and aquatic birds; their predilection site is within the small intestine of the definitive host. Only two species, *Macracanthorhynchus hirudinaceus,* the thorny-headed worm of swine, and *Oncicola canis,* the canine acanthocephalan, are important to veterinary medicine.

TECHNICIAN'S NOTE Only two species of acanthocephalans are important to veterinary medicine. Most species parasitize marine fish, freshwater fish, and aquatic birds.

KEY MORPHOLOGIC FEATURES

Members of the phylum Acanthocephala are important parasites of domesticated and wild animals. Adult acanthocephalans are internal parasites, living in the small intestine of their vertebrate hosts. Acanthocephalans are typically elongate, cylindric worms, tapered on both ends. One acanthocephalan (*M. hirudinaceus*) can measure up to 70 cm in length. Acanthocephalans are dioecious; that is, they have separate sexes. Female acanthocephalans are typically larger than their male counterparts. The colloquial names *thorny-headed worm* and *spiny-headed worm* are derived from the fact that acanthocephalans possess a retractable proboscis, or "nose," on the anterior end (Figure 9-1). This proboscis is covered with tiny backward-facing spines and serves as an organ of attachment (Figure 9-2). The proboscis embeds in the small intestinal mucosa and allows the acanthocephalan parasite to attach to the host, similar to the scolex of the true tapeworm. It is in this enteric site that acanthocephalans feed; however, these are unusual parasites in that they lack a mouth. Instead, these strange-looking helminths have a trait that is similar to that of tapeworms: They do not possess an alimentary tract (a gut or intestinal tract). As a result, acanthocephalans must absorb nutrients through their body surface, or tegument.

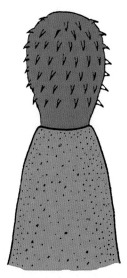

FIGURE 9-1 Anterior end of *Macracanthorhynchus hirudinaceus*, the thorny-headed worm of swine. This colloquial name is derived from acanthocephalans' possessing a retractable proboscis, or nose, on the anterior end.

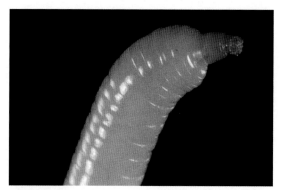

FIGURE 9-2 Proboscis of *Macracanthorhynchus hirudinaceus* is covered with tiny backward-facing spines and serves as an organ of attachment.

> **TECHNICIAN'S NOTE** Acanthocephalans attach or imbed in the small intestine of their host with a proboscis covered with tiny backward-facing spines. They absorb their nutrients through their body walls.

Another important organ system in the acanthocephalan is the reproductive tract. As with all helminths, acanthocephalans have a tremendous reproductive potential—one adult female worm can produce in excess of a quarter million eggs per day! These eggs pass out of the definitive host within its feces and embryonate in the external environment.

LIFE CYCLE OF THE THORNY-HEADED WORM

The typical acanthocephalan has a unique life cycle. Because adult acanthocephalans are found attached to the small intestinal mucosa, the eggs are voided in the feces of the definitive host. The egg is spindle-shaped and has a shell of three layers (Figure 9-3). This egg contains the larval acanthocephalan, or acanthor. The intermediate host, usually some type of arthropod (e.g., dung beetle), ingests the egg, and the acanthor larva hatches in that intermediate host. Within the intermediate host, the larva develops to the next stage, the acanthella. The acanthella develops into the cystacanth stage, which has an inverted proboscis. The definitive host ingests the arthropod intermediate host. Within the intestine of the definitive host, the acanthella everts its proboscis and attaches to the wall of the small intestine. This juvenile acanthocephalan grows to the adult stage, and the life cycle begins again (Figure 9-4).

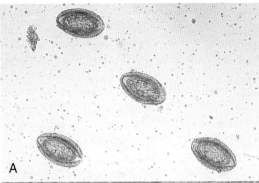

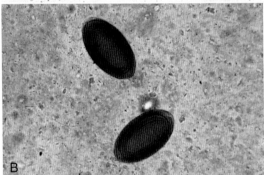

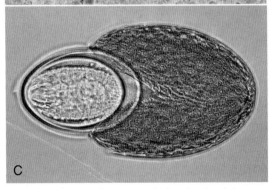

FIGURE 9-3 Egg of *Macracanthorhynchus hirudinaceus* is spindle-shaped and has a shell of three layers. The egg contains the larval acanthocephalan, or acanthor.

TECHNICIAN'S NOTE The adult female acanthocephalan can produce 250,000 eggs per day. The eggs are ingested by an arthropod and develop into an acanthor larva, then an acanthella to a cystacanth stage. The arthropod is ingested by the new host, and the acanthella everts its proboscis to imbed in the intestinal mucosa.

ACANTHOCEPHALANS OF IMPORTANCE IN VETERINARY PARASITOLOGY

M. hirudinaceus and *O. canis* are the acanthocephalans of importance in veterinary medicine.

Macracanthorhynchus hirudinaceus
Parasite: *Macracanthorhynchus hirudinaceus*
Host: Pigs
Location of Adult: Small intestinal mucosa
Intermediate Host: Dung beetle
Distribution: Worldwide
Derivation of Genus: Large thorny nose
Transmission Route: Ingestion of infective dung beetle
Common Name: Thorny-headed worm of swine
Zoonotic: No

M. hirudinaceus, the thorny-headed worm of swine, is the acanthocephalan found attached to the lining of the small intestine of pigs (Figure 9-5). Because of its attachment to the intestinal mucosa, the parasite has the potential to perforate the intestine, thus causing peritonitis and possible death. This parasite has the dubious distinction of having the longest scientific name among all the parasites of wild and domesticated animals. During postmortem examination the prosector (pathologist) might, at first glance, make a diagnosis of swine roundworm, *Ascaris suum* (see Chapter 4). On closer examination, however, it is apparent that the parasite is firmly attached to the mucosa of the small intestine rather than free within the lumen. *A. suum* does not attach to the mucosa but remains within the lumen of the small intestine. *M. hirudinaceus* can grow up to 70 cm in length, although the males average up to 10 cm in length and the females up to 35 cm, and these worms are 4 to 10 mm thick. The proboscis is tiny and is covered with six rows of six hooks each. These backward-facing hooks are used to anchor the adult parasite to the mucosa. The eggs of *M. hirudinaceus* are 40 to 65 μm × 67 to 110 μm and have a three-layered shell; the second shell is brown and pitted (Figure 9-3) and can be found using standard fecal flotation prodecures. Because humans seldom intentionally eat dung beetles (the intermediate host of *M. hirudinaceus*),

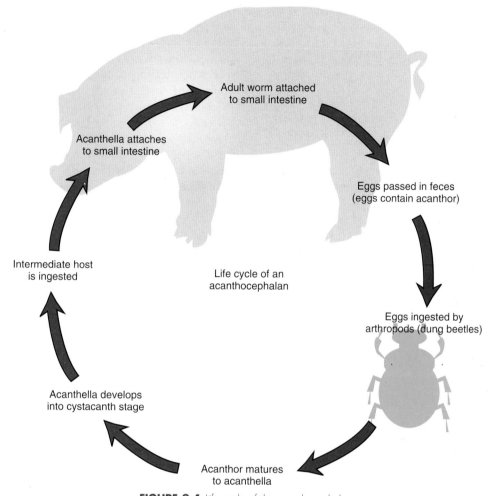

Adult worm attached
to small intestine

Acanthella attaches
to small intestine

Eggs passed in feces
(eggs contain acanthor)

Intermediate host
is ingested

Life cycle of an
acanthocephalan

Eggs ingested by
arthropods (dung beetles)

Acanthella develops
into cystacanth stage

Acanthor matures
to acanthella

FIGURE 9-4 Life cycle of the acanthocephalan.

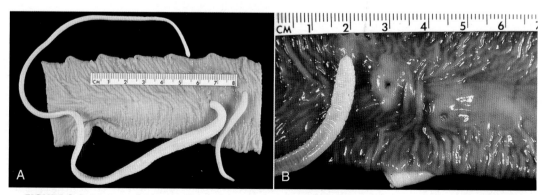

FIGURE 9-5 *Macracanthorhynchus hirudinaceus*, the thorny-headed worm of swine, is found attached to the lining of the small intestine of pigs.

this acanthocephalan is seldom identified as a zoonotic parasite.

POSTMORTEM EXAMINATION On postmortem examination, one may confuse *Macracanthorhynchus hirudinaceus* with *Ascaris suum*. On closer examination, the worm will be found to be firmly attached to the mucosal lining rather than being free within the lumen of the intestine.

Oncicola canis

Parasite: *Oncicola canis*
Host: Dogs
Location of Host: Small intestinal mucosa
Intermediate Host: Dung beetle
Distribution: North and South America
Derivation of Genus: Strain mass
Transmission Route: Ingestion of infective dung beetle
Common Name: Thorny-headed worm of dogs
Zoonotic: No

O. canis, the thorny-headed worm of dogs, is the acanthocephalan found attached to the lining of the small intestine of dogs. This is a tiny acanthocephalan, only 14 mm in length. The body is tapered posteriorly, and on the anterior end is the characteristic proboscis armed with hooks. As with *M. hirudinaceus*, these are backward-facing hooks used to anchor the adult parasite to the mucosa of the small intestine. With their proboscis embedded within the small intestinal wall, they often penetrate through to the peritoneum. Perforation of the intestinal wall leading to peritonitis and death is possible. The eggs of *O. canis* are brown and oval, approximately 65 × 45 μm, and can be found with standard fecal flotation procedures.

TECHNICIAN'S NOTE This parasite is an acanthocephalan but it is very rare to find this parasite, *Oncicola canis*, in the dog.

Although the phylum Acanthocephala is extremely small with regard to domesticated animals, veterinarians should understand its importance, especially with regard to the swine industry.

CHAPTER NINE TEST

MATCHING—Match the term with the correct phrase or term.

A. Acanthocephalans

B. Proboscid with backward-facing spines

C. Tegument

D. Dung beetle

E. Acanthocephalan egg

F. Acanthor

G. Acanthella and cystacanth

H. *Macracanthorhynchus hirudinaceus*

I. *Oncicola canis*

J. Acanthocephalan pathology

1. Larval acanthocephalan stages within the intermediate host

2. Three-layered shell

3. "Feeding organelle" that absorbs nutrients through the body surface

4. Organ of attachment; holdfast organelle

5. Larval acanthocephalan stage within the egg

6. Thorny-headed worm of dogs

7. Thorny-headed worm of swine

8. Thorny-headed or spiny-headed worms

9. Usual intermediate host for an acanthocephalan

10. Attachment to the wall of the small intestine

QUESTIONS FOR THOUGHT AND DISCUSSION

1. *Macracanthorhynchus hirudinaceus,* the swine acanthocephalan, is often confused with *Ascaris suum,* the swine ascarid. Compare and contrast these two important swine parasites relative to their size, location within the host, pathologic findings/conditions, description of the eggs (ova), and life cycle.

2. What two features or qualities do acanthocephalans have in common with true tapeworms?

10 The Protozoans

LEARNING OBJECTIVES

After studying this chapter, the reader should be able to do the following:

• Identify the four basic types of protozoans.

• Describe how the four different groups of protozoans move.

KEY TERMS

Cilia	Flagellum	Protozoans	Sarcomastigophorans
Ciliophoran	Pathogenicity	Pseudopodia	Trophozoite

Only two kingdoms of living creatures have members that are true parasites of domesticated animals. These parasites belong to the kingdom Animalia and the kingdom Protista. Most of the parasites of domesticated animals belong to the Animalia kingdom (flukes, tapeworms, roundworms, thorny-headed worms, arthropods, and leeches). The rest of the animal parasites belong to the kingdom Protista. This kingdom contains the unicellular, or one-celled, organisms (better known as the protozoans).

Most protozoans are free-living organisms; however, those protozoans that are parasitic may produce significant pathology in domesticated animals and humans. Within the kingdom Protista are several phyla, which contain (1) flagellated protozoans, (2) ameboid protozoans, (3) apicomplexans, and (4) ciliated protozoans. These phyla contain the primary protozoans that may cause significant pathology in domesticated animals and humans.

> ⬛ *TECHNICIAN'S NOTE* The parasitic protozoans are categorized in several phyla: **sarcomastigophorans** (subphylum flagellated and subphylum ameboid), apicomplexan, and ciliated (**ciliophoran**) protozoans.

CHARACTERISTICS OF THE PROTOZOANS

Protozoans are unicellular organisms; that is, they are one-celled organisms. Protozoans vary greatly in size, form, and structure; most are microscopic, and a very few are macroscopic, that is, visible to the naked eye. The kingdom Protista is divided into several phyla. These phyla differ in the manner in which the protozoans move within their tiny micro-environments. In veterinary parasitology, the most important phyla are Sarcomastigophora (containing the flagellates and amoebae), Ciliophora (containing the ciliates), and Apicomplexa (containing the coccidia, malarial organisms, and piroplasms).

> ⫿ *TECHNICIAN'S NOTE*   Protozoans are single-celled organisms or parasites.

MASTIGOPHORA (FLAGELLATES)

Kingdom: Protista
    Phylum: Sarcomastigophora
        Subphylum: Mastigophora (flagellates)

The flagellates are those protozoans that possess at least one flagellum (a long whiplike or lashlike appendage) in their trophozoite, or moving, form. This flagellum allows the protozoan to move about in a fluid medium. As a result of this activity, parasitic flagellates live in the liquid world of the host's blood, lymphatic fluid, or cerebrospinal fluid. Flagellates are often pear-shaped or bullet-shaped and are able to swim in their host's body fluids, meeting very little resistance. These flagellates vary greatly in pathogenicity (disease-causing potential). Some flagellates are highly pathogenic, whereas others appear to cause little or no harm to the host. Some important genera of parasitic flagellates of domestic animals are *Leishmania, Trypanosoma, Trichomonas, Histomonas,* and *Giardia* species. Figure 10-1 is a diagram of a representative flagellate, *Tritrichomonas foetus,* a flagellated protozoan of the reproductive tract of cattle.

SARCODINA (AMOEBAE)

Kingdom: Protista
    Phylum: Sarcomastigophora
        Superclass: Sarcodina (amoebae)

The amoebae are protozoans that move via pseudopodia ("false feet"). Amoebae have two forms: the motile trophozoite form and the resistant cyst

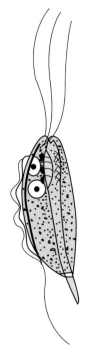

FIGURE 10-1 Diagram of the representative flagellate, *Tritrichomonas foetus,* a flagellated protozoan of the reproductive tract of cattle. Note the three anterior flagella, undulating membrane, and trailing posterior flagellum.

form. In their motile trophozoite form, amoebae glide or flow along a solid surface, usually the surface at the bottom of the liquid medium. Amoebae are amorphous (poorly defined, or bloblike, in shape). As with the flagellates, the amoebae vary greatly in their pathogenicity. Some amoebae are highly pathogenic, whereas others appear to cause little or no harm to the host. Amoebae demonstrate a resistant cyst form that allows them to survive in adverse conditions in the external environment.

The most important parasitic amoeba of humans is *Entamoeba histolytica. Entamoeba coli,* a non-pathogenic amoeba, may also be found in humans and pigs. Figure 10-2 is a diagram of the motile trophozoite stage of a representative amoeba, *E. histolytica,* an amoeboid protozoan. Figure 10-3 is a diagram of the resistant cyst stage of *E. histolytica.*

> ⫿ *TECHNICIAN'S NOTE*   *Entamoeba histolytica* is the most important amebic protozoan in humans.

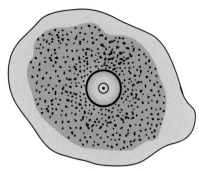

FIGURE 10-2 Diagram of the motile trophozoite stage of a representative amoeba, *Entamoeba histolytica*, an ameboid protozoan, with characteristic nucleus and bull's-eye nucleolus.

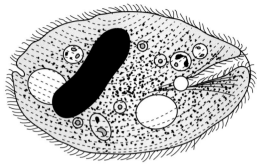

FIGURE 10-4 Diagram of the motile trophozoite form of a representative ciliate, *Balantidium coli*, a ciliated protozoan of the intestinal tract of pigs.

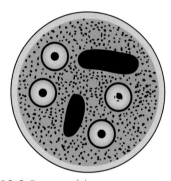

FIGURE 10-3 Diagram of the resistant cyst stage of a representative amoeba, *Entamoeba histolytica*, with thick cyst wall, four nuclei, and dark chromatoid bodies.

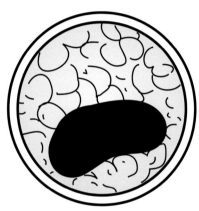

FIGURE 10-5 Diagram of the resistant cyst stage of *Balantidium coli*, with thick cyst wall and large, dark nucleus.

CILIOPHORA (CILIATES)

Kingdom: Protista
   Phylum: Ciliophora (ciliates)

Ciliates are protozoans that are covered with tiny, short hairs over most of their body surface. These tiny hairs are called cilia, thus the name ciliates. Ciliates move with these beating, undulating hairs. As with amoebae, ciliates demonstrate two forms: the motile trophozoite form and the resistant cyst form. In their trophozoite, or moving, form, ciliates dart and twirl speedily in liquid media. Ciliates come in a variety of sizes and shapes, but all are covered with these tiny hairs. Figure 10-4 is a diagram of the motile trophozoite form of a representative ciliate, *Balantidium coli*, a ciliated

protozoan of the intestinal tract of pigs. Some amoebae, such as *B. coli* and *Ichthyophthirius multifiliis*, are highly pathogenic to their hosts, whereas other ciliates, such as those in the rumen of the cow or sheep or the cecum of the horse, have beneficial roles. As with amoebae, ciliates demonstrate a resistant cyst form that allows them to survive in adverse conditions in the external environment. Figure 10-5 is a diagram of the resistant cyst stage of *B. coli*. The ciliates are unique among the protozoans in that they possess two types of nuclei: a macronucleus and a micronucleus.

TECHNICIAN'S NOTE Some ciliate protozoan parasites can have beneficial roles in their hosts.

APICOMPLEXA (APICOMPLEXANS)

Kingdom: Protista
   Phylum: Apicomplexa (apicomplexans)

Of the protozoans, the apicomplexans are the most diverse and the most complicated. The apicomplexans are parasites of almost every animal phylum. In domesticated animals, they are found primarily in the epithelium of the intestine, within blood cells, and within cells of the reticuloendothelial system. The life cycles of these protozoans vary among the genera that affect domesticated animals; however, they do have a common trait in that their life cycles are complex and intimately integrated into the physiology of the host's body. The locomotory organelles of the flagellates, amoebae, and ciliates (i.e., flagella, pseudopodia, and cilia, respectively) are discernible. In contrast, the locomotory organelles of the apicomplexans are not visible to the naked eye; their locomotory organelles are internal. The apicomplexans are often banana-, comma-, or boomerang-shaped (Figure 10-6) and move via undulations. Some of the most important genera of parasitic apicomplexans of domestic animals are *Eimeria, Cystoisospora, Toxoplasma, Sarcocystis, Cryptosporidium, Plasmodium, Haemoproteus, Leukocytozoon, Babesia,*

Theileria, Cytauxzoon, and *Hepatozoon.* These protozoans are perhaps the most diverse, complicated members of the Protista kingdom.

> **TECHNICIAN'S NOTE**   The apicomplexan parasites do not have visible locomotory organelles but move via undulations. Some of the most commonly seen apicomplexans are *Eimeria* and *Cystoisospora.*

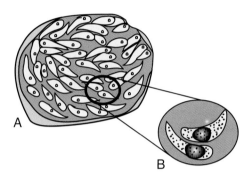

FIGURE 10-6 A, Diagram of a cyst containing banana-, comma-, or boomerang-shaped sporozoites typical of apicomplexans of domestic animals, for example, *Eimeria, Isospora, Toxoplasma, Sarcocystis, Cryptosporidium, Plasmodium, Haemoproteus, Leukocytozoon, Babesia,* and *Theileria* species. **B,** Note the enlarged banana-, comma-, or boomerang-shaped sporozoites.

CHAPTER TEN TEST

MATCHING—Match the term with the correct phrase or term.

A. Protozoans

B. Sarcomastigophorans

C. Ciliophorans

D. Apicomplexans

E. Flagellum

F. Trophozoite

G. Pathogenicity

H. Pseudopodia

I. Cilia

J. Locomotory organelles of apicomplexans and piroplasms

1. Tiny, short, moving hairs over most of the body surface

2. Disease-causing potential

3. Organelles of internal movement, not visible to the naked eye

4. A long whiplike or lashlike appendage

5. *Balantidium coli* and *Ichthyophthirius multifiliis*

6. Unicellular, or one-celled, organisms

7. Flagellates and amoebae

8. False feet of amoebae

9. Moving or motile form

10. Coccidia, malarial organisms

QUESTIONS FOR THOUGHT AND DISCUSSION

1. Discuss the different ways in which protozoans move.

2. Most of the parasites affecting domestic and wild animals are in the kingdom Animalia. Why do you think that protozoans are included in a separate kingdom, Protista?

11 Common Protozoans That Infect Domestic Animals

OUTLINE

LEARNING OBJECTIVES

After studying this chapter, the reader should be able to do the following:

- Remember the scientific names and the corresponding common names for the major protozoan parasites affecting domestic animals, laboratory animals, and fish.
- Recognize cyst and trophozoite forms of protozoans infecting the gastrointestinal tract when presented with a definitive host.

- Recognize intra- and extra-erythrocytic forms of the hemoprotozoans when presented with a definitive host.
- Recognize the significance of protozoans that are zoonotic parasites.

KEY TERMS

Canine piroplasm
Cyst stage
Endosome
Equine protozoal
  myeloencephalitis (EPM)

Gamonts
Hemoprotozoan
Ichthyophthiriosis
Infectious enterohepatitis or
  blackhead

Phlebotomine sand flies
Ring form
Trophozoite

This chapter is a continuation of Chapter 10 in that it details the common protozoans that infect domestic animals. The parasitic protozoans are discussed in the same order as in Chapter 10: flagellates, amoebae, ciliates, and apicomplexans. These parasites are discussed in the same system-by-system manner, that is, those infecting the gastrointestinal tract, the circulatory system and peripheral blood, and the urogenital system. These parasites are discussed in the following species of domesticated animals: dogs and cats, ruminants (i.e., cattle and sheep), horses, pigs, pet and aviary birds, domestic fowl, rabbits, mice, rats, hamsters, guinea pigs, and fish.

DOGS AND CATS

GASTROINTESTINAL TRACT

Protozoans that infect the gastrointestinal tract of dogs and cats are flagellates, amoebae, ciliates, and apicomplexans.

Flagellates

Parasite: 🅩 *Giardia* species
Host: Dogs, cats, horses, ruminants, and exotic species
Location: Intestinal mucosa
Distribution: Worldwide
Derivation of Genus: Named after the famous protozoologist Alfred Giard
Transmission Route: Ingestion of oocysts
Common Name: *Giardia*
Zoonotic: *Giardia* assemblage A: Yes; all other assemblages: No

Giardia species are flagellated protozoans often recovered from the feces of dogs and cats with diarrhea. They may also be recovered from animals with normal stools. These parasites occur in two morphologic forms: a rarely observed, motile feeding stage (the **trophozoite**) and a frequently observed, resistant **cyst stage**.

The motile trophozoite stage is pear-shaped and dorsoventrally flattened and possesses four pairs of flagella. This stage is 9 to 21 μm × 5 to 15 μm. Two nuclei and a prominent adhesive disk are present

on the anterior portion of the trophozoite, suggesting to the observer that a pair of eyes is "staring back." Figure 11-1 presents the motile trophozoite form of the *Giardia* species.

The mature cysts of *Giardia* species are oval and are 8 to 10 μm × 7 to 10 μm. They have a refractile wall and four nuclei. Immature cysts, which represent recently encysted motile forms, contain only two nuclei. Figure 11-2 presents a cyst of the *Giardia* species. In dogs, diarrhea may begin as early as 5 days after exposure to *Giardia*, with cysts first appearing in the feces at 1 week.

TECHNICIAN'S NOTE The trophozoites of *Giardia* species are typically seen in animals with diarrhea rather than formed stool.

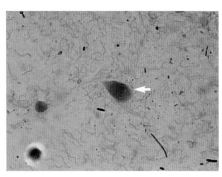

FIGURE 11-1 Motile trophozoite of *Giardia* species is pear-shaped and dorsoventrally flattened and possesses four pairs of flagella. Two nuclei and a prominent adhesive disk are present on the anterior portion of the trophozoite, suggesting a pair of eyes staring back.

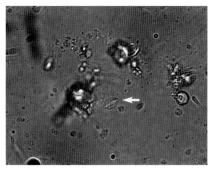

FIGURE 11-2 Mature cysts of *Giardia* species are oval and possess a refractile wall and four nuclei. Immature cysts, which represent recently encysted motile forms, contain only two nuclei.

Recent advances in molecular biology have changed the way *Giardia* species are named. Currently, *Giardia* is referred to in terms of assemblages rather than species. Assemblages A and B are associated with human beings, whereas assemblages C and D constitute the organisms found in dogs. Those organisms associated with cows, sheep, goats, horses, pigs, etc., are grouped in assemblage E. Assemblage F encompasses the forms found in cats, whereas assemblage G includes the organisms found in rodents. Although *Giardia* seems to be more species specific than once thought, assemblage A (that affecting humans) has been found in dogs and cats. This means there can still be a source of zoonotic infection from animals. However, it is more common that people are infected with *Giardia* by other people. Figure 11-3 shows the life cycle of *Giardia* species (Bowman, 2009).

Diagnosis of *Giardia* species is by standard fecal flotation. Zinc sulfate (specific gravity, 1.18) and Sheather sugar solution are considered the best flotation media for recovering cysts. Cysts are often distorted, with a semilunar appearance. The motile trophozoite occasionally can be found on direct

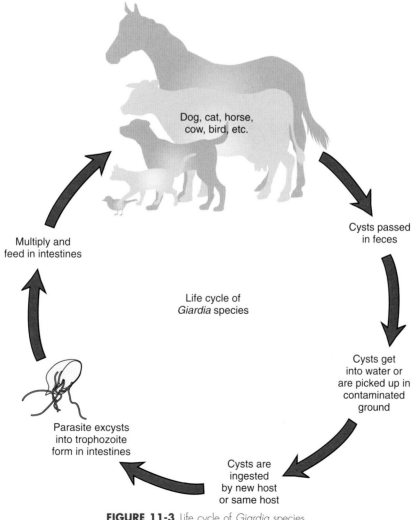

Dog, cat, horse, cow, bird, etc.

Multiply and feed in intestines

Cysts passed in feces

Life cycle of *Giardia* species

Cysts get into water or are picked up in contaminated ground

Parasite excysts into trophozoite form in intestines

Cysts are ingested by new host or same host

FIGURE 11-3 Life cycle of *Giardia* species.

smear of fresh feces using isotonic saline. Lugol iodine stain may be used to visualize the internal structures of both cysts and trophozoites. Fecal immunodiagnostic tests are also frequently used. Using immunodiagnostic tests in conjunction with fecal flotation tests provides the best protocol for diagnosing *Giardia* infection.

> **TECHNICIAN'S NOTE** The cysts are hard to find in diarrheic samples, thus immunodiagnostic tests may be helpful with a definitive diagnosis.

Amoebae
Parasite: ⚡ *Entamoeba histolytica*
Host: Canines, felines, primates, and humans
Location: Large intestines
Distribution: Worldwide but rare in the United States
Derivation of Genus: Internal amoeba

Transmission Route: Ingestion of cysts
Common name: *Entamoeba*
Zoonotic: Yes

Entamoeba histolytica, the etiologic agent that produces amebic dysentery (an extremely severe dysentery) in humans, may also produce sporadic infections in dogs. These cases usually have been acquired by association with infected humans. *E. histolytica* may produce acute or chronic diarrhea in dogs. Cats are rarely infected; most infections have been experimental.

E. histolytica occurs in two morphologic forms: a motile feeding stage (the trophozoite) and an environmentally resistant cyst stage. The motile trophozoite of *E. histolytica* ranges in size from 10 to 60 μm and has a single spherical nucleus that is 4 to 7 μm with a tiny pinpoint center, a structure called an endosome (Figure 11-4). The mature cysts are round and are 5 to 20 μm. They have a

CASE PRESENTATION 11-1

Setting up the Scenario
Mr. Amazon brought his 8-year-old, male-neutered German shorthaired pointer, Cherokee, to the veterinary clinic for an annual physical examination and routine vaccinations. Dr. Joseph performed the examination and administered the necessary vaccinations while the veterinary technician performed a heartworm test and fecal centrifugation analysis. The technician reported finding *Giardia* assemblage C or D cysts in the stool sample. Dr. Joseph prescribed a 5-day course of fenbendazole followed by a 5-day course of metronidazole.

What Information Must the Veterinary Technician Convey to Mr. Amazon?
The technician educated Mr. Amazon on canine giardiasis.

"Mr. Amazon, Cherokee has been diagnosed as having an intestinal protozoan parasite called *Giardia.* This is a one-celled parasite that lives in the small intestine and can cause diarrhea in dogs. You may remember the often-repeated story about traveler's diarrhea being contracted in Mexico by drinking contaminated water. This diarrhea is often

referred to as *Montezuma's revenge* and is often associated with *Giardia,* the protozoan parasite producing this illness. The parasite can be spread by a dog drinking water containing cysts of *Giardia* or ingesting cysts in soil contaminated by them. It is important that responsible dog owners clean up feces from the yard to prevent infection from their dog to any other dog that might become exposed.

You should also know that dogs can serve as a reservoir for the *Giardia* species found in humans or in an assemblage or groupings of this parasite. Although the human form does not harm or cause disease to your dogs, dogs are capable of transmitting this parasite to you or to members of your family. Whenever anyone comes in contact with dog feces, that person's hands must be thoroughly washed with soap and hot water.

Dr. Joseph is sending you home with two different antiprotozoals that will treat *Giardia.* Do you have any questions before you leave?"

The technician noted the discussion had taken place and that the zoonotic potential of the protozoan had been noted in the patient's record.

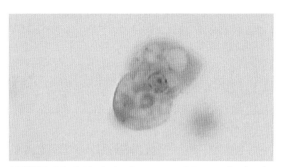

FIGURE 11-4 Motile feeding stage of *Entamoeba histolytica,* the trophozoite stage. Note the single spherical nucleus with a tiny pinpoint center, or endosome.

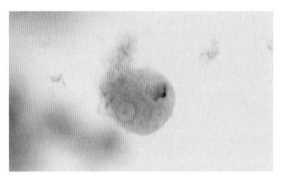

FIGURE 11-5 Cyst of *Entamoeba histolytica.* The cyst may demonstrate as many as four nuclei. Immature cysts, which represent recently encysted motile forms, contain only one nucleus.

thin refractile wall and may demonstrate as many as four nuclei, each with its own endosome. Immature cysts, which represent recently encysted motile forms, contain only one nucleus (Figure 11-5).

> **TECHNICIAN'S NOTE** *Entamoeba histolytica* is the parasite that causes amebic dysentery in humans.

Diagnosis of *E. histolytica* is by standard fecal flotation, which may be used to demonstrate both cyst and trophozoite forms. In a formed stool usually the cyst form is found; however, in diarrheic stool both the cyst and the trophozoite forms may be observed. The direct smear technique may be used to observe motile forms in warm, freshly passed diarrheic stools. Lugol iodine stain may be used to

visualize the internal structures of both cysts and trophozoites. Zinc sulfate may be used to concentrate cysts. If infection with *E. histolytica* is suspected in a human, a human pathology laboratory should be consulted for assistance with diagnosis. Because *E. histolytica* is primarily a human pathogen, great care should be taken with suspect feces.

E. histolytica also can be a significant problem in primates such as monkeys and chimpanzees. Great care should be taken when handling suspect feces. Infection in monkeys has great public health significance.

> **TECHNICIAN'S NOTE** *Entamoeba histolytica* is primarily a human parasite.

Ciliates
Parasite: **Z** *Balantidium coli*
Host: Canines and swine
Location: Cecum and colon of canines and large intestine of swine
Distribution: Worldwide
Derivation of Genus: Small bag
Transmission Route: Ingestion of cysts
Common Name: *Balantidium*
Zoonotic: Yes (per *The Merck Veterinary Manual*)

Balantidium coli is the ciliated protozoan found occasionally in the cecum and colon of dogs. This parasite has been associated with diarrhea in dogs. *B. coli* is more intimately associated with pigs (see the section on swine protozoan parasites).

Apicomplexans
Parasite: *Cystoisospora* species (formerly *Isospora* species)
Host: Canines, felines, and swine
Location: Small intestines
Distribution: Worldwide
Derivation of Genus: Equal seeds; sac same spore
Transmission Route: Ingestion of oocysts
Common Name: Coccidia
Zoonotic: No

Cystoisospora species (coccidians) are protozoan parasites of the small intestine of dogs and cats. They produce a clinical syndrome known as coccidiosis, caused by inflammation of the intestine, one of the most commonly diagnosed protozoan diseases in puppies and kittens. It produces loose stool to a watery diarrhea. Coccidiosis is rarely a problem in mature animals. The oocyst is the diagnostic stage observed in a fecal flotation of fresh feces; it is unsporulated in fresh feces and varies in size and shape among the common *Cystoisospora* species. Figure 11-6 shows an unsporulated oocyst, and Figure 11-7 shows a sporulated oocyst. The canine coccidians and their measurements are *Cystoisospora canis*, 34 to 40 μm × 28 to 32 μm; *Cystoisospora ohioensis*, 20 to 27 μm × 15 to 24 μm; and *Cystoisospora burrowsi*, 10 to 14 μm × 7.5 to 9 μm. The feline coccidians and their measurements are *Cystoisospora felis*, 38 to

51 μm × 27 to 29 μm, and *Cystoisospora rivolta*, 21 to 28 μm × 18 to 23 μm. Figure 11-8 shows the life cycle of *Cystoisospora* species. The prepatent period varies among species, but it is usually 7 to 14 days.

> **TECHNICIAN'S NOTE** *Cystoisospora* species are some of the most commonly diagnosed parasites in puppies and kittens.

CASE PRESENTATION 11-2

Setting up the Scenario

Ms. Dunleavy brought her new 8-week-old female kitten, Clarisse, to her first kitten appointment for a through physical examination and routine vaccinations. The technician recorded the kitten's weight, collected a fecal sample, and trimmed Clarisse's nails. (Question: Can a kitten's nails be trimmed at 8 weeks?) Dr. Dundee performed a physical examination and administered first vaccinations to Clarisse while the technician performed the fecal centrifugation analysis. The technician reported finding oocysts of *Cystoisospora felis* in the fecal sample. Dr. Dundee diagnosed Clarisse as having coccidia and prescribed an effective antiprotozoal compound.

What Information Must the Veterinary Technician Convey to Ms. Dunleavy?

The technician explained the following to Ms. Dunleavy: "Clarisse has been diagnosed as having protozoans commonly called *coccidia*. Dr. Dundee is sending you home with an effective antiprotozoal for Clarisse. Coccidia or *C. felis* are common protozoan (single-celled) parasites found in young kittens and puppies. Coccidia commonly cause diarrhea, but this particular feline protozoan is not a parasite that humans can get from cats. This parasite is usually controlled by your kitten's body, but it will take time for Clarisse to develop immunity to the parasite. Therefore Dr. Dundee is going to treat the parasite so that Clarisse will not have diarrhea. The antiprotozoal agent should clear up the parasitic infection very quickly.

Do you have any questions regarding *C. felis*?"

The technician noted in the patient's record that the discussion had taken place and that the protozoan parasite lacked zoonotic potential.

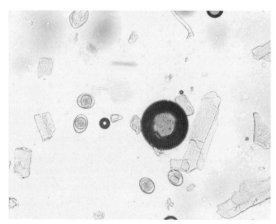

FIGURE 11-6 Unsporulated oocysts of *Cystoisospora* species. *Cystoisospora canis* (large oocysts) and *Cystoisospora burrowsi* (small oocysts) are present.

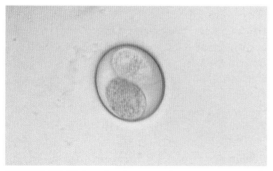

FIGURE 11-7 Sporulated oocyst of *Cystoisospora rivolta* from older feces.

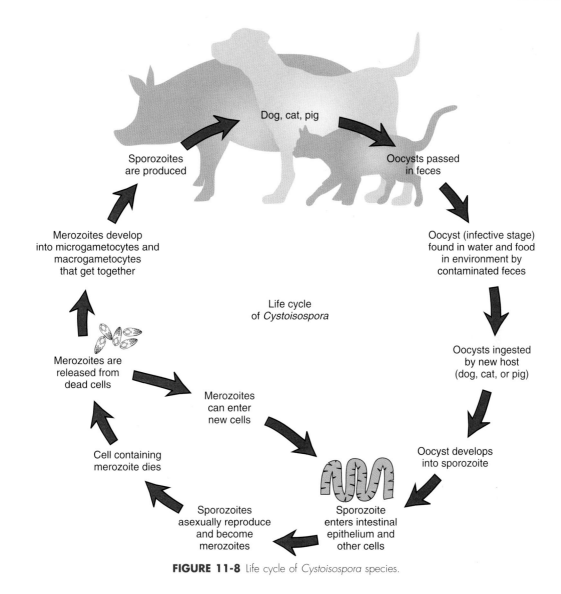

FIGURE 11-8 Life cycle of *Cystoisospora* species.

Parasite: 2 *Toxoplasma gondii*
Host: Definitive host is the feline; can also occur in other animals and humans as an incidental parasite.
Location: Intestines
Distribution: Worldwide
Derivation of Genus: Bow body
Transmission Route: Ingestion of sporulated oocysts

Common Name: *Toxoplasma*
Zoonotic: Yes

Toxoplasma gondii is an intestinal coccidian of cats. Its oocysts are usually diagnosed using a standard fecal flotation solution. Oocysts of *T. gondii* are unsporulated in fresh feces and measure 10 × 12 μm (Figure 11-9). Several

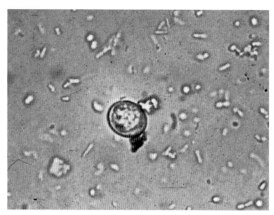

FIGURE 11-9 Unsporulated oocyst of *Toxoplasma gondii*, an intestinal coccidian of cats, from fresh feline feces. Its oocysts measure 10 × 12 μm.

immunodiagnostic tests using whole blood or serum are available for diagnosis of *T. gondii*. The prepatent period is highly variable, ranging from 5 to 24 days, and depends on the infection route. Figure 11-10, *A*, shows the life cycle of *T. gondii* in

the feline host, and Figure 11-10, *B*, shows the life cycle in the nonfeline host. Because this parasite can use humans (and many other warm-blooded vertebrates) as intermediate hosts, *T. gondii* is a very important zoonotic parasite.

T. gondii can be a significant pathogen in humans (particularly the pregnant woman and her developing fetus). It is important to discuss this parasite with clients. Great care should be taken when handling suspect feces. Infection in cats has great public health significance.

> **TECHNICIAN'S NOTE** The feline sheds *Toxoplasma gondii* oocysts for only up to 2 weeks of its life.

Parasite: **Z** *Cryptosporidium* species
Host: Canines, felines, bovines, ovines, swine, avians, guinea pigs, snakes, and mice
Location: Small intestine

CASE PRESENTATION 11-3

Setting up the Scenario
Ms. Vance came into the veterinary clinic with her cat, and she was crying. Ms. Vance had come to the clinic to have her cat euthanized. Jerry is a 3-year-old male, neutered, domestic shorthaired cat. Ms. Vance was led into the examination room and questioned regarding her cat's "medical problem." Ms. Vance replied that she recently found out she was expecting a baby and that her obstetrician had informed her that she needed to get rid of Jerry because the cat might transmit the deadly protozoan parasite *Toxoplasma gondii* to her unborn baby. Dr. Cotton had the technician run a fecal flotation and performed a physical examination on Jerry. The technician reported that there were no protozoan oocysts or helminth ova observed during the analysis of the fecal specimen. Dr. Cotton told Ms. Vance to remain calm and that there were a few preventive measures that she might implement so that Jerry could remain in her home and not have to be euthanized. Dr. Cotton had the technician explain the life cycle of

toxoplasmosis to Ms. Vance and detail the measures that might be taken to prevent human infection.

What Information Must the Veterinary Technician Convey to Ms. Vance?
The technician explained the following to Ms. Vance:

"*T. gondii* is a protozoan parasite that causes toxoplasmosis, a disease that can be transmitted to humans, especially during pregnancy. Your physician is right to be so worried about the possibility of this disease being transmitted to you from your cat. Only cats can serve as definitive hosts, capable of transmitting the parasite to other animals. However, cats pass the parasite only during about a 2-week time period in their lives. We did not observe any protozoan oocysts or helminth eggs during the examination of Jerry's stool sample. Although it is true that a mother being exposed for the first time during pregnancy can have problems, this is not a common occurrence. Most humans have already been exposed to the parasite, and their immune systems are programmed to prevent further infection. In addition, there are several techniques that might be used to prevent exposure to this parasite.

1. Have someone else (e.g., your husband or other family members or friends) clean and empty the litter box. If this is not possible, you should wear gloves while cleaning the litter box. The litter box should be cleaned daily to remove any developing oocysts from the home environment. It takes approximately 48 hours for the oocysts to become infective to animals including humans; the oocysts are undergoing a process called *sporulation*. If the litter box is changed daily, the oocyst will not develop in the presence of a pregnant woman, and the feces will not become infective for toxoplasmosis.

2. Hands should be thoroughly washed with soap and warm water, especially after the litter box has been cleaned, after working in garden soil, and after playing with children in a sandbox. Outdoor cats prefer flower and vegetable gardens and sandboxes as sites in which to defecate. Even if one does not own a cat, one can still become exposed to toxoplasmosis during normal day-to-day activities. Precautions should always be taken to avoid infection.

3. If Jerry is kept inside the house away from mice and rats, it will not be possible for him to become exposed to this parasite. Cats enjoy preying on rodents and other small creatures that are capable of serving as intermediate hosts when they are eaten by the cat.

4. Sandboxes must be covered after each and every episode of use to prevent cats from using the play area as their litter box. Gardens should be securely fenced and patrolled for the same reason. Both of these options may prove difficult, but precautions must be taken to prevent exposure.

5. Hands should be thoroughly washed with soap and warm water during the food preparation process, especially after handling raw meat. Raw muscle may contain one of the life cycle developmental stages of *Toxoplasma* that can become encysted within animal muscle (and therefore become contagious to people).

6. Another way that humans can become infected with *T. gondii* is by ingesting poorly cooked meat. Although cats are the only animals that shed the oocysts in their feces, other animals can become infected by ingesting the tissues stages within meat. This infective encysted form in the muscle can easily be transmitted in raw meat. Make sure that meat is not consumed in either a raw or undercooked state. Cats should never be fed raw or undercooked meat.

7. The kitchen and dining room should never be considered an acceptable place to locate a cat's litter box. Cat feces should never be in close proximity to food preparation/consumption areas.

Do you have any other questions regarding *T. gondii*?"

Ms. Vance left the clinic with a big smile on her face and Jerry in her arms. The technician noted that the discussion regarding this pathogenic protozoan had taken place and that the zoonotic potential had been noted in the patient's record.

Distribution: Worldwide
Derivation of Genus: Hidden small seeds
Transmission Route: Ingestion of oocysts
Common Name: Cryptosporidia, "Crypto"
Zoonotic: Yes

Cryptosporidium species is another coccidian-like parasite that parasitizes the mucosal cells of the small intestine of a variety of animals and causes inflammation of those cells. These animals include cows, pigs, dogs, cats, birds, and guinea pigs. *Cryptosporidium* species in snakes and mice and some species in cows parasitize the stomach and abomasum (cows). There is also a species of *Cryptosporidium* that parasitizes humans. In most cases of infection, diarrhea is the major clinical sign. The sporulated oocysts in the feces are oval to spherical and measure only 4 to 6 μm. Diagnosis is by

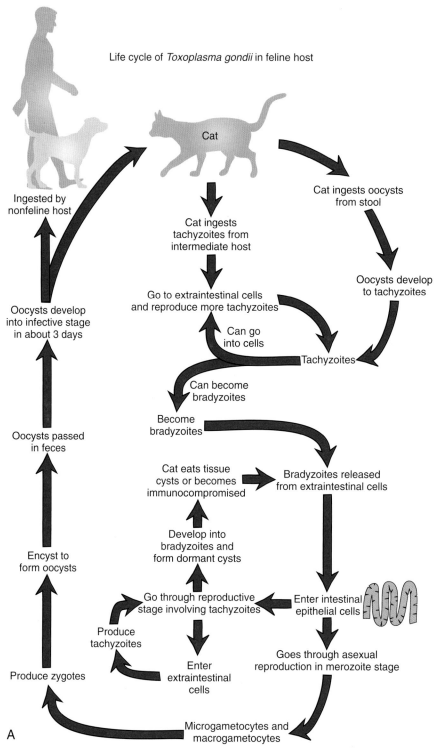

FIGURE 11-10 A, Life cycle of *Toxoplasma gondii* for feline hosts.

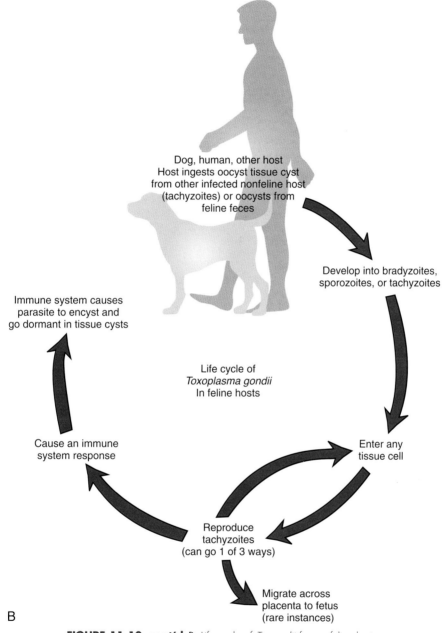

FIGURE 11-10, cont'd B, Life cycle of *T. gondii* for nonfeline hosts.

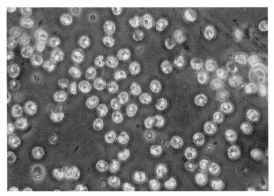

FIGURE 11-11 Numerous oocysts of *Cryptosporidium*, a coccidian parasite that parasitizes the small intestine of dogs and cats. Sporulated oocysts in feces are oval to spherical and measure 3 to 5 μm. Diagnosis is by standard fecal flotation. Oocysts are extremely small and may be observed just under the coverslip, not in the same plane of focus as other oocysts and parasite ova. Examination of fresh fecal smears using special stains (modified acid-fast stain) is also helpful.

standard fecal flotation. The oocysts are extremely small and may be observed just under the coverslip, not in the same plane of focus as other oocysts and parasite eggs (Figure 11-11). Examination of fresh fecal smears using special stains (modified acid-fast stain) is also helpful. ELISA (enzyme-linked immunoassay) tests are also being used to diagnose this parasite.

Because humans may become infected with *Cryptosporidium* species, feces suspected of harboring this protozoan should be handled with great care. *Cryptosporidium* is a zoonotic parasite. *Cryptosporidium parvum* is the most common zoonotic species. However, *Cryptosporidium canis*, *Cryptosporidium felis*, *Cryptosporidium meleagridis* (birds), *Cryptosporidium muris* (mice), and *Cryptosporidium suis* (pigs) have been seen in humans.

> **TECHNICIAN'S NOTE** Feces suspected of containing *Cryptosporidium* oocysts should be handled with great care.

Parasite: *Sarcocystis* species
Host: Canines and felines
Location: Small intestine
Distribution: Worldwide

Derivation of Genus: Flesh cyst
Transmission Route: Ingestion of the muscle of horses, pigs, and ruminants
Common Name: Sarcocystis
Zoonotic: No

Sarcocystis species are the final coccidian parasites cited here that are found in the small intestine. Several species infect dogs and cats, and identification of an individual species can be quite difficult. The oocysts of *Sarcocystis* species are sporulated when passed in the feces. Each oocyst contains two sporocysts, each with four sporozoites. These individual oocysts measure 12 to 15 μm × 8 to 12 μm and may be recovered in standard fecal flotation of fresh feces. The oocysts are ingested by a ruminant, horse, or pig depending on the specific species of *Sarcocystis*. The oocysts excyst and go through multiple asexual reproductive stages before encysting in the muscles of the intermediate host. The muscle tissue of the intermediate host must be ingested to complete the maturation to the oocyte stage in the final host species, canine or feline.

> **TECHNICIAN'S NOTE** There are seven species of *Sarcocystis* that infect dogs and five species that infect cats. Each of the species has a different intermediate host.

CIRCULATORY SYSTEM AND BLOOD

Protozoans that infect the circulatory system and blood of dogs and cats are flagellates and apicomplexans.

Flagellates

Parasite: **Z** *Trypanosoma cruzi*
Host: Humans and occasionally canines
Location: Peripheral blood
Distribution: Primarily in Central and South America but occasionally in the southern United States
Derivation of Genus: Borer body
Transmission Route: Ingestion of intermediate host, reduviid bug, or feces of reduviid bug left on mucous membranes of the final host
Common Name: Trypanosome
Zoonotic: Yes

Trypanosoma cruzi is a hemoprotozoan (a protozoan found circulating in the peripheral blood). It is found primarily in Central and South America; however, it is occasionally reported in dogs in the southern half of the United States. This trypanosome is extracellular; it is not found within the red blood cell (RBC) itself. It "swims" within the blood. This swimming stage is called a trypomastigote and is 16 to 20 µm in length, approximately 3 to 10 times as long as an RBC is wide. It is banana-shaped and possesses a lateral, undulating membrane and a thin whiplike tail (the flagellum) that is used for swimming. These parasites are also transmitted by blood-feeding arthropods called reduviid bugs, or "kissing bugs" (see Chapter 13). *T. cruzi* also has a resting cyst stage (the amastigote stage) that may be found encysted within cardiac muscle and other tissues such as the esophagus. The encysted amastigote stage lacks the undulating flagellum of the swimming trypomastigote stage.

The trypomastigote stage of *T. cruzi* may be found swimming within the peripheral blood and may be demonstrated in direct blood smears. The amastigote stage must be confirmed using histopathologic sectioning. Suspect tissues should be submitted to a histopathology laboratory for diagnosis by a veterinary pathologist or parasitologist.

> **TECHNICIAN'S NOTE** The trypomastigote stage of *Trypanosoma cruzi* can be found in a peripheral blood smear.

Parasite: Z *Leishmania* species
Host: Canines
Location: Reticuloendothelial cells of the capillaries and spleen, as well as other internal organs and white blood cells (WBCs)
Distribution: Worldwide but rarely seen in North America
Derivation of Genus: Named after the famous physician William Leishman
Transmission Route: Bite by an infective intermediate host, phlebotomine sand flies
Common Name: *Leishmania*
Zoonotic: Yes

Leishmania species is another hemoprotozoan (blood protozoan). The parasite is found primarily in areas other than North America; however, it is occasionally reported in dogs that have traveled or were born overseas. It is rarely diagnosed in dogs that have never left the United States. This flagellate is intracellular and found within reticuloendothelial cells of the capillaries, spleen, and other internal organs and in monocytes, polymorphonuclear leukocytes, and macrophages. Instead of having a flagellum and being called the *trypomastigote stage,* as with *T. cruzi,* this parasite lacks the flagellum and is called the *amastigote stage. Leishmania* is transmitted by blood-feeding arthropods called phlebotomine sand flies (see Chapter 13).

The amastigote stage of *Leishmania* must be confirmed using histopathologic sectioning of infected organs. Suspect tissues should be submitted to a histopathology laboratory for diagnosis by a veterinary pathologist or parasitologist.

> **TECHNICIAN'S NOTE** *Leishmania* species are rarely seen in dogs in North America.

Apicomplexans
Parasite: *Babesia canis*
Host: Canine
Location: Within RBCs
Distribution: Europe, Africa, Asia, North and South America
Derivation of Genus: Named after the famous bacteriologist Victor Babès
Transmission Route: Bite of an infective intermediate host, tick
Common Name: *Babesia* or canine piroplasm
Zoonotic: No

Babesia canis is an intracellular parasite found within the RBCs of dogs. It has been referred to as the canine piroplasm. The parasite demonstrates pear-shaped organisms within canine RBCs. This protozoan parasite is spread by the bite of infected ticks. Diagnosis is by observing basophilic, pear-shaped organisms within RBCs in stained blood smears (Figure 11-12). This parasite causes damage by residing within the RBCs. Common symptoms include pale mucous membranes, icterus, hemoglobinuria, depression, hemoglobinemia, weakness, splenomegaly, fever, and anorexia.

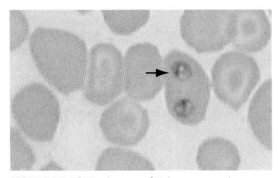

FIGURE 11-12 Trophozoites of *Babesia canis* within canine red blood cells.

> 📎 *TECHNICIAN'S NOTE*   *Babesia canis* can be broken down into three subspecies that denote in which country the species is found. *Babesia canis canis* is found in Europe, *Babesia canis vogeli* is found in Northern Africa and North America, and *Babesia canis rossi* is found in Southern Africa (Bowman, 2009).

Parasite: *Cytauxzoon felis*
Host: Feline
Location: Within RBCs
Distribution: Africa and the United States
Derivation of Genus: Hollow vessel-increasing animal
Transmission Route: Bite from an infective intermediate host, tick
Common Name: *Cytauxzoon*
Zoonotic: No

Cytauxzoon felis is another intracellular parasite that has been reported in the RBCs of cats in sporadic sites (Missouri, Arkansas, Georgia, and Texas) throughout the United States and Africa. It also produces piroplasms; however, these bodies have been described as being in the shape of a "bejeweled ring" and are referred to as the ring form in stained blood smears (Figure 11-13). This disease is spread by ticks, and its prognosis is poor. Diagnosis is made by observing the bejeweled-ring piroplasms within the RBCs in stained blood smears. Common symptoms include fever, icterus, anemia, dehydration, and death. As with *B. canis, C. felis* causes damage by inflammation within the RBCs.

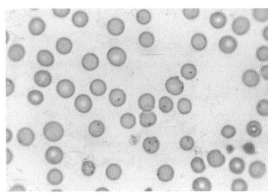

FIGURE 11-13 Ring form of *Cytauxzoon felis* in stained feline red blood cells.

> 📎 *TECHNICIAN'S NOTE*   *Cytauxzoon felis* is diagnosed by finding the bejeweled ring form in the RBCs in stained blood smears.

Parasite: *Hepatozoon canis* and *Hepatozoon americanum*
Host: Canines
Location: Gamonts are found within WBCs, whereas schizonts are found in the endothelial cells of the spleen, bone marrow, and liver.
Distribution: United States, Africa, Asia, and southern Europe
Derivation of Genus: Liver animal
Transmission Route: Ingestion of infective intermediate host, *Rhipicephalus sanguineus* tick for *H. canis* and *Amblyomma maculatum* tick for *H. americanum*
Common Name: *Hepatozoon*
Zoonotic: No

Hepatozoon canis and *Hepatozoon americanum* are intracellular, malaria-like parasites affecting dogs. The blood forms (the gamonts) of these protozoan parasites are found in the leukocytes. (Leukocytes containing gamonts of *H. canis* are common in peripheral blood smears, whereas those of *H. americanum* are rare.) Schizonts are found in the endothelial cells of the spleen, bone marrow, and liver. The gamonts are surrounded by a delicate capsule and stain pale blue with a dark reddish-purple nucleus. Numerous pink granules are found in the cytoplasm of the leukocyte. The "onion skin" tissue

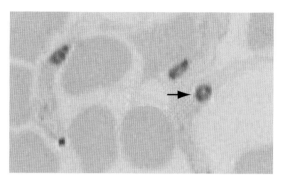

FIGURE 11-14 The onion skin tissue cysts of *Hepatozoon americanum* are found in the skeletal muscle of dogs.

cysts of *H. americanum* are found in the skeletal muscle of dogs (Figure 11-14). This is an unusual parasite in that the dog becomes infected by ingestion of an infected tick, *Amblyomma maculatum. H. canis* is well adapted to its canine host and varies from being subclinical to producing mild disease. *H. americanum* produces a violent and frequently fatal course of disease; it is theorized to have crossed the species barrier from a wild animal host to the domestic dog.

> **TECHNICIAN'S NOTE** Almost all intracellular malaria-like parasites are transmitted by the bite of an arthropod (a mosquito or a mite), but *Hepatozoon* species are spread by the ingestion of an arthropod.

RUMINANTS (CATTLE AND SHEEP)

GASTROINTESTINAL TRACT
Protozoans that infect the gastrointestinal tract of ruminants are ciliates and apicomplexans.

Ciliates
Nonpathogenic ciliates live in the rumen of all ruminants, including cattle and sheep. These are mutualists; in this type of symbiotic relationship both individuals benefit from the association. The cow provides a warm, moist, particulate medium in which the ciliates live; the ciliates, in exchange, aid in digestion by breaking down cellulose. Sometimes ciliates may be observed in the diarrheic feces of cattle and sheep. These ciliates may be recovered on

fecal flotation. Similar ciliates occur in the cecum of the horse and are often recovered from diarrheic feces.

Apicomplexans
Parasite: *Eimeria* species, *Eimeria bovis,* and *Eimeria zuernii*
Host: Ruminants
Location: Cecum and colon
Distribution: Worldwide
Derivation of Genus: Named after the famous zoologist Gustav Eimer
Transmission Route: Ingestion of oocysts
Common Name: Coccidia
Zoonotic: No

Ruminants serve as host to many species of the coccidian parasite *Eimeria*. It is often difficult to identify the individual species of *Eimeria* because their oocysts are similar in size and shape. The life cycle is similar to that of *Cystoisospora* species (see Figure 11-8) and causes damage by inflammation of the intestinal cells. The two most common species of coccidia in cattle are *Eimeria bovis* and *Eimeria zuernii;* they can be differentiated on standard fecal flotation. Oocysts of *E. bovis* are oval, have a micropyle (opening), and measure 20 × 28 μm; the oocysts of *E. zuernii* are spherical, lack the micropyle, and measure 15 to 22 μm × 13 to 18 μm. When oocysts are recovered on fecal flotation, the observation is usually noted as coccidia. The coccidian oocysts of ruminants can be partially differentiated by size and appearance and cause diarrhea and possibly neurologic signs, such as muscle tremors, convulsions, and blindness (Figure 11-15).

> **TECHNICIAN'S NOTE** Individual species of *Eimeria* can be partially differentiated by oocyst size and appearance.

Parasite: ⓩ *Cryptosporidium* species (discussed in greater detail in canine and feline section)
Host: Canines, felines, bovines, swine, avians, guinea pigs, snakes, and mice
Location: Small intestine
Distribution: Worldwide

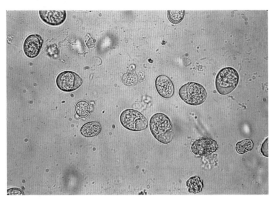

FIGURE 11-15 Unsporulated oocysts of *Eimeria* species recovered from fresh goat feces.

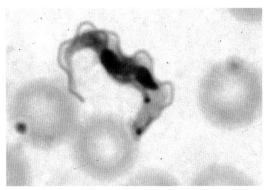

FIGURE 11-16 *Trypanosoma* species in bovine blood smear. (From Bowman: *Georgis' Parasitology for Veterinarians*, ed 10, 2013, Elsevier.)

Derivation of Genus: Hidden small seeds
Transmission Route: Ingestion of sporulated oocyst
Common Name: *Cryptosporidium;* Crypto
Zoonotic: Yes

The *Cryptosporidium* species is another coccidian that parasitizes the small intestine of a variety of animals including cattle, sheep, and goats. The sporulated oocysts in the feces are colorless and transparent and measure only 3 to 5 µm. Diagnosis is by standard fecal flotation and stained fecal smears. Because humans may become infected with *Cryptosporidium* species, feces suspected of harboring this protozoan should be handled with great care. These oocysts are often recovered using Sheather sugar solution. (See Figure 11-11 for features of the oocysts of *Cryptosporidium* species.)

> **TECHNICIAN'S NOTE** Feces suspected of being infected with *Cryptosporidium* should be handled with great care because of the potential for zoonosis.

CIRCULATORY SYSTEM AND BLOOD

Protozoans that infect the circulatory system and blood are flagellates and apicomplexans.

Flagellates
Parasite: 🅩 *Trypanosoma* species (see general discussion in canine and feline section)

Host: Ruminants
Location: Peripheral blood
Distribution: Primarily in Central and South America but occasionally in the southern United States
Derivation of Name: Borer body
Transmission Route: Bite of infective fly
Common Name: Trypanosome
Zoonotic: Yes

Trypanosoma species are hemoprotozoans found in the peripheral blood of many ruminants. This trypanosome has a long narrow body, a dark nucleus, an anterior flagellum, and a sail-like undulating membrane (Figure 11-16). These protozoans may be observed among the RBCs in a thin blood smear. *Trypanosoma* species are not pathogenic and are very common but are seldom seen in a routine smear.

> **TECHNICIAN'S NOTE** These parasites are very common in ruminants but are rarely seen on a routine blood smear.

Apicomplexans
Parasite: *Babesia bigemina*
Host: Bovines
Location: Within RBCs
Distribution: Europe, Africa, Asia, North and South America
Derivation of Genus: Named after the famous bacteriologist Victor Babès

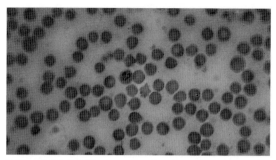

FIGURE 11-17 Trophozoites of *Babesia bigemina* within bovine red blood cells. Piroplasms are characteristically pear-shaped and lie in pairs, forming an acute angle within the erythrocyte.

Transmission Route: Bite of an infective *Boophilus annulatus* tick
Common Name: *Babesia*
Zoonotic: No

Babesia bigemina is an intracellular parasite found within the RBCs of cattle. This parasite is a large piroplasm that causes damage by residing within the RBC, is 4 to 5 μm in length × about 2 μm wide, and can be observed in a stained blood smear. These piroplasms are characteristically pear-shaped and lie in pairs, forming an acute angle within the erythrocyte (Figure 11-17). The intermediate host for this protozoan parasite is the tick *Boophilus annulatus* (see Chapter 13). Common symptoms include fever, depression, icterus, anorexia, hemoglobinuria, pale mucous membranes, weakness, and splenomegaly.

> **TECHNICIAN'S NOTE** If diagnosed, both the protozoan and its tick intermediate host should be reported to state and federal authorities.

UROGENITAL SYSTEM

Parasite: *Tritrichomonas foetus*
Host: Bovine
Location: Prepuce of bulls and vagina, cervix, and uterus of cows
Distribution: Worldwide but becoming rare where artificial insemination is used
Derivation of Genus: Three hair unit

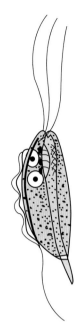

FIGURE 11-18 Diagram of *Tritrichomonas foetus*. This flagellated protozoan is pear-shaped and approximately 10 to 25 μm long, with a sail-like undulating membrane, a trailing posterior flagellum, and three rapidly moving, anterior whip-like flagella.

Transmission Route: Sexual transmission
Common Name: *Trichomonas*
Zoonotic: No

Tritrichomonas foetus is a protozoan parasite residing in the reproductive tract of cattle. These protozoans reside in the prepuce of infected bulls and in the vagina, cervix, and uterus of infected cows. In the cow, the parasite causes physiologic disturbance leading to abortion. *T. foetus* is pear-shaped and approximately 10 to 25 μm long, with a sail-like undulating membrane and three rapidly moving, anterior whiplike flagella (Figure 11-18). In fresh specimens they move actively with a jerky movement. Diagnosis is by finding these protozoans in fluid freshly collected from the stomach of an aborted fetus, from uterine discharge, or from washing of the vagina and prepuce. Fluid material should be centrifuged at 2000 rpm for 5 minutes. The supernatant is then removed and a drop of sediment transferred to a glass slide for microscopic examination for the moving organisms. Several slides should be examined. For more accurate diagnosis, fluid material from the sources just mentioned can be cultured in special media. A specialized parasitology laboratory should be consulted for information on these techniques.

> **TECHNICIAN'S NOTE** *Tritrichomonas foetus* is typically spread through a herd by the bull.

HORSES

GASTROINTESTINAL TRACT

Protozoan parasites that infect horses are flagellates, ciliates, and apicomplexans.

Flagellates

Parasite: *Giardia* assemblage E (*Giardia* is discussed in the canine and feline section)
Host: Horses, cows, sheep, goats, and pigs
Location: Small intestine
Distribution: Worldwide
Derivation of Name: Named after the famous biologist Alfred Giard
Transmission Route: Ingestion of oocysts
Common Name: *Giardia*
Zoonotic: No (only assemblage A is zoonotic)

Giardia assemblage E is a flagellated protozoan of low incidence in horses. The trophozoites and cysts of this parasite are morphologically similar to those of the species found in dogs and cats (see Figure 11-1). *Giardia* invades the small intestine and causes chronic diarrhea. Normal flotation techniques rarely detect *Giardia,* but zinc sulfate and Sheather sugar solution will float the cysts.

Ciliates

As with the rumen ciliates of cattle and sheep, nonpathogenic ciliates live in the cecum of the horse. These mutualists live in the warm, moist, particulate-rich medium of the cecum. Sometimes ciliates may be observed in the diarrheic feces of horses and are often recovered on fecal flotation.

Apicomplexans

Parasite: *Eimeria leuckarti*
Host: Equine

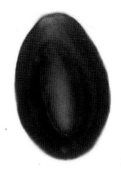

FIGURE 11-19 Unsporulated oocyst of *Eimeria leuckarti* (350×).

Location: Small intestine
Distribution: Worldwide
Derivation of Genus: Named after the German zoologist Gustav Eimer
Transmission Route: Ingestion of oocysts
Common Name: Coccidia
Zoonotic: No

Eimeria leuckarti is the coccidian found in the small intestine of horses, particularly young ones, in the United States. Infections are usually asymptomatic and self-limiting but can cause inflammation of the intestinal cells. Horses rapidly become immune to further infection. This protozoan demonstrates unique oocysts that are quite large, 80 to 87 μm × 55 to 60 μm, and dark brown, with a thick wall and a distinct micropyle at the narrow end (Figure 11-19). These oocysts can be recovered on fecal flotation using saturated sodium nitrate (1:360) and saturated sugar solution (1:320); however, they also may be easily recovered using fecal sedimentation. The oocysts of *E. leuckarti* are the largest coccidian oocysts. They are frequently described in histopathologic examination.

> **TECHNICIAN'S NOTE** *Eimeria leuckarti* infections are typically asymptomatic and self-limiting.

CIRCULATORY SYSTEM AND BLOOD

Apicomplexans are the protozoans that infect the circulatory system and blood of horses.

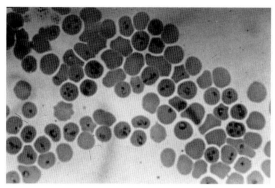

FIGURE 11-20 Basophilic, pear-shaped trophozoites of *Babesia equi* in red blood cells in stained equine blood smear. Trophozoites of *B. equi* may be round, ameboid, or pyriform (pear-shaped). Four organisms may be joined, giving the effect of a Maltese cross. Individual organisms are 2 to 3 μm long.

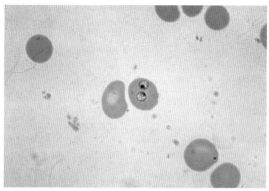

FIGURE 11-21 Trophozoites of *Babesia caballi* in red blood cells in stained equine blood smear. These piroplasms are pyriform, round or oval, and 2 to 4 μm long. They occur characteristically in pairs at acute angles to each other.

Apicomplexans

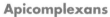

Parasite: *Theileria* (formerly *Babesia*) *equi* and *Babesia caballi*
Host: Equine
Location: Within RBCs
Distribution: Europe, Africa, Asia, North and South America
Derivation of Genus: Named after the famous bacteriologist Victor Babès
Transmission Route: Bite by infective tick
Common Name: Equine piroplasm
Zoonotic: No

Theileria equi and *Babesia caballi* are intracellular parasites found within the erythrocytes of horses. They are also referred to as the *equine piroplasms*. The parasites cause damage by residing in the RBCs. These parasites are spread by the bite of infected ticks. Diagnosis is by observing basophilic, pear-shaped trophozoites in RBCs in stained blood smears. Trophozoites of *T. equi* may be round, ameboid, or pyriform (pear-shaped). Four organisms may be joined, giving the effect of a Maltese cross (Figure 11-20). Individual organisms are 2 to 3 μm long. Trophozoites of *B. caballi* are pyriform, round, or oval and 2 to 4 μm long. They occur characteristically in pairs at acute angles to each other (Figure 11-21). Common symptoms include fever, depression, icterus, anorexia, hemoglobinuria, pale mucous membranes, weakness, and splenomegaly.

TECHNICIAN'S NOTE *Babesia* and *Theileria* use different tick intermediate hosts.

UROGENITAL SYSTEM

The protozoans that infect the urogenital system of horses are apicomplexans.

Apicomplexans

Parasite: *Klossiella equi*
Host: Equine
Location of Adult: Kidneys
Distribution: Worldwide
Derivation of Genus: Little organism; named after a parasitologist, Kloss
Transmission Route: Ingestion of oocysts in urine
Common Name: *Klossiella*
Zoonotic: No

Klossiella equi is a nonpathogenic coccidian infecting the kidney of horses. Oocysts can occasionally be found during histopathologic examination of the kidney and in urine sediment. There is no marked inflammatory response to infection with *Klossiella* in the horse.

TECHNICIAN'S NOTE Pathologic effects due to inflammation have been reported only in immune-compromised horses.

NERVOUS SYSTEM

Apicomplexans are the protozoans that infect the nervous system of horses.

Apicomplexans

Parasite: *Sarcocystis neurona*
Host: Equine
Location: Schizogonous, or asexual, stage found in the nervous system
Distribution: North, Central, and South America
Derivation of Genus: Flesh cyst
Transmission Route: Ingestion of oocysts from opposum feces
Common name: (*Sarcocystis*)
Zoonotic: No

Sarcocystis neurona is sporadically found in the asexual, or schizogonous, stage of development in the nervous system, particularly the spinal cord, of horses. This stage can invade the central nervous system, producing a condition called equine protozoal myeloencephalitis (EPM). This disease most often affects standardbreds and thoroughbreds. Clinical signs are caused mainly by destruction of neurons. Clinical signs are ataxia, weakness, stumbling, muscle wasting, and disorientation. *S. neurona* oocysts are ingested from food or water that has been contaminated with opossum feces. EPM can resemble many other equine neurologic diseases, including wobbler syndrome, the neurologic form of herpesvirus infection, rabies, West Nile virus infection, and other equine viral encephalitis diseases (e.g., eastern and western equine encephalitis). These developmental stages cannot be seen antemortem. Diagnosis of this parasite is by histopathologic examination. Tissues suspected of harboring developmental stages of *S. neurona* should be submitted to a histopathology laboratory for diagnosis by a veterinary pathologist or parasitologist.

S. neurona causes encephalomyelitis in many species of mammals and is the most important cause of neurologic disease in horses. Its complete life cycle is unknown, particularly its development and localization in the opossum intermediate host or the equine aberrant host.

> ◖TECHNICIAN'S NOTE *Sarcocystis neurona* can invade the central nervous system of the horse and cause equine protozoal myeloencephalitis.

SWINE

GASTROINTESTINAL TRACT

Protozoans that infect the gastrointestinal tract of swine are ciliates and apicomplexans.

Ciliates

Parasite: ⊘ *Balantidium coli* (also see discussion in canine section)
Host: Swine and occasionally canines
Location: Large intestine
Distribution: Worldwide
Derivation of Name: Small bag
Transmission Route: Ingestion of oocysts
Common Name: *Balantidium*
Zoonotic: Yes (per *The Merck Veterinary Manual*)

B. coli is the ciliated protozoan found in the large intestine of swine. Although it is often observed during microscopic examination of fresh diarrheic feces, it is generally considered to be nonpathogenic. Two morphologic stages can be found in feces: the cyst stage and the trophozoite stage. Both stages may vary in size. This is a very large protozoan parasite. The trophozoites may be 150 × 120 μm, with a sausage- to kidney-shaped macronucleus. *B. coli* is covered with numerous rows of cilia and moves about the field with lively motility. The cyst is spherical to ovoid, 40 to 60 μm in diameter, and has a slight greenish-yellow color. Both of these stages may be easily recognized by microscopic examination of the intestinal contents of fresh, diarrheic feces by fecal flotation and fecal direct smear. Figure 11-22 demonstrates the trophozoite stage of *B. coli* recovered on fecal flotation, and Figures 11-23 and 11-24 demonstrate *B. coli* in histopathologic sections.

Apicomplexans

Parasite: *Cystoisospora suis* (see also discussion of *Cystoisospora* spp. in the canine and feline section)

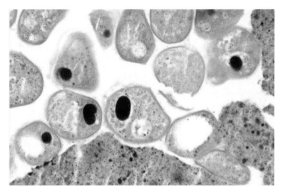

FIGURE 11-22 Motile trophozoite stage of *Balantidium coli*, a ciliated protozoan found in the large intestine of swine, is often observed during microscopic examination of fresh diarrheic feces. It is covered with numerous rows of cilia and moves about the field of view with lively motility.

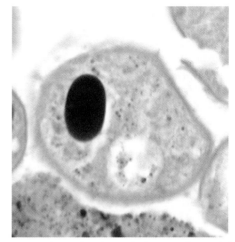

FIGURE 11-24 *Balantidium coli* of swine in histopathologic section. This photomicrograph was taken at higher magnification than Figure 11-23.

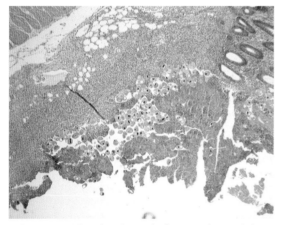

FIGURE 11-23 *Balantidium coli* of swine in histopathologic section. This photomicrograph was taken at low magnification. Note that *B. coli* is quite large and easily visible *(arrows)*.

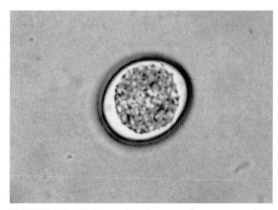

FIGURE 11-25 Unsporulated oocyst of swine coccidian, *Cystoisospora suis*, recovered from swine feces (560×).

Host: Swine
Location: Small intestine
Distribution: Worldwide
Derivation of Genus: Bladder same spore
Transmission Route: Ingestion of oocysts
Common Name: Coccidia
Zoonotic: No

Cystoisospora suis is the coccidian that parasitizes the small intestine of swine, especially young piglets. The merozoite stage causes inflammation in the small intestine. Oocysts are usually found on flotation of fresh feces. They are subspherical, lack a micropyle, and measure 18 to 21 μm. Common symptoms include diarrhea, dehydration, and weight loss. Postmortem diagnosis in piglets exhibiting clinical signs but not shedding oocysts can be achieved by direct smear of the jejunum stained with Diff-Quik. Diagnosis is by observation of the banana-shaped merozoites. The prepatent period is 4 to 8 days. (Figure 11-25 shows features of the oocyst of *C. suis*.)

TECHNICIAN'S NOTE The prepatent period for *Cystoisospora suis* is a short 4 to 8 days.

Parasite: ⓩ *Cryptosporidium* species (also see discussion in canine and feline section)
Host: Canines, felines, bovines, swine, avians, guinea pigs, snakes, and mice
Location: Small intestine
Distribution: Worldwide
Derivation of Genus: Hidden small seeds
Transmission Route: Ingestion of oocyst
Common Name: *Cryptosporidium*, Crypto
Zoonotic: Yes

The *Cryptosporidium* species is another coccidian that parasitizes the small intestine of a variety of animals, including swine. The sporulated oocysts in the feces are colorless and transparent and measure only 3 to 5 μm. Diagnosis is by standard fecal flotation and stained fecal smears. Because humans may become infected with *Cryptosporidium* species, feces suspected of harboring this protozoan should be handled with great care. (See Figure 11-11 for features of the oocysts of *Cryptosporidium* species.)

> ▌**TECHNICIAN'S NOTE** *Cryptosporidium* species are transferred from host to host by ingestion of oocysts. Because humans are hosts, feces suspected of containing the oocysts should be handled with great care.

PET AND AVIARY BIRDS AND OTHER DOMESTIC FOWL

GASTROINTESTINAL TRACT

Protozoans that infect the gastrointestinal tract of birds are flagellates and apicomplexans.

Flagellates
Parasite: *Giardia psittaci* (see also discussion at beginning of chapter)
Host: Avians
Location of Adults: Intestinal mucosa
Distribution: Worldwide
Derivation of Genus: Named after the famous protozoologist Alfred Giard
Transmission Route: Ingestion of oocysts

Common Name: *Giardia*
Zoonotic: No (only assemblage A is zoonotic)

Giardia psittaci is the most common protozoan seen in pet bird practices. This flagellated parasite is most often found in cockatiels, budgerigars, and lovebirds. The feces of affected birds often become voluminous and chunky, with a pea-soup consistency. Fresh saline mounts can demonstrate the motile trophozoites, with the characteristic "falling leaf" motility. Allergic skin conditions may be associated with giardiasis in cockatiels. It may be difficult to demonstrate *Giardia* in some of these cases.

The fecal trichrome stain can enhance visualization of *Giardia* species (Figure 11-26). Other stains used to enhance visualization of this flagellate include Lugol iodine, Gram iodine, and Wright stain. Other stains, such as acid-fast stain or Gram stain, may incidentally demonstrate trophozoites (Figure 11-27).

Parasite: *Histomonas meleagridis*
Host: Turkeys, peafowl, chickens, and pheasants
Location: Liver
Distribution: Worldwide
Derivation of Genus: Tissue unit
Transmission Route: Ingestion of intermediate host ova, *Heterakis gallinarum*, or direct ingestion of ova
Common Name: "Blackhead"
Zoonotic: No

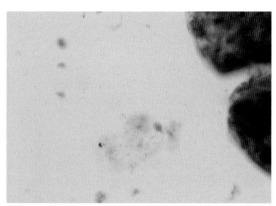

FIGURE 11-26 *Giardia* trophozoites (trichrome stain) from feces of a cockatiel.

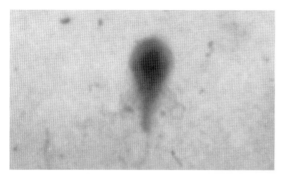

FIGURE 11-27 *Giardia* trophozoite showing flagellar detail in Gram-stained fecal smear. This was an incidental finding because Gram stain is not the stain of choice for flagellates.

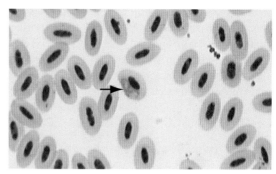

FIGURE 11-28 *Trichomonas gallinae* in the crop wash from a dove.

Histomonas meleagridis infects turkeys, chickens, pheasants, and peafowl, causing a fatal liver disease called infectious enterohepatitis, or blackhead. The oocysts are ingested directly from infective feces or within the intermediate host ova, *Heterakis gallinarum*. *H. gallinarum* ova can survive for extended periods of up to years in the environment. Within several days of being ingested, the oocysts are released by the intermediate host ova, reproduce in the cecum, and migrate to the liver where they cause inflammation and necrosis of liver cells. Diagnosis is usually by necropsy and histopathologic examination of the liver. Suspect tissues should be submitted to a histopathology laboratory for diagnosis by a veterinary pathologist or parasitologist. Suspicion of infection is increased by finding on fecal flotation the eggs of the cecal worm, *H. gallinarum,* which serves as the intermediate host for this parasite.

> **TECHNICIAN'S NOTE** If *Heterakis gallinarum* ova are found on fecal flotation, *Histomonas meleagridis* should also be suspected.

Parasite: *Trichomonas gallinae*
Host: Pigeons, doves, poultry, and raptors that feed on pigeons
Location of Adult: Crop
Distribution: North America and countries with doves and pigeons
Derivation of Genus: Hair unit

Transmission Route: Direct contact with contaminated water or an infected bird
Common Name: *Trichomonas*
Zoonotic: No

Trichomonas gallinae is frequently found in crop washes and crop swabs of pigeons, doves, and poultry. Occasionally this parasite is associated with mortality in finches. In North America trichomoniasis appears to be rare in psittacine birds but has been reported in budgerigars. *T. gallinae* does not produce oocysts, so only direct contact with contaminated water from an infected bird or direct contact with an infected bird from fighting or feeding will result in transfer of the parasite. *T. gallinae* produces nodules in the crop that can cause cell death and obstructions. The parasite is best demonstrated by a direct saline smear of crop contents and is characterized by four anterior flagella. An air-dried smear can be stained with Wright stain. The parasite assumes an oval shape, staining blue with a red axostyle (Figure 11-28).

> **TECHNICIAN'S NOTE** A severe infection of *Trichomonas gallinae* can result in the parasite spreading to the esophagus and even to the liver.

Apicomplexans

Coccidial infections are rare in pet birds, although *Cystoisospora* and *Eimeria* have been reported. Coccidia are often observed in poultry and pigeons. A common error made by inexperienced veterinary technicians is to mistake normal urate crystals for coccidia. *Cryptosporidium* species has been reported in cockatiels. This tiny apicomplexan parasite is difficult to visualize in fecal samples and is usually diagnosed by histopathologic examination of the small intestine. Suspect tissues should be submitted to a histopathology laboratory for diagnosis by a veterinary pathologist or parasitologist.

CIRCULATORY SYSTEM AND BLOOD

Protozoans that infect the circulatory system and blood of birds are flagellates and apicomplexans.

Flagellates

Parasite: *Trypanosoma* species (see discussion in canine and feline section)
Host: Cockatoos
Location of Adult: Peripheral blood
Distribution: Worldwide
Derivation of Genus: Borer body
Transmission Route: No definitive intermediate hosts have been identified for birds
Common Name: Trypanosome
Zoonotic: Yes

Trypanosoma species is occasionally found in cockatoos and rarely produces clinical disease. As with the trypanosomes of mammals, this swimming, flagellated protozoan does not infect the RBCs. It has a very distinctive appearance, with a posterior flagellum and an undulating membrane (Figure 11-29).

> **TECHNICIAN'S NOTE** *Trypanosoma* species are not a major concern in cockatoos because they rarely produce clinical disease.

Apicomplexans

Parasite: *Haemoproteus* species
Host: Cockatoos, green-winged macaws, and some species of conures
Location: Within RBCs
Distribution: Worldwide
Derivation of Genus: Many forms in the blood
Transmission Route: Bite by an infected *Culicoides* species or *Chrysops* species of fly
Common Name: *Haemoproteus*
Zoonotic: No

Haemoproteus species is often found within the RBCs of the white species of cockatoos, green-winged macaws, and some species of conures. This blood parasite is rarely associated with clinical disease such as anemia but can destroy RBCs if anemia is associated with the clinical disease. *Haemoproteus* is characterized by a bluish, sausage-shaped body in the cytoplasm of the RBC; sometimes the body is overlain with blue dots (Figure 11-30). It infects a variety of wild waterfowl and can cause death in these birds.

> **TECHNICIAN'S NOTE** Some species of *Haemoproteus* infect turtles and lizards.

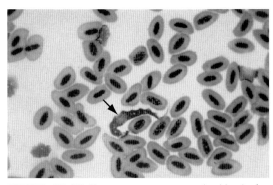

FIGURE 11-29 *Trypanosoma* species in the blood of a cockatoo.

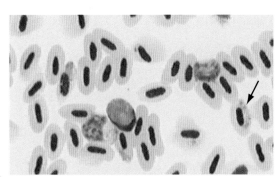

FIGURE 11-30 *Haemoproteus* is normally seen as a sausage-shaped body within the cytoplasm of the avian red blood cell.

Parasite: *Plasmodium* species
Host: Avians
Location: Within RBCs
Distribution: Worldwide
Derivation of Genus: Any thing formed
Transmission Route: Bite of infected mosquito
Common Name: Avian malaria
Zoonotic: No

Plasmodium species is the etiologic agent of avian malaria. It can cause mortality in canaries in some parts of the United States. This may be the result of the transmission of a local passerine strain by the mosquito intermediate host to susceptible canaries. The organism may not be observable in the peripheral blood cells; many of the developmental stages of *Plasmodium* species occur in internal organs, such as the liver and spleen, and can cause inflammation in these organs. A "signet ring" form, in which the body of the organism displaces the nucleus of the RBC, is the most frequently observed form (Figure 11-31), which can cause cell destruction leading to anemia. Diagnosis of infections with *Plasmodium* species is also by organ impression smears and histopathologic examination of the liver and the spleen. Tissues suspected of harboring developmental stages of *Plasmodium* should be submitted to a histopathology laboratory for confirmation by a veterinary pathologist or parasitologist. Polymerase chain reaction tests have also been developed for testing of *Plasmodium* species.

Parasite: *Leucocytozoon* species
Host: Raptors
Location: Within WBCs
Distribution: Worldwide
Derivation of Genus: White cell organism
Transmission Route: Bite of infected black flies, *Simulium* species
Common Name: *Leucocytozoon*
Zoonotic: No

Leucocytozoon species infects the white blood cells of raptors—birds of prey such as owls, hawks, and falcons. The presence of this large protozoan organism greatly distorts the shape and appearance of the WBC. A variety of forms can be present and can be associated with occasional leukocytosis and disease. The most common morphology of this protozoan is the fusiform, or spindle, shape (Figure 11-32). Most infections are subclinical, but deaths have been reported.

> **TECHNICIAN'S NOTE** The *Leucocytozoon* parasite distorts the WBC to the point that it may not be recognized as such.

Parasite: *Aegyptianella* species
Host: Pet birds

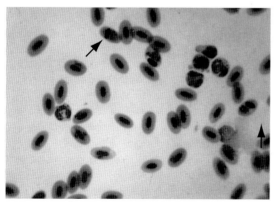

FIGURE 11-31 *Plasmodium* displacing the nucleus of an erythrocyte in the blood of a canary.

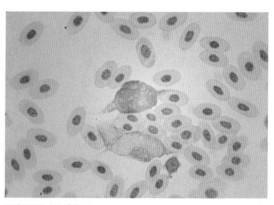

FIGURE 11-32 *Leucocytozoon* species in an avian peripheral blood smear.

Location of Adult: Within RBCs
Distribution: Primarily in the Mediterranean areas
Derivation of Genus: Little organism from Egypt
Transmission Route: Bite of an argasid tick
Common Name: *Aegyptianella*
Zoonotic: No

Aegyptianella species is occasionally found in pet birds such as the African gray parrot. This protozoan causes few clinical problem. The organism infects the RBCs, appearing as a marginated dot on the cells.

RESPIRATORY SYSTEM

The protozoans that infect the respiratory system of birds are apicomplexans.

Apicomplexans
Parasite: *Cystoisospora serini*
Host: Canaries and finches
Location: Lung, liver, and spleen
Distribution: Worldwide
Derivation of Genus: Same bladder organism
Transmission Route: Ingestion of oocyst during sexual stage
Common Name: Coccidia or atoxoplasmosis
Zoonotic: No

Cystoisospora (formerly *Atoxoplasma*) *serini* is a protozoan coccidial parasite of canaries and finches (Figure 11-33). *C. serini* can affect several organs,

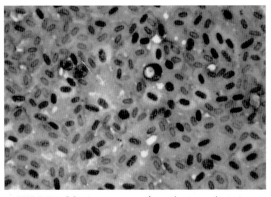

FIGURE 11-33 *Cystoisospora* (formerly *Atoxoplasma*) *serini* in a mononuclear cell on a lung impression smear from a canary (Wright stain).

causing respiratory signs related to inflammation of those organs. The parasite goes through a sexual cycle in the intestinal mucosa, at which time oocysts can be passed in the feces. However, few oocysts are typically seen after the sexual cycle has passed. An asexual cycle occurs in the liver, lungs, and spleen causing inflammation to these organs. This parasite is best visualized on organ impression smears of the lung, liver, and spleen.

> **TECHNICIAN'S NOTE** *Cystoisospora serini* causes atoxoplasmosis in canaries and finches.

RABBITS

GASTROINTESTINAL TRACT

The protozoans that infect the gastrointestinal tract of rabbits are apicomplexans.

Apicomplexans
Parasite: *Eimeria irresidua, Eimeria magna, Eimeria media,* and *Eimeria perforans*
Host: Lagomorph (rabbit)
Location: Small intestine; *E. media* also affects the large intestine
Distribution: Worldwide
Derivation of Genus: Organism named after German zoologist Gustav Eimer
Transmission Route: Ingestion of oocysts
Common Name: Coccidia of rabbits
Zoonotic: No

Numerous species of *Eimeria* can infect rabbits. Most infect the intestine, causing intestinal coccidiosis, and one species, *Eimeria stiedae*, affects the bile ducts within the liver. The more pathogenic varieties of *Eimeria* species that affect the intestine are discussed in this section, and *E. stiedai* is considered separately. The intestinal coccidia of rabbits include *Eimeria irresidua, Eimeria magna, Eimeria media,* and *Eimeria perforans*. All species of *Eimeria* infect the small intestine; *E. media* may also affect the large intestine.

The oocysts of *E. irresidua* are 38 × 26 μm and ovoid. The wall of the oocyst is smooth and light yellow. There is a wide micropyle, with no polar

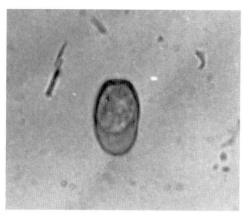

FIGURE 11-34 Unsporulated oocyst of the rabbit intestinal coccidian *Eimeria magna.*

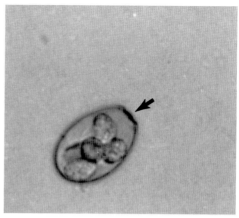

FIGURE 11-35 Oocyst of *Eimeria magna* after sporulation. *Arrow* indicates a micropyle. Round darkened body in the center of the oocyst is a residuum. Four lighter oval bodies are sporocysts.

granules or residuum. Sporocysts within the oocyst are also ovoid, with both a body and a residuum. Antemortem diagnosis depends on recognition of the mature oocyst along with clinical signs, which may include severe hemorrhagic diarrhea, excessive thirst, and dehydration caused by inflammation of the intestines. Postmortem indications include inflammation of the intestines and sloughing of the lining of the intestine.

> **TECHNICIAN'S NOTE** *Eimeria irresidua, Eimeria magna, Eimeria media,* and *Eimeria perforans* all infect the small intestine, whereas *Eimeria stiedai* infects the bile ducts.

The mature oocyst of *E. magna* is 35 × 24 µm and ovoid, with a distinctive dark, yellow-brown wall (Figure 11-34). A wide micropyle appears built up around the rim, with no micropyle cap. Oocysts and sporocysts contain a residuum (Figure 11-35). The sporocysts are ovoid and have a body. *E. magna,* like *E. irresidua,* is highly pathogenic. Clinical signs include weight loss, anorexia, and mucoid diarrhea. Necropsy signs include inflammation and sloughing of the lining of the intestine.

E. *media* oocysts are ovoid and 31 × 18 µm, with a smooth wall and a light-pink color. There is a micropyle and a residuum. Sporocysts within the mature oocyst are ovoid, with a body and a residuum. *E. media* is moderately pathogenic and may

cause enteritis and diarrhea caused by inflammation of the intestines. At necropsy, the intestinal wall may be edematous and contain gray foci of necrosis.

Parasite: *Eimeria stiedae*
Host: Lagomorph (rabbit)
Location: Bile ducts
Distribution: Worldwide
Derivation of genus: Organism named after German zoologist Gustav Eimer
Transmission Route: Ingestion of oocysts
Common Name: Coccidia of rabbits
Zoonotic: No

E. *stiedae* is a highly pathogenic coccidian that affects the bile ducts of rabbits. It causes variable mortality, which is highest in young rabbits. Oocysts of *E. stiedae* are 35 × 20 µm and ovoid, with a flattened pole at the micropyle end. The wall is smooth and yellow. There is no polar granule or residuum. Sporocysts are ovoid, with a body and a residuum.

Light infections with *E. stiedae* usually produce no clinical signs. Heavier infections may cause blockage of the bile ducts and impaired liver function, resulting in icterus and a distended abdomen caused by liver enlargement. Diarrhea or constipation and anorexia may be noted. At necropsy, white, dilated nodules are likely to be seen in the liver. Hyperplastic bile ducts contain a yellow-green creamy material in which oocysts may be seen in impression smears when examined microscopically. Transmission of *E. stiedae* is by ingestion of sporulated oocysts passed in the feces. The prepatent period is 15 to 18 days. As in all *Eimeria* species, there is no cross-species contamination or public health significance.

TECHNICIAN'S NOTE *Eimeria stiedae* is a highly pathogenic coccidian of rabbits.

MICE

GASTROINTESTINAL TRACT

Protozoans that infect the gastrointestinal tract of mice are flagellates and apicomplexans.

Flagellates

A few flagellates may be found by direct smear or fecal flotation from the mouse. They include *Giardia* assemblage G, *Spironucleus muris, Tetratrichomonas microti,* and *Tritrichomonas muris.*

Parasite: *Tetratrichomonas microti* and *Tritrichomonas muris*
Host: Mouse
Location: Small intestine, cecum, and colon
Distribution: Worldwide
Derivation of Genus: Four hair unit, three hair unit
Transmission Route: Ingestion of oocysts
Common Name: Flagellates of mice
Zoonotic: No

T. microti and *T. muris* are generally considered nonpathogenic in the mouse. Tritrichomonads and tetratrichomonads have three and four anterior flagella, respectively. Both genera have a trailing caudal flagellum. These trichomonads are frequently found in the small intestine, cecum, and colon of the mouse. Mice with diarrhea, regardless of the cause, often have numerous tritrichomonads and tetratrichomonads on fecal smear and flotation because the diarrheic fluid medium secondarily provides an optimal habitat for the multiplication

of these intestinal protozoans. Transmission of these trichomonads is by ingestion of organisms passed in the feces. *T. microti* is approximately 22 × 10 μm, and *T. muris* is approximately 7 × 5 μm.

TECHNICIAN'S NOTE *Tetratrichomonas microti* and *Tritrichomonas muris* are commonly found in diarrhea because diarrhea supplies an optimal habitat for multiplication.

Parasite: *Giardia* assemblage G and *Spironucleus muris*
Host: Rodents (*Giardia* assemblage G), mice
Location: Proximal small intestine
Distribution: Worldwide
Derivation of Genus: Named after the famous biologist Alfred Giard (*Giardia*)
Transmission Route: Ingestion of oocyst
Common Name: *Giardia* (*Giardia* spp.), flagellates of mice (*S. muris*)
Zoonotic: No (only assemblage A is zoonotic)

Giardia and *S. muris* are the most common mouse flagellates and demonstrate the greatest potential for pathogenicity. Both *S. muris* and *Giardia* occur in the proximal small intestine and can produce enteritis related to inflammation, particularly in young weanling mice. The location of these flagellates in the intestines is proportional to the severity of the enteritis produced; the more severe the enteritis, the farther back (more distally) in the intestinal tract they are found. *Giardia* assemblage G appears similar to other *Giardia* species. The trophozoite is pyriform (pear-shaped), with two nuclei at the anterior end. Eight flagella emerge in symmetric pairs from different locations cranially to caudally in the organism. *Giardia* species may be suspected when motile forms are observed on a direct smear at 100× (high-dry) magnification. *Giardia* species are identified by staining the direct fecal smear with Lugol iodine, which enhances the detail of the cranial nuclei and flagella.

Transmission of *Giardia* is by ingestion of cysts that have been passed in the feces. *Giardia* has also been found in the rat and hamster; therefore the owner of multiple species should be made aware of the possibility of cross-contamination. Although other species of *Giardia* are pathogenic to humans, the *Giardia* species found in rodents and rabbits have no known zoonotic potential.

S. muris appears somewhat similar to *Giardia* species except that the trophozoite of *S. muris* is uniformly slender, unlike the widened anterior end of *Giardia* species. *S. muris* has two anterior nuclei. There are three pairs of anterior flagella and one pair of trailing caudal flagella.

> **TECHNICIAN'S NOTE** *Spironucleus muris* appears similar to *Giardia* assemblage G on fecal flotation, but the trophozoite is uniformly slender compared with the widened anterior end of *Giardia* species on direct smear.

Apicomplexans
Parasite: *Eimeria falciformis, Eimeria ferrisi,* and *Eimeria hansonorum*
Host: Mice
Location: *E. falciformis* and *E. hansonorum* (small intestines); *E. ferrisi* (cecum)
Distribution: Worldwide
Derivation of Genus: Named after German biologist Gustav Eimer
Transmission Route: Ingestion of oocysts
Common Name: Coccidia of mice
Zoonotic: No

Several species of *Eimeria* infect mice, including *Eimeria falciformis, Eimeria ferrisi,* and *Eimeria hansonorum*. *E. falciformis* and *E. hansonorum* infect the small intestine, whereas *E. ferrisi* is found in the cecum. Although mixed infections can occur, little is known concerning the pathogenicity of *E. ferrisi* and *E. hansonorum*.

E. falciformis is common in wild mouse populations. Oocysts are 14 to 26 µm × 11 to 24 µm, round to oval, smooth, and colorless. There is no micropyle or residuum. Sporocysts are oval and have a residuum and a small body. There are two sporozoites per sporocyst and four sporocysts per sporulated oocyst. Oocysts of *E. ferrisi* and *E. hansonorum* appear similar to those of *E. falciformis,* except they are small, 16 to 18 µm, and more spherical. *E. ferrisi* has a small body on the sporocysts, whereas *E. hansonorum* has a broad body.

Oocysts of *Eimeria* species can be detected by fecal flotation. As in coccidial infections in other species, finding oocysts on fecal flotation does not necessarily mean that *Eimeria* species is a primary cause of the disease. Diagnosis is made by considering clinical signs usually caused by inflammation, enteric lesions, and identification of the coccidia in histopathologic section. Again, tissues suspected of harboring developmental stages of murine coccidiosis should be submitted to a histopathology laboratory for confirmation by a veterinary pathologist or parasitologist.

> **TECHNICIAN'S NOTE** Finding *Eimeria* species oocysts does not mean that this organism is the primary cause of a disease.

Clinical signs, if seen, are usually in younger animals that have developed little to no immunity and may include diarrhea, catarrhal enteritis, anorexia, hemorrhage, and epithelial sloughing.

As with other species of *Eimeria*, transmission is by ingestion of sporulated oocysts that have been passed in the feces. Oocysts passed in the feces sporulate in about 3 days. *Eimeria* species are host specific and thus are not considered zoonotic parasites.

UROGENITAL SYSTEM
The protozoans that infect the urogenital system of mice are apicomplexans.

Apicomplexans
Parasite: *Klossiella muris*
Host: Mice
Location: Kidneys
Distribution: Worldwide
Derivation of Genus: Little organism found by a researcher named Kloss
Transmission Route: Ingestion of oocysts
Common Name: *Klossiella*
Zoonotic: No

Klossiella muris is a relatively nonpathogenic coccidian that occurs mainly in the kidneys of both wild and laboratory mice. This parasite has also been found in different stages of its life cycle in the adrenal and thyroid glands and in the brain, lung, and spleen. The oocyst of *K. muris* matures in the endothelial cells that line the arterioles and capillaries associated with the glomeruli of the kidney. At maturity, the oocyst is 40 μm in diameter. The oocyst grows and divides to form sporoblasts, which eventually rupture the host's endothelial cells and pass through the urine as sporocysts. Other mice are then infected by ingestion of sporulated oocysts.

K. muris cannot be detected antemortem. On postmortem examination, the kidneys may appear enlarged and have small gray necrotic areas on the surface. Histopathologic examination reveals that most of the necrotic areas are at the corticomedullary junction. Infection with *K. muris* is usually diagnosed from gross and microscopic lesions, including finding the organism in renal tissue. Tissues suspected of harboring developmental stages of renal coccidiosis should be submitted to a histopathology laboratory for confirmation by a veterinary pathologist or parasitologist.

Transmission of *K. muris* is by ingestion of the sporulated sporocysts passed in the urine. Because wild mice can carry this parasite, strict sanitation and prevention of wild mouse access to the pet population are necessary to control this parasite. *K. muris* is species specific and is not a zoonotic parasite.

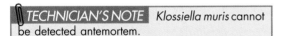

TECHNICIAN'S NOTE *Klossiella muris* cannot be detected antemortem.

RATS

GASTROINTESTINAL TRACT

The protozoans that infect the gastrointestinal tract of rats are flagellates and apicomplexans.

Flagellates

Although somewhat less susceptible than mice, rats may be infected with the flagellates discussed previously in the mouse section: *Giardia* assemblage G, *S. muris*, *T. microti*, and *T. muris*. Identification, detection, clinical signs, and transmission in rats are similar to those discussed for the mouse.

Apicomplexans

Parasite: *Eimeria nieschultzi*
Host: Rats
Location: Intestines
Distribution: Worldwide
Derivation of Genus: Named after zoologist Gustav Eimer
Transmission Route: Ingestion of oocysts
Common Name: Coccidia of rats
Zoonotic: No

Eimeria nieschultzi is an intestinal coccidian uncommon in laboratory rats but common in wild rats. The sporulated oocyst of *E. nieschultzi* is oval, 16 to 26 μm × 13 to 21 μm, with no residuum. It has a smooth or colorless wall with no micropyle. The sporulated oocyst contains four oval sporocysts, each with a small Stieda body and a residuum.

Antemortem, *E. nieschultzi* may be detected by finding the oocysts in fecal flotations or direct fecal smears. However, diagnosis is usually based on identification of the organism histopathologically in sections of the intestinal epithelium. Clinical signs of *E. nieschultzi* infections are usually seen in young rats less than several months of age. Signs include diarrhea, weakness, emaciation, and possibly death due to inflammation of the intestines. Rats become infected with *E. nieschultzi* by ingestion of sporulated oocysts in the feces. *E. nieschultzi* is species specific and therefore is not considered a potential cross-contaminant or zoonotic problem.

TECHNICIAN'S NOTE *E. nieschultzi* is uncommon in pet rats but is common in wild rats.

HAMSTERS

GASTROINTESTINAL TRACT

The protozoans that infect the gastrointestinal tract of hamsters are flagellates.

Flagellates

Hamsters typically carry numerous intestinal flagellates without showing clinical signs. These parasites can be observed in fecal flotations or direct smear preparations. These flagellates include

Giardia species, *S. muris, Tetranucleus microti,* and *T. muris (criceti)*. Infected hamsters may serve as a source of infection for more susceptible rodents, such as in the transmission of *S. muris* to mice.

The identification, detection, clinical signs, transmission, and public health significance of this parasite in hamsters are similar to those discussed for the mouse.

> **TECHNICIAN'S NOTE** Hamsters carry numerous intestinal flagellates but do not tend to show clinical signs of these protozoans.

GUINEA PIGS

GASTROINTESTINAL TRACT

The protozoans that infect the gastrointestinal tract of guinea pigs are flagellates, amoebae, and apicomplexans.

Flagellates

Parasite: *Giardia* assemblage G
Host: Rodents
Location of Adult: Proximal small intestine
Distribution: Worldwide
Derivation of Genus: Named after the famous zoologist Alfred Giard
Common Name: *Giardia*
Zoonotic: No (only assemblage A is zoonotic)

Trophozoites of *Giardia* assemblage G are similar to those previously described. The body is pyriform, or pear-shaped. Two nuclei lie at the anterior end, and four pairs of flagella emerge at various points of the body. Trophozoites are 8 to 15 μm $\times$ 6.5 μm. Cysts are about the same size as the trophozoites and contain two to four nuclei.

Cysts or trophozoites of *Giardia* may be detected in a direct fecal smear or possibly in a fecal flotation preparation. If fecal flotation is used, zinc sulfate solution is preferred because sugar and salt solutions may distort the cysts. Diarrheic animals should be examined by direct smear for the presence of motile trophozoites; cyst forms will not be present.

There are no specific clinical signs in infected guinea pigs; however, mucoid diarrhea has been reported in other infected rodents. *Giardia* assemblage G is not considered a public health problem.

> **TECHNICIAN'S NOTE** *Giardia* assemblage G is not considered a public health hazard.

Parasite: *Tritrichomonas caviae*
Host: Guinea pig
Location: Cecum
Distribution: Worldwide
Derivation of Genus: Three hair unit
Transmission Route: Ingestion of oocysts
Common Name: Flagellate of guinea pigs
Zoonotic: No

Tritrichomonas caviae is of little or no pathologic significance in the guinea pig. As with *T. muris, T. caviae* has three anterior flagella and a trailing posterior flagellum. *T. caviae* measures 10 to 22 μm $\times$ 6 to 11 μm and is larger than *Giardia caviae*. It has an undulating membrane that extends the length of its body. These trichomonads are usually found in the cecum of the guinea pig. The veterinary technician should be aware that in cases of protracted diarrhea produced by another pathogen, *T. caviae* protozoans proliferate secondarily because of the fluid medium produced by the diarrhea. *T. caviae* therefore may be observed on direct fecal smear, particularly in animals exhibiting clinical signs of diarrhea.

T. caviae is transmitted between guinea pigs by ingestion of the trophozoites passed in the feces of carrier animals. *T. caviae* is not seen in other species of animals and is not considered a public health hazard.

> **TECHNICIAN'S NOTE** *Tritrichomonas caviae* typically proliferate (as a secondary infection) in the presence of another pathogen causing diarrhea as a result of the fluid medium produced by the diarrhea.

Amoebae

Parasite: *Entamoeba caviae*
Host: Guinea pigs

Location: Cecum
Distribution: Worldwide
Derivation of Genus: Internal amoeba
Transmission Route: Ingestion of oocysts
Common Name: Amoeba of guinea pigs
Zoonotic: No

Entamoeba caviae is a relatively common non-pathogenic cecal organism in guinea pigs; it is mentioned in this chapter to make the veterinary technician aware that it should be disregarded as a pathogenic organism. The most frequently observed form of this protozoan is the motile trophozoite. Cysts are infrequently observed on concentration with zinc sulfate flotation medium. Mature cysts are 11 to 27 µm and have eight nuclei. The trophozoites are most often found in a direct fecal smear and measure 10.5 to 20 µm in diameter. The appearance of these trophozoite stages can be enhanced by staining the direct fecal smear with Lugol iodine.

Entamoeba caviae is transmitted by ingestion of infective cyst forms that have been passed in the feces of chronic carrier guinea pigs. *Entamoeba caviae* is species specific and is not considered to be of zoonotic significance.

> **TECHNICIAN'S NOTE** *Entamoeba caviae* is nonpathogenic and can be found on fecal flotation and direct fecal smears.

Apicomplexans

Parasite: *Eimeria caviae*
Host: Guinea pigs
Location: Large intestine
Distribution: Worldwide
Derivation of Genus: Named after zoologist Gustav Eimer
Transmission Route: Ingestion of oocysts
Common Name: Coccidia of guinea pigs
Zoonotic: No

Eimeria caviae is a typical coccidian, with an oval to slightly subspherical oocyst that is 13 to 26 µm × 12 to 23 µm. Oocyst walls are brown and have no micropyle or polar granule. However, oocysts

contain a residuum, as do sporocysts. *Eimeria caviae* is commonly found in the guinea pig's large intestine, particularly the ascending or proximal colon.

Eimeria caviae can be detected by fecal flotation. Repeated flotation should be done 4 to 5 days apart for 2 to 3 weeks. Diagnosis is made more consistently postmortem, at which time intestinal scrapings placed in saline may be examined microscopically for both intracellular intestinal stages and oocysts of *Eimeria caviae*.

Eimeria caviae is generally nonpathogenic, but young animals stressed by poor nutrition and husbandry may show clinical signs. Clinical signs are limited to diarrhea seen 11 to 13 days after exposure related to inflammation of the intestine. The diarrhea ceases after a few days if the animal is not reinfected. Diarrhea may continue if reinfection occurs. As with the other protozoans of guinea pigs, *Eimeria caviae* is species specific and is not considered of zoonotic significance.

> **TECHNICIAN'S NOTE** *Eimeria caviae* is essentially nonpathogenic but can cause symptoms in young stressed animals with poor nutrition and husbandry.

Parasite: 🅩 *Cryptosporidium wrairi*
Host: Guinea pigs
Location of Adult: Tips of the intestinal villi of the ileum
Distribution: Worldwide
Derivation of Genus: Hidden small seeds
Transmission Route: Ingestion of oocysts
Common Name: *Cryptosporidium* or Crypto
Zoonotic: Yes

Cryptosporidium wrairi of guinea pigs is similar to *C. parvum* and *C. muris* of mice. However, *C. wrairi* is considered a distinct species. *C. wrairi* is most often seen lining the tips of the intestinal villi in the ileum of young guinea pigs. Examination of fresh mucosal scrapings by phase-contrast microscopy may provide the best results in the detection and identification of *C. wrairi*. Examination of paraffin-embedded materials is least satisfactory, especially when formalin is used as a fixative. The organisms appear to be extracellular but actually are within the microvilli of the intestinal epithelial cells. The only clinical sign of *C. wrairi* infection is weight loss. Younger guinea pigs at 250 to 300 g are most likely to carry the parasite. Older animals seem to be resistant or to have developed immunity to *C. wrairi*. *C. wrairi* is not found in other species of animals and is not considered a public health problem.

> **TECHNICIAN'S NOTE** Examination of fresh mucosal scrapings of the intestinal villi is the preferred diagnostic test for *Cryptosporidium wrairi*.

FISH

SKIN

Protozoans that infect the skin of fish are ciliates.

Ciliates
Parasite: *Ichthyophthirius multifiliis*
Host: Freshwater and ornamental fish
Location: Skin, gills, fins, and eyes
Distribution: Worldwide
Derivation of Genus: Fish louse with many children
Transmission Route: Contact with infective stage of life cycle

Common Name: Ciliate of fish
Zoonotic: No

Ichthyophthirius multifiliis is a ciliate that infects the skin, gills, fins, and eyes of many freshwater tropical and ornamental fish in home aquaria and in hatcheries. This ciliated protozoan causes a skin disease called ichthyophthiriasis, or more commonly, *ich*. Ich is characterized by the formation of tiny white spots (the thin-walled trophozoite stage just beneath the epidermis) over many of the exposed surfaces of the fish. These parasites may be from 100 to 1000 µm in diameter, so they are grossly visible to the observer. Diagnosis is by observation of typical lesions; however, it is possible to perform skin scrapings on infected fish to reveal characteristic ciliates. *Cryptocaryon irritans*, a similar parasite, affects warm water marine (saltwater) fish. Other ciliates infecting fish include *Chilodonella, Tetrahymena*, and *Piscinoodinium*. As with *I. multifiliis*, there are marine counterparts for these genera. For details of these and other protozoan parasites of both freshwater and marine fish, a fish disease textbook should be consulted.

> **TECHNICIAN'S NOTE** *Ichthyophthirius multifiliis* is diagnosed by observation of typical lesions and skin scrapings.

CHAPTER ELEVEN TEST

MATCHING—Match the scientific name of each parasite with the correct name, phrase, or term.

A. *Giardia* species

B. *Entamoeba histolytica*

C. *Balantidium coli*

D. *Cystoisospora* species in dogs and cats

E. *Toxoplasma gondii*

F. *Trypanosoma cruzi*

G. *Babesia canis*

H. *Cytauxzoon felis*

I. *Hepatozoon americanum*

J. Rumen ciliates

1. Very large ciliated protozoan found in the large intestine of swine

2. Feline piroplasm—bejeweled ring within stained red blood cells of cats

3. Onion skin tissue cysts found in skeletal muscle of dogs transmitted by ingestion of the tick *Amblyomma maculatum*

4. Intestinal protozoan of cats (only definite host); zoonotic parasite

5. Most commonly diagnosed clinical condition in puppies and kittens (coccidiosis)

6. Mutuals of cattle

7. Hemoprotozoan of Central and South America with two forms: trypomastigote and amastigote (zoonotic parasite)

8. Canine piroplasm; basophilic, pear-shaped organism within canine red blood cells

9. Amebic dysentery in humans

10. Oval cysts with a refractile wall and two to four nuclei; may be distorted to semilunar appearance on standard fecal flotation

MATCHING—Match the scientific name of each parasite with the correct name, phrase, or term.

AA. *Eimeria bovis, Eimeria zuernii*

BB. *Cryptosporidium* species

CC. *Babesia bigemina*

DD. *Tritrichomonas foetus*

EE. Cecal ciliates of horses

FF. *Eimeria leuckarti*

GG. *Theileria equi*

HH. *Klossiella equi*

II. *Sarcocystis neurona*

JJ. *Klossiella muris*

1. Protozoan parasite residing in the reproductive tract of cattle

2. Equine piroplasms; pear-shaped organisms that may join, giving the effect of a Maltese cross

3. Equine protozoal myeloencephalitis

4. Piroplasm of cattle transmitted by the tick *Boophilus annulatus*

5. Coccidiosis in cattle

6. Oocysts found on histopathologic examination of the horse kidney and in urine sediment

7. Nonpathogenic coccidian found in the kidneys of wild and laboratory rats

8. Colorless sporulated oocyst; 3 to 5 μm in diameter on fecal flotation (zoonotic parasite)

9. Mutuals of horses

10. Unique oocysts that are the largest of the coccidians

MATCHING—Match the scientific name of each parasite with the correct name, phrase, or term.

AAA. *Cystoisospora suis*

BBB. *Histomonas meleagridis*

CCC. *Trichomonas gallinae*

DDD. *Haemoproteus* species

EEE. *Plasmodium* species of birds

FFF. *Leukocytozoon* species

GGG. *Eimeria stiedae*

HHH. *Trichomonas caviae*

III. *Ichthyophthirius multifiliis*

JJJ. *Leishmania* species

1. Intracellular flagellate (amastigote) found within reticuloendothelial cells of capillaries, spleen, etc.; transmitted by phlebotomine sand flies; zoonotic parasite

2. Ciliate affecting the skin, gills, fins, and eyes of freshwater, tropical, and ornamental fish in home aquaria

3. Avian malaria

4. Cecal ciliate of guinea pigs; usually nonpathogenic but may be observed in diarrheic conditions

5. Bluish sausage-shaped body within the cytoplasm of the avian red blood cell

6. Infectious enterohepatitis; blackhead in turkeys; intermediate host *Heterakis gallinarum*

7. Greatly distorts the shape of the avian white blood cell

8. Coccidian that parasitizes the small intestine of swine, especially young piglets

9. Found within crop washes and crop swabs of pigeons, doves, and poultry

10. Coccidiosis within the bile ducts of the liver of rabbits

QUESTIONS FOR THOUGHT AND DISCUSSION

1. Which protozoan parasites have life cycles that involve arthropods that serve as intermediate hosts? What is the significance of these relationships?

2. What are the four kinds of protozoans that affect domesticated animals? Give three examples of parasites for each of these groups.

12 Introduction to the Arthropods

OUTLINE

LEARNING OBJECTIVES

After studying this chapter, the reader should be able to do the following:

- Describe the key morphologic features of all arthropods.
- Identify four reasons arthropods are important.
- Detail the importance of crustaceans in veterinary parasitology.
- Detail the importance of insects in veterinary parasitology.

- Describe the key morphologic features of insects.
- Compare complex metamorphosis versus simple metamorphosis of insects.
- Identify the members of different orders of insects.
- Describe the key morphologic features of mites and ticks.

KEY TERMS

Abdomen	Coleoptera	Hemiptera	Mandibulata
Acariasis	Complex	Hemocoel	Metamorphosis
Acarines	metamorphosis	Hemolymph	Simple
Anoplura	Crustaceans	Hymenoptera	metamorphosis
Arthropod	Dictyoptera	Idiosoma	Siphonaptera
Capitulum	Dioecious	Insects	Terminal anus
Chelicerata	Diptera	Lepidoptera	Thorax
Chitin	Head	Mallophaga	Ventral mouth

ARTHROPODA

The phylum Arthropoda is one of the largest phyla. There are more than a million species of arthropods, including the extinct trilobites, spiders, mites, ticks, crabs, crayfish, lobsters, water fleas, copepods, millipedes, centipedes, and other insects. The insects include the cockroaches, beetles, bedbugs, fleas, bees, ants, wasps, mosquitoes, butterflies, moths, grasshoppers, lice, silverfish, and dragonflies. With more than 900,000 species, insects are by far the largest class within the phylum Arthropoda.

> **TECHNICIAN'S NOTE** The insects are the largest class in the phylum Arthropoda, with more than 900,000 species.

KEY MORPHOLOGIC FEATURES

The name arthropod means "jointed foot" (*arthro* means "joint," and *pod* means "foot"). All adult arthropods have jointed appendages. All arthropods are covered with a chitinous exoskeleton that is composed of segments. Chitin is a hard (yet elastic) body covering that envelops the entire body of all arthropods. Whenever you step on a cockroach, the chitin makes the "crunch" sound. Arthropods have a hemocoel, a body cavity filled with hemolymph. Hemolymph is a bloodlike fluid that bathes the internal organs of an arthropod. When a flying insect hits the windshield of a speeding car and "splats," hemolymph is the fluid that creates the splat. Arthropods have a very simple circulatory system composed of a heartlike dorsal tube. This dorsal tube is actually a primitive heart that pumps the hemolymph to the arthropod's head. The digestive system of arthropods begins with a ventral mouth and ends with a terminal anus. Arthropods possess a variety of respiratory systems; they may use gills, book lungs, or tracheal tubes as respiratory organs. Arthropods have complex nervous and excretory systems. However, the most important organ system of the arthropods is the reproductive system. Arthropods have separate sexes; they are dioecious. Reproduction is by means of eggs. Arthropods have a tremendous reproductive capacity.

> **TECHNICIAN'S NOTE** Arthropods are dioecious and use eggs for reproduction. They have a tremendous capacity for reproduction.

DIVISIONS OF THE PHYLUM ARTHROPODA

The phylum Arthropoda is made up of the following subphyla: Trilobitomorpha (the extinct trilobites), Onychophora (onychophorans, or "living fossils"), Tardigrada (water bears), Pycnogonida (sea spiders), Chelicerata (mites, ticks, spiders, scorpions, and others), and Mandibulata (crustaceans, centipedes and millipedes, and insects). Most of the arthropods important to veterinary parasitology are members of Chelicerata and Mandibulata.

Members of the phylum Arthropoda are important because (1) they may serve as causal agents themselves, (2) they may produce venoms or toxic substances, (3) they may serve as intermediate hosts for protozoan and helminth parasites, and (4) they may serve as vectors for bacteria, viruses, spirochetes, rickettsiae, chlamydial agents, and other pathogens.

> **TECHNICIAN'S NOTE** Arthropods are extremely important ectoparasites because they can act as parasites themselves, can serve as intermediate hosts for other parasites, can produce toxins or venoms, or can serve as vectors for bacteria, viruses, spirochetes, rickettsiae, and other pathogens.

CRUSTACEA (AQUATIC ARTHROPODS)

Phylum: Arthropoda
   Subphylum: Mandibulata
      Class: Crustacea (aquatic arthropods)

Members of the class Crustacea are always aquatic. Crustaceans are important because they serve as intermediate hosts for many helminth parasites, including flukes (e.g., *Paragonimus kellicotti*), tapeworms (e.g., *Spirometra mansonoides*), and roundworms (e.g., *Dracunculus insignis*). Crustaceans also serve as causal agents because they are ectoparasites of many fish, amphibians, and exotic reptiles.

MYRIAPODA (CENTIPEDES AND MILLIPEDES)

Phylum: Arthropoda
   Subphylum: Mandibulata
      Class: Myriapoda (centipedes and millipedes)

Members of the class Myriapoda are represented by centipedes and millipedes. Myriapodans are important because they produce venoms and toxic substances. Centipedes and millipedes are usually slow-moving arthropods. For defense mechanisms, they are capable of producing venoms and toxic substances that can sting, blind, paralyze, burn, or even kill.

INSECTA (INSECTS)

Phylum: Arthropoda
   Subphylum: Mandibulata
      Class: Insecta (insects)

As mentioned earlier, the class Insecta has the largest number of members (more than 900,000 species) in the phylum Arthropoda. This is also the most diverse group. Members of the class Insecta are important because (1) they may serve as causal agents themselves, (2) they may produce venoms or toxic substances, (3) they may serve as intermediate hosts for protozoan and helminth parasites, and (4) they may serve as vectors for bacteria, viruses, spirochetes, rickettsiae, chlamydial agents, and other pathogens. Examples of all of these important pathogenic mechanisms are covered in Chapter 13.

KEY MORPHOLOGIC FEATURES

As members of the phylum Arthropoda, insects share the following morphologic characteristics: a segmented body with three pairs of segmented legs, bilateral symmetry, a chitinous exoskeleton, a dorsal heart, a ventral nerve cord, a digestive system from

mouth to anus, an excretory system, and a reproductive system. As with all other arthropods, insects are dioecious (they, too, have separate sexes) and demonstrate a tremendous reproductive capacity.

> TECHNICIAN'S NOTE All insects have the same morphologic characteristics: segmented body with three pairs of segmented legs, bilateral symmetry, chitinous exoskeleton, dorsal heart, ventral nerve cord, digestive system from mouth to anus, excretory system, and reproductive system.

The body of all adult insects is divided into three basic body sections: the head, thorax, and abdomen. The head is on the anterior, or front end, of the insect; the head contains the insect's brain, its antennae, the ventrally directed mouthparts, and the eyes (if eyes are present; some insects are eyeless). The thorax is the middle body section. The thorax of the adult insect always has three pairs of legs and may have either one or two pairs of wings; however, many insects, such as lice and fleas, are wingless. The abdomen is the posterior, or the hind, section of the insect. It often contains the reproductive organs but has no ventral, segmented appendages (e.g., mouthparts of the head, legs of the thorax).

> TECHNICIAN'S NOTE The insect body is divided into the head, thorax, and abdomen.

To achieve the size and development of the adult insect, the young insect must undergo changes in size, form, and structure. This series of changes is called metamorphosis. For purposes of this text, there are two types of metamorphosis: simple metamorphosis and complex metamorphosis. Simple metamorphosis consists of three developmental stages: the egg stage, the nymphal stage, and the adult stage. In this form of metamorphosis the nymphal stage resembles the adult stage in form except that it is smaller and is not sexually mature (and therefore cannot reproduce). In winged insects the wings may be absent in the nymphal stage. An example of an insect that undergoes simple metamorphosis is the cockroach.

Complex metamorphosis consists of four developmental stages: the egg stage, the larval stage, the pupal stage, and the adult stage. None of these developmental stages bears a resemblance to any of the others. The egg stage does not resemble the larval stage, which in turn does not resemble the pupal stage, which in turn does not resemble the adult stage. The larval stage is described as *worm-like*. To reach the adult stage the insect must develop through the pupal stage, which is a resting stage. The adult stage emerges from the pupal stage and eventually becomes sexually mature and reproduces, producing large numbers of offspring.

> **TECHNICIAN'S NOTE** The insect goes through a simple or complex metamorphosis as it progresses through its life cycle. The metamorphosis depends on the species of the insect.

ORDERS OF INSECTA

With regard to veterinary parasitology, the class Insecta is further divided into nine orders. The orders of greatest significance in parasitology are Dictyoptera (cockroaches and grasshoppers), Coleoptera (beetles), Lepidoptera (moths and butterflies), Hemiptera (true bugs), Hymenoptera (ants, bees, wasps, yellow jackets, and other stinging insects), Anoplura (sucking lice), Mallophaga (chewing lice), Diptera (two-winged flies), and Siphonaptera (fleas). Each of the orders within the class Insecta and its relative importance in veterinary medicine is discussed in detail in Chapter 13.

ACARINA (MITES AND TICKS)

Phylum: Arthropoda
    Subphylum: Chelicerata
        Order: Acarina (mites and ticks)

The subphylum Mandibulata comprises crustaceans, centipedes and millipedes, and insects. The members of the subphylum Chelicerata include mites, ticks, spiders, and scorpions. Within this subphylum are members of the class Arachnida, order Acarina, the mites and the ticks. Mites and ticks are often referred to as acarines, and infestation with mites or ticks is referred to as acariasis.

> **TECHNICIAN'S NOTE** Ectoparasites cause infestations rather than infections. Infestation with mites and ticks is called *acariasis*.

Mites and ticks are *not* insects; they are acarines. They are morphologically different from insects. First, the body segmentation of mites and ticks is different from that of insects. Insects are divided into head, thorax, and abdomen; mites and ticks, however, have lost all the external signs of body segmentation and are divided into two body components, the capitulum (the mouthparts, or a fusion of the head and thorax) and the idiosoma (the abdomen). Discussions in this text refer to the two basic body parts of mites and ticks as the *mouthparts* and the *abdomen*. Although insects may have antennae, wings, and compound eyes, acarines lack these structures. The mouthparts of the mites and ticks have two basic functions: sucking blood or tissue fluids and attaching or holding on to the host. The following organ systems are represented in mites and ticks: digestive, excretory, respiratory, nervous, and reproductive systems. As with insects, mites and ticks are dioecious (have separate sexes) and possess a tremendous reproductive capacity.

In contrast to insects, mites and ticks do not undergo metamorphosis. There are four developmental stages in the life cycle of acarines: the egg stage, the larval stage, the nymphal stage, and the adult stage. The major difference among these life stages is that the larval acarine has three pairs of legs (or six legs), whereas both nymphal and adult acarines have four pairs of legs (or eight legs). Only the adult stage is capable of sexual reproduction.

> **TECHNICIAN'S NOTE** Mites and ticks do not go through a metamorphosis as insects do. Instead, their four life stages resemble each other with the exception of the number of pairs of legs possessed at each stage of development. Only the adult is capable of sexual reproduction.

Mites and ticks are significant in veterinary medicine and are discussed in detail in Chapter 13.

CHAPTER TWELVE TEST

MATCHING—Match the term with the correct phrase or term.

A. Arthropods	1. Beetles
B. Chitin	2. Ants, bees, wasps, yellow jackets, and other stinging insects
C. Dioecious	3. Centipedes and millipedes
D. Mandibulata	4. Jointed appendages
E. Chelicerata	5. Two-winged flies
F. Myriapoda	6. Egg, larva, pupa, and adult
G. Body sections of insects	7. Fleas
H. Simple metamorphosis	8. Having separate sexes; both male and female
I. Complex metamorphosis	9. Crustaceans, centipedes, millipedes, and insects
J. Dictyopterans	10. True bugs
K. Coleopterans	11. Causal agents, venom producers, intermediate hosts, vectors
L. Lepidopterans	12. The blood of most arthropods
M. Hemipterans	13. Mites and ticks collectively
N. Hymenopterans	14. Sucking lice
O. Anoplurans	15. Hard, elastic covering that envelops the bodies of all arthropods
P. Mallophagans	16. Mites, ticks, spiders, scorpions, etc.
Q. Dipterans	17. Head, thorax, and abdomen
R. Siphonapterans	18. TREMENDOUS!
S. Capitulum	19. Developmental stages in the life cycle of a mite or tick
T. Idiosoma	20. Mouthparts of a mite or tick
U. Acarines	21. Infestation with either mites or ticks
V. Acariasis	22. Moths and butterflies
W. Egg, larva, nymph, adult	23. Cockroaches and grasshoppers
X. Importance of arthropods	24. Egg, nymph, and adult
Y. Reproductive potential for arthropods	25. Chewing lice
Z. Hemolymph	26. Abdomen of a mite or tick

QUESTIONS FOR THOUGHT AND DISCUSSION

1. Compare and contrast insects and acarines. How are they similar? How are they different?

2. There are many diverse orders within the class Insecta. How does each of these orders integrate into the ways in which arthropods are important? These facts will become evident after studying the following chapter.

13 Arthropods That Infect and Infest Domestic Animals

OUTLINE

LEARNING OBJECTIVES

After studying this chapter, the reader should be able to do the following:

- Describe the subclass Mandibulata and the subclass Chelicerata.
- Identify the three types of arthropodan parasites that are reportable to the USDA (United States Department of Agriculture).
- Identify and give examples of arthropods that serve as causal agents themselves.
- Identify and give examples of arthropods that serve as producers of venoms or toxic substances.
- Identify and give examples of arthropods that serve as intermediate hosts for tapeworms, flukes, and especially nematodes.

- Identify and give examples of arthropods that serve as vectors of diseases.
- Compare and contrast the following disease entities in domestic animals: pediculosis, myiasis, siphonapterosis, and acariasis.
- Compare and contrast facultative myiasis and obligatory myiasis.
- Compare and contrast localized and generalized demodicosis.
- Compare and contrast insects and acarines.
- Identify the major arthropodan parasites of domestic animals (when given the host and the location within that host).

KEY TERMS

Acariasis
Adult stage
American dog tick or
  wood tick
Aragasid or soft tick
Arthropodology
Biting housefly or
  stable fly
Borreliosis

Brown dog tick
Buffalo gnat
Chelicerae
Chelicerata
Coleopterans
Continental rabbit
  tick
Crustaceans
Demodicosis

Dictyopterans
Diptera
Egg stage
Empodia
Face fly
Facultative myiasis
Flea dirt or flea frass
Foot and tail mites
Fowl tick

Gadding
Generalized
  demodicosis
Gulf Coast tick
Hippoboscid fly
Horn fly
Horse bots or
  stomach bots
Hymenopterans

KEY TERMS—cont'd

Hypostome
Inornate
Insects
Ixodid or hard ticks
Lepidopterans
Localized form of
 demodicosis
Lone star tick
Mallophaga
Mandibulata
Myiasis
Myriopoda
Nasal bots or nasal
 bot flies
New World sand flies

Nit
Northern mite of
 poultry
No-see-ums, punkies,
 sand flies
Nymph
Obligatory myiasis
Ornate
Ox warbles, cattle
 grubs
Palps
Pedicels or stalks
Pediculosis
Pedipalps
Periodic parasite

Psoroptidae family
Queensland itch,
 sweat itch, sweet
 itch, summer
 dermatitis
Reportable parasite
Reportable parasites
 (this is NOT a
 repeat)
Sarcoptidae family
Scabies
Scaly leg
Screwworm fly
Scutum
Seed ticks

Sheep ked
Siphonapterans
Siphonapterosis
Spinose ear tick
Spiracular plate
Texas cattle fever tick
 or North American
 tick
Tick paralysis
Tropical rat mite
Walking dandruff
Wolves, warbles

The study of arthropods is referred to as arthropodology. Arthropods, members of the phylum Arthropoda, are important in veterinary parasitology for several reasons. Arthropods (1) serve as causal agents themselves by producing pathology or disease in domesticated or wild animals (or in humans); (2) serve as intermediate hosts for **helminths** (flukes, tapeworms, and roundworms) and **protozoans** (single-celled organisms) that infect domesticated or wild animals (or humans); (3) serve as vectors for bacteria, viruses, spirochetes, chlamydial agents, and other pathogens that produce disease in domesticated or wild animals (or humans); and (4) produce venoms and other substances that may be toxic to domesticated or wild animals (or humans). From one to four of these important criteria are true for each group of arthropods.

> **TECHNICIAN'S NOTE** Arthropods can serve as agents of disease; intermediate hosts for other parasites; and vectors for bacterial, viral, spirochete, chlamydial, and other pathogenic diseases and can produce venoms or other substances that may be toxic to animals and humans.

The phylum Arthropoda is broken down into several subphyla, two of which are important in veterinary parasitology. These two subphyla are the Mandibulata (crustaceans, myriopodans, and insects) and the Chelicerata (mites, ticks, spiders, and scorpions).

CRUSTACEANS

Kingdom: Animalia
 Phylum: Arthropoda (arthropods)
  Subphylum: Mandibulata (possess mandibulate mouthparts)
   Class: Crustacea (aquatic crustaceans)

Crustaceans are important in veterinary medicine for several reasons. First, crustaceans may be causal agents themselves when they serve as ectoparasites of fishes and amphibians. Tiny, microscopic crustaceans, such as the *Argulus* species (Figure 13-1), parasitize the skin and gills of aquatic animals and can produce significant pathology. Crustaceans such as crabs can also be important as causal agents when they are swallowed by dogs that frequent beaches; in this scenario, crustaceans act as foreign bodies within the stomach or other portions of the gastrointestinal tract. Crustaceans may also serve as

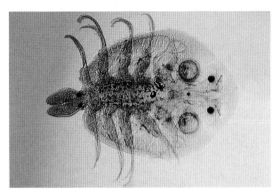

FIGURE 13-1 Tiny, microscopic *Argulus* species parasitizes the skin and gills of fish.

intermediate hosts for certain helminth parasites of domesticated animals. For example, the crayfish serves as the intermediate host for *Paragonimus kellicotti,* the lung fluke of dogs and cats. Certain aquatic copepods serve as first intermediate hosts for *Diphyllobothrium latum* and *Spirometra mansonoides,* pseudotapeworms of dogs and cats. Finally, certain freshwater crustaceans serve as the intermediate host for *Dracunculus insignis,* the guinea worm, a subcutaneous parasite of dogs.

> **TECHNICIAN'S NOTE** *Argulus* species of crustaceans parasitize the gills and skin of aquatic animals, whereas other crustacean species act as intermediate hosts to several types of parasites.

MYRIOPODANS

Kingdom: Animalia
   Phylum: Arthropoda (arthropods)
      Subphylum: Mandibulata (possess mandibulate mouthparts)
         Class: Myriopoda (centipedes and millipedes)

The class Myriopoda comprises the centipedes and the millipedes (myriopodans). This strange class of arthropods is important because its members produce venoms or toxic substances.

Parasite: Centipedes
Host: None

Location: Free in the environment
Distribution: Truly poisonous centipedes in jungles and dense vegetation worldwide with the exception of North America
Derivation of Name: Hundred legged
Common Name: Centipede
Transmission Route: Not transmitted

Centipedes are usually small terrestrial arthropods, predatory on creatures smaller than themselves. Centipedes have one pair of legs for every body segment. On the anterior end, they possess poison claws that connect to large poison glands. Centipedes often subdue their prey with these poison claws. It is important to note, however, that most of the truly poisonous centipedes are restricted to the jungles and areas of dense vegetation throughout the world and *not* to the continent of North America. Some pet stores sell exotic varieties of centipedes, and veterinarians are infrequently asked to "treat" these exotic arthropods; however, a medical arthropodologist (or entomologist) might be consulted. Great care should be taken when handling all centipedes because they can bite. The bite of some of the larger centipede varieties has been likened to the sting of a hornet.

> **TECHNICIAN'S NOTE** Centipedes have one pair of legs for every body segment, whereas millipedes have two pairs of legs for every body segment.

Parasite: Millipedes
Host: None
Location: Free in the environment
Derivation of common Name: Thousand legged
Distribution: Truly poisonous millipedes in jungles and dense vegetation worldwide with exception of North America
Transmission Route: Not transmitted
Common Name: Millipede

Millipedes are also small terrestrial arthropods. Whereas centipedes are predatory on smaller creatures, millipedes are vegetarians. Millipedes have two pairs of legs for every body segment; remember that centipedes have only one pair. Beneath each pair of legs are repugnatorial glands that contain caustic substances capable of burning the skin. Millipedes are able to "squirt" these caustic, irritating substances onto the skin of any creature that might threaten them. As with the centipedes most of the truly poisonous millipedes are restricted to the jungles and areas of dense vegetation throughout the world and *not* to the continent of North America. Some tribal people in these jungle areas grind up caustic millipedes and dip their arrow tips into the "juice" to make poisonous arrows. Although centipedes are sold as exotic pets in some pet stores, millipedes do not make good family pets.

INSECTS

Kingdom: Animalia
    Phylum: Arthropoda (arthropods)
        Subphylum: Mandibulata (possess mandibulate mouthparts)
            Class: Insecta (insects)

A major portion of this chapter discusses the orders of the class Insecta and their place in veterinary parasitology. The following orders are discussed:

Class: Insecta
    Order: Dictyoptera (cockroaches)
    Order: Coleoptera (beetles)
    Order: Lepidoptera (butterflies and moths)
    Order: Hymenoptera (ants, bees, and wasps)
    Order: Hemiptera (true bugs)
    Order: Mallophaga (chewing or biting lice)
    Order: Anoplura (sucking lice)
    Order: Diptera (two-winged flies)
    Order: Siphonaptera (fleas)

DICTYOPTERA (COCKROACHES)

Cockroaches or dictyopterans are members of the order Dictyoptera. These disgusting creatures are perhaps the most commonly occurring insects that may actively "infest" a veterinary clinic. Because of their voracious feeding habits and their close association with stored food products (e.g., dried dog and cat food), cockroaches are often associated with the nocturnal environment of the veterinary clinic.

Cockroaches habitually disgorge portions of their partly digested food and also defecate wherever they roam and feed. Under the proper circumstances, cockroaches may be incriminated in the natural transmission of pathogenic organisms such as *Salmonella* species to both humans and domesticated animals.

COLEOPTERA (BEETLES)

Members of the order Coleoptera, coleopterans or beetles, are important because they may serve as intermediate hosts for certain parasites of domesticated animals. Dung beetles serve as intermediate host for *Spirocerca lupi*, the roundworm that produces esophageal nodules in dogs, and for *Gongylonema* species, a roundworm found in the tissues of the oral cavity and esophagus of goats and swine. Beetles can also serve as the intermediate host for the swine acanthocephalan *Macracanthorhynchus hirudinaceus*.

> **TECHNICIAN'S NOTE** Dung beetles are intermediate hosts to several parasites including *Spirocerca lupi* in dogs and *Gongylonema* species in goats and swine.

Parasite: Blister beetles
Host: None
Location: Free in the environment
Distribution: Continental United States and Canada
Derivation of Genus: Based on individual type of beetle
Transmission Route: Usually ingested
Common Name: Blister beetles

Certain types of beetles, commonly called **blister beetles**, produce within their tissues a toxic substance called **cantharidin** (Figure 13-2). If these beetles are ingested by a mammalian host, they can produce a blistering of the skin, the oral mucosa, and the epithelium lining the alimentary tract. These beetles often infest the earth immediately below alfalfa hay, and when the hay is harvested, the beetles may be collected and subsequently fed to horses. When horses ingest these beetles, a fatal colic often results. Blister beetles have been referred

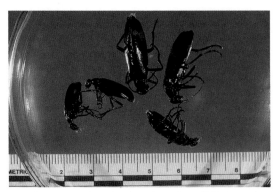

FIGURE 13-2 Blister beetles often infest alfalfa hay. They contain cantharidin, a toxic substance that produces colic in horses.

to as *Spanish fly,* a type of aphrodisiac or "love potion"; however, blister beetles are caustic and will burn living tissues and should not be used as an aphrodisiac.

> **TECHNICIAN'S NOTE** Blister beetles produce a toxic substance that is caustic and will burn living tissue and are often found below alfalfa hay.

LEPIDOPTERA (BUTTERFLIES AND MOTHS)

Members of the order Lepidoptera, or lepidopterans, have two life cycle stages—the adult stage and the larval, or caterpillar, stage—that may be pathogenic to domestic animals. Some moths and butterflies in certain parts of Southeast Asia feed on the lachrymal (lacrimal) secretions (tears) of domestic and wild animals. These are exotic creatures, not native to North America. Some moths and butterflies from these exotic regions also have been known to suck blood.

Several species of larval moths and butterflies found in North America are covered with tiny, urticating, or stinging, hairs. Because caterpillars are often slow moving, these hairs serve as defense mechanisms against their predators. These stinging hairs cause significant stings in humans and domestic animals.

HYMENOPTERA (ANTS, BEES, AND WASPS)

The veterinarian should remember three basic facts about ants, bees, wasps, and hornets (members of the order Hymenoptera, or hymenopterans). First, "fire ants" are indigenous to the southeastern United States and can bite and sting almost any domesticated animal. "Downer cows" and newborn animals (weak, young lambs and calves and hatchling chicks) are particularly at risk to the perils of fire ants. Fire ants can attack any animal with which they come in contact. Second, bees, wasps, and hornets can sting domestic animals, particularly curious dogs and cats. These are minor envenomizations, seldom resulting in the death of an animal. Third, after being released in Brazil, Africanized honeybees, or "killer bees," have spread throughout South America and have crossed the border separating Texas and Mexico. Each year, these bees invade farther into the United States. Almost any domestic animal (and humans) can be at risk of inadvertently disturbing a ground hive containing these bees and arousing its inhabitants. Death often results from thousands of stings from these killer bees. Bees and wasps can cause anaphylactic reactions in allergic animals and humans. If not treated, these reactions can be severe enough to cause death.

If the veterinary diagnostician suspects that ants, bees, wasps, or hornets are causing problems, the intact hymenopteran should be collected in a sealed container containing 10% formalin or ethyl alcohol and submitted to an entomologist for identification.

> **TECHNICIAN'S NOTE** The hymenopterans can bite and/or sting domesticated animals, causing mild envenomization to death depending on the species and number of bites or stings and the reaction by the animal's or human's body.

HEMIPTERA (TRUE BUGS)

Parasite: Reduviid bugs
Host: Dogs and humans
Location: On host's lips and skin of the mouth when feeding
Distribution: Species can be found worldwide
Derivation of Genus: None found
Transmission Route: Periodic parasite
Common Name: Kissing bugs

The veterinary diagnostician should remember the following basic facts about true bugs (members of the order Hemiptera). There are two groups of hemipterans that are of veterinary importance: reduviid bugs (kissing bugs) and bedbugs. **Reduviid bugs** are periodic parasites; that is, they make frequent visits to the host to obtain a blood meal. Kissing bugs serve as intermediate hosts for *Trypanosoma cruzi*, a protozoan parasite that can produce a rare disease called **Chagas disease** in humans and dogs. This disease is also called **South American trypanosomiasis** and is rarely diagnosed in the United States. *T. cruzi* infects a variety of internal organs; its infective stages swim in the blood of an infected host. Kissing bugs take blood meals from infected hosts and incubate the parasite in their intestinal tracts. The parasites are then transmitted to uninfected mammals as the bugs defecate. After taking a blood meal from a host, a kissing bug turns around and defecates on the feeding site. This inoculates the infective trypanosomes into the uninfected host. Kissing bugs play a key role in the transmission of Chagas disease.

> *TECHNICIAN'S NOTE* Reduviid bugs are an intermediate host to *Trypanosoma cruzi*.

Parasite: *Cimex lectularius*
Host: Humans, rabbits, poultry, and pigeons
Location: On the host when feeding
Distribution: North America, Europe, and Central Asia
Derivation of Genus: Latin for *bug*
Transmission Route: Periodic parasite
Common Name: Bedbug

Bedbugs, *Cimex lectularius,* are the second type of hemipteran important in veterinary parasitology. Bedbugs are dorsoventrally flattened, wingless hemipterans with a three-segmented proboscis tucked under the thorax and ventral "stink glands" producing a characteristic "bedbug odor" that often infests human dwellings. They have operculated ova that are deposited on mattresses, in wall cracks and crevices, and under peeling wallpaper. They are periodic parasites, making frequent visits to the

host to obtain a blood meal. Bedbugs are nocturnal feeders. They are diagnosed by the identification of wingless adult hemipterans, characteristic bedbug odor, and identification of operculated ova in the host environment. Although bedbugs are most often incriminated as human parasites, they may also be found in rabbit colonies, poultry houses, and pigeon colonies, preying on domesticated animals (Figure 13-3). Unlike kissing bugs, bedbugs do not serve as intermediate hosts for pathogenic agents that infect humans or domestic animals.

> *TECHNICIAN'S NOTE* After feeding, the bedbug turns around and defecates onto the former feeding site. This act should set up a scenario for transmission of human pathogens, but the bedbug does not serve as a vector or intermediate host.

If the veterinary diagnostician suspects that reduviid bugs or bedbugs may be causing problems, the

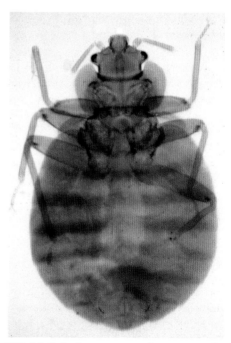

FIGURE 13-3 Bedbugs are periodic parasites of rabbit colonies, poultry houses, and pigeon colonies. (From Bowman: *Georgis' Parasitology for Veterinarians,* ed 10, 2013, Elsevier.)

intact hemipteran should be collected and stored in 10% formalin or ethyl alcohol and submitted to an entomologist for identification.

> **TECHNICIAN'S NOTE** The bedbug is making a comeback as a significant periodic parasite of humans. It has been found in many "high-priced" hotels, condominiums, and apartments in New York City.

Parasite: *Rhodnius* species, *Panstrongylus* species, and *Triatoma* species
Host: Dogs, humans, opossums, cats, guinea pigs, armadillos, rats, raccoons, and monkeys
Location of Adult: Lips and skin of the mouth when feeding (periodic parasites)
Distribution: South America, Central America, and parts of southwestern and western United States (i.e., Texas, Arizona, California, New Mexico)
Derivation of Genus: *Rhodnius*, rose; *Panstrongylus*, all round; *Triatoma*, cut into three
Transmission Route: Fly or move from host to host
Common Name: Kissing bugs

Rhodnius, Panstrongylus, and *Triatoma* species are known as the kissing bugs because they like to feed on **mucocutaneous** junctions such as those between the lips and the skin of the mouth. They appear to be "kissing" the host. The adults have three body portions: head, thorax, and abdomen. These species are winged hemipterans capable of flying. They have a three-segment proboscis reflexed back (tucked) under the thorax. The ova can be found in the environment of the host but are not usually observed. Kissing bugs are periodic parasites and voracious blood-feeders. They do not reside upon the host but frequent the host to obtain a blood meal. The kissing bugs serve as intermediate hosts for *T. cruzi*, a protozoan parasite. These parasites reside in the host's environment and travel to the host to obtain their blood meal. They transmit *T. cruzi* to dogs and humans but may feed on other mammalian hosts. These other hosts may serve as reservoirs for *T. cruzi*. Humans infected with *T. cruzi* develop a disease called *Chagas disease*.

Diagnosis is made by identifying the kissing bug within the host's environment, such as within the thatched roof of a hut and in cracks and crevices of mud walls.

> **TECHNICIAN'S NOTE** After feeding on the host's blood, the kissing bug turns around and defecates onto its former feeding site. This act sets up transmission of the infective forms of *Trypanosoma cruzi* to uninfected hosts.

MALLOPHAGA (CHEWING OR BITING LICE) AND ANOPLURA (SUCKING LICE)

Lice are some of the most prolific ectoparasites of domesticated and wild animals. There are two orders of lice: Mallophaga, the chewing or biting lice, and **Anoplura**, the sucking lice. Lice are dorsoventrally flattened, wingless insects. As insects, lice have bodies with three divisions: (1) the head, with mouthparts and antennae; (2) the thorax, with three pairs of legs and a noticeable lack of wings; and (3) the abdomen, the portion that bears the reproductive organs. These body divisions and their relationship to each other are important in diagnostic veterinary parasitology.

> **TECHNICIAN'S NOTE** Lice are dorsoventrally flattened and wingless insects with three distinctive body parts: head, thorax, and abdomen.

Parasite: Mallophagan species
Host: Mammals and birds
Location of Parasite: In and among the hairs and feathers of the respective hosts
Distribution: Worldwide
Derivation of Genus: Wool eaters
Transmission Route: Animal-to-animal contact
Common Name: Chewing lice
Zoonotic: No

Members of the order Mallophaga (chewing or biting lice) are usually smaller than members of the order Anoplura (sucking lice). Mallophagans are

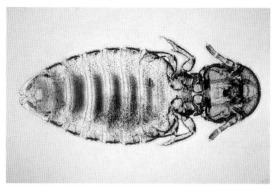

FIGURE 13-4 *Damalinia bovis*, the bovine-biting, chewing louse.

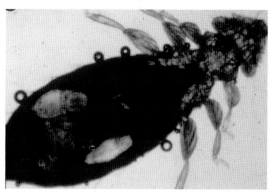

FIGURE 13-6 *Menacanthus stramineus*, the avian body louse.

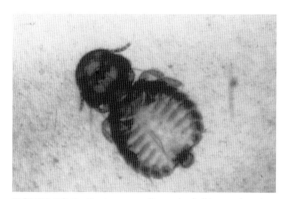

FIGURE 13-5 *Goniocotes gallinae*, the fluff louse of poultry.

usually yellow and have a large rounded head. The mouthparts are mandibulate and are adapted for chewing or biting. Characteristically the head of every chewing louse is wider than the widest portion of the thorax. On the thorax are the three pairs of legs, which may be adapted for clasping or for moving rapidly among feathers or hairs. Chewing (biting) lice may parasitize birds, dogs, cats, cattle, sheep, goats, and horses. Chewing lice of cattle and fowl include *Damalinia bovis* (Figure 13-4), *Goniocotes gallinae* (Figure 13-5), and *Menacanthus stramineus* (Figure 13-6).

> **TECHNICIAN'S NOTE** Chewing lice are found on both birds and mammals; however, they are species specific, and there is no crossover between species of animals.

Parasite: Anopluran species
Host: Domestic animals except cats and birds
Location of Parasite: Clinging to the host's hair
Distribution: Worldwide
Derivation of Genus: Unarmed tail
Transmission Route: Animal-to-animal contact
Common Name: Sucking lice
Zoonotic: No

Members of the order Anoplura (sucking lice) are larger than chewing lice. These lice range from red to gray; the color usually depends on the amount of blood that has been ingested from the host. Anoplurans have three body portions: the head, thorax, and abdomen. The adult anoplurans are wingless. In contrast to the large-headed mallophagans, anoplurans have a head that is narrower than the widest part of the thorax. Their mouthparts are of the piercing type and are adapted for sucking. Their pincerlike claws are adapted for clinging to the host's hairs. Interestingly, although they are found on many species of domestic animals, sucking lice do not parasitize birds or cats. Sucking lice of sheep, swine, monkeys, and dogs are species specific and include, respectively, *Solenopotes capillatus* (Figure 13-7), *Haematopinus suis* (Figure 13-8), *Pedicinus obtusus* (Figure 13-9), and *Linognathus setosus* (Figure 13-10).

> **TECHNICIAN'S NOTE** Sucking lice are species specific and do not parasitize birds or cats. However, they can attach to other species to carry them from one host to another.

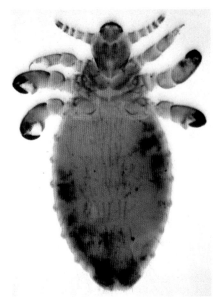

FIGURE 13-7 Sucking louse *Solenopotes capillatus* of sheep. (From Bowman: *Georgis' Parasitology for Veterinarians*, ed 10, 2013, Elsevier.)

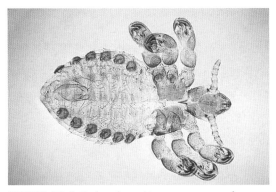

FIGURE 13-8 Sucking louse *Haematopinus suis* of swine.

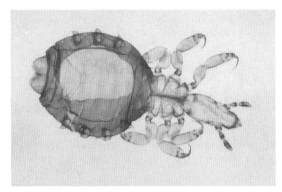

FIGURE 13-9 Sucking louse *Pedicinus obtusus* of monkeys.

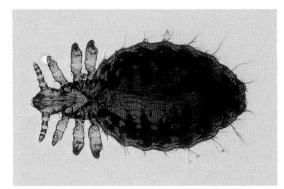

FIGURE 13-10 Sucking louse *Linognathus setosus* of dogs.

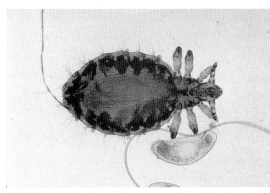

FIGURE 13-11 *Linognathus setosus.* Gravid female sucking louse and associated nit on hair shaft collected from a dog. Nits are oval, white, and usually found cemented to the hair or feather shaft of the definitive host.

Anoplurans and mallophagans have a life cycle consisting of three developmental stages. The egg stage, which is also called a nit, is tiny, approximately 0.5 to 1 mm in length. Nits are oval and white and are usually found cemented to the hair or feather shaft. Figure 13-11 shows *L. setosus*, a gravid female sucking louse and an associated nit collected from a dog. Nits hatch about 5 to 14 days after being laid by the adult female louse. Thousands of nits can be cemented by female lice to the hair coat of domesticated animals (Figure 13-12). The **nymphal stage** is similar in appearance to the adult louse. However, the nymph is smaller and lacks functioning reproductive organs and genital openings. There are three nymphal stages, each progressively larger than its predecessor. The nymphal stage lasts from 2 to

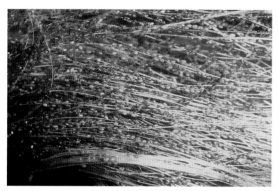

FIGURE 13-12 Thousands of nits can be cemented by female lice to the hair coat of domesticated animals. This calf's tail contains thousands of nits.

3 weeks. The adult stage is similar in appearance to the nymphal stage except that it is larger and has functional reproductive organs (Figure 13-13). The male and female lice copulate, the female louse lays eggs, and the life cycle begins again, taking 3 to 4 weeks to complete. Nymphal and adult stages may live no longer than 7 days if removed from the host. Eggs hatch within 2 to 3 weeks during warm weather but seldom hatch off the host.

Lice usually are transmitted by direct contact, but all life stages may be transmitted by **fomites**, inanimate objects such as blankets, brushes, and other grooming equipment. Lice are easily transmitted among young, old, and malnourished animals. Veterinarians often cannot determine why certain animals in a flock or herd are heavily infested, whereas others have only a few lice.

> TECHNICIAN'S NOTE Sucking and chewing lice have three body portions: head, thorax, and abdomen. Chewing lice have a head that is wider than the thorax, whereas sucking lice have a head that is narrower than the thorax.

Infestation by lice (either mallophagan or anopluran) is referred to as pediculosis (Figure 13-14). Sucking lice can ingest blood to such a degree that they produce severe anemia in the parasitized host; fatalities can occur, especially in young animals. The packed cell volume can decrease as much as 10% to 20%. As many as a million lice may be found on a severely infested animal. Infested animals become more susceptible to other diseases and parasites and may succumb to stresses not ordinarily pathologic to uninfested animals. When animals are poorly fed and kept in overcrowded conditions, they often become severely infested with lice and quickly become anemic and unthrifty.

Careful examination of the hair coat or feathers of infested animals easily reveals the presence of adult lice and their accompanying nits. Hair clippings also serve as a good source for collecting lice. For those animals with a thick hair coat, pediculosis may be overlooked. A handheld magnifying lens or a binocular headband magnifier (e.g., OptiVI-SOR™) may assist in isolation of adult or nymphal lice crawling through or clinging to hair or feathers or tiny nits cemented to individual hairs.

When lice or nits are isolated, they may be collected with tiny thumb forceps and placed within a drop of mineral oil on a glass microscope slide. A coverslip should be placed over the specimen, and the slide should be examined using the 4× or 10× objective of the microscope (Figure 13-15).

Identification of a louse to the genus and specific epithet is quite difficult. It is better to identify the specimen as being anopluran (sucking) versus mallophagan (chewing or biting). The veterinary diagnostician should remember that the head of every chewing louse is wider than the widest portion of its thorax. The typical sucking louse has a head that is narrower than the widest part of the thorax.

> TECHNICIAN'S NOTE Identification of lice to specific species is very difficult and should therefore be limited to identifying the louse as an anopluran or a mallophagan.

Lice of Mice, Rats, Gerbils, and Hamsters
Parasite: *Polyplax serrata*
Host: Mouse
Location of Parasite: Within hair coat
Distribution: Worldwide
Derivation of Genus: Many plates
Transmission Route: Direct contact between mice
Common Name: Mouse louse
Zoonotic: No

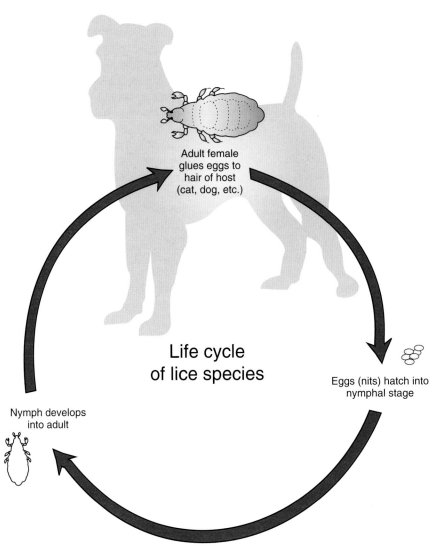

Adult female
glues eggs to
hair of host
(cat, dog, etc.)

Life cycle
of lice species

Eggs (nits) hatch into
nymphal stage

Nymph develops
into adult

FIGURE 13-13 Life cycle of the lice species.

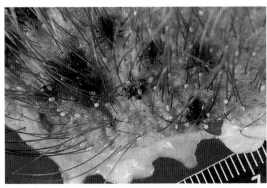

FIGURE 13-14 Pediculosis can be defined as infestation by either chewing or sucking lice; in this case, *Haematopinus suis* infestation in a pig.

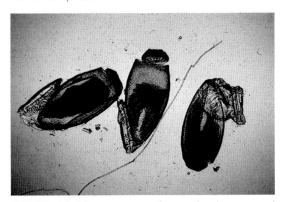

FIGURE 13-15 Appearance of operculated nits viewed with compound microscope.

Polyplax serrata is the house mouse louse. This louse is an anopluran (sucking louse), with mouthparts morphologically adapted for sucking blood from its host. Anoplurans are generally more debilitating than mallophagans (chewing lice). *P. serrata* is 0.6 to 1.5 mm long. It is a slender, yellow brown-to-white louse with a head that is narrower than the widest part of the thorax. As with most lice, *P. serrata* is large enough to be detected by careful visual inspection of the hair coat or by microscopic examination of pulled hairs. The adult stage of *P. serrata* is most likely found on the forebody of the mouse. Oval nits may be seen attached near the base of the hair shafts.

Clinical signs associated with infestation by *P. serrata* include restlessness, pruritus, anemia, unthrifty appearance, and death. The diagnostician should not attribute dermal signs to pediculosis unless a louse or a nit is detected. The dermal signs may be the result of other causes, such as concurrent infestation with mites. Therefore it is wise to examine an animal or hair sample thoroughly rather than ceasing when a single parasite has been identified.

> **TECHNICIAN'S NOTE** Clinical signs of *Polyplax serrata* include restlessness, pruritus, anemia, unthrifty appearance, and even death; however, dermal signs should not be attributed to pediculosis unless lice or nits are found.

P. serrata is transmitted by direct contact between mice. Because lice are species specific, cross-contamination of other species housed in the same area and transmission to humans are not considerations. However, *P. serrata* may serve as a vector for several rickettsial organisms and should therefore be handled with caution.

Parasite: *Polyplax spinulosa*
Host: Rat
Location of Adult: Within the hair coat
Distribution: Worldwide
Derivation of Genus: Many plates
Transmission Route: Direct animal-to-animal contact
Common Name: Rat louse
Zoonotic: No

As with *P. serrata* in the mouse, *Polyplax spinulosa* in the rat is an anopluran louse (sucking louse). *P. spinulosa* is similar to *P. serrata,* also having a narrow head compared with the thorax. Similarly, its mouthparts are adapted for sucking blood from the rat.

P. spinulosa may be detected by gross visual examination of the midbody and shoulders of the rat. Hair may be pulled from these areas and examined for nits, nymphs, and adults. Nits are often found attached to the base of the hair shafts. Nymphs resemble small, pale adult lice. Clinical signs include restlessness, pruritus, anemia, debilitation, and potentially death. Transmission of the rat louse is by direct contact. Ivermectin has been used successfully to treat lice in rodents. Because lice are species specific, transmission to other animals or humans is not a concern. *P. spinulosa* is a vector responsible for the spread of *Haemobartonella muris* and *Rickettsia typhi* between rats. *R. typhi* also can be transmitted from infected rats to humans by rat fleas.

> **TECHNICIAN'S NOTE** *Polyplax spinulosa* is the vector of transmission for *Haemobartonella muris* and *Rickettsia typhi* in rats.

Parasite: *Hoplopleura meridionidis*
Host: Gerbil
Location of Adult: Within the hair coat
Distribution: Not found
Derivation of Genus: Unknown
Transmission Route: Direct animal-to-animal contact
Common Name: Gerbil louse
Zoonotic: No

The louse found on the common pet store gerbil is *Hoplopleura meridionidis*. It is interesting that there are no records of lice reported from either the common pet store hamster, *Cricetus*, or the common laboratory hamster, *Mesocricetus auratus.*

> **TECHNICIAN'S NOTE** *Hoplopleura meridionidis* of gerbils is similar to the lice of rats and mice. There have been no reports of lice from the pet store hamster or the laboratory hamster.

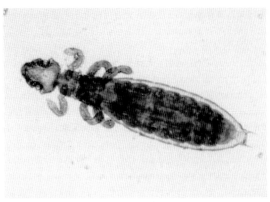

FIGURE 13-16 *Gliricola porcelli,* the slender, commonly found guinea pig louse.

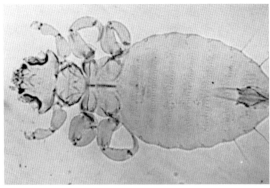

FIGURE 13-17 *Gyropus ovalis* is more oval than *Gliricola porcelli,* and its head is much broader.

Lice of Guinea Pigs

Parasite: *Gliricola porcelli* and *Gyropus ovalis*
Host: Guinea pig
Location of Adult: Within the hair coat
Distribution: Predominantly South and North America
Derivation of Genus: Unknown
Transmission Route: Direct animal-to-animal contact
Common Name: Guinea pig lice
Zoonotic: No

Gliricola porcelli and *Gyropus ovalis* are the lice of guinea pigs. Both species belong to the order Mallophaga (chewing lice). These lice differ from those of the order Anoplura (sucking lice) by their wide, triangular heads. Chewing lice have a strong pair of mandibles, which are used to abrade skin and obtain cutaneous fluids. *G. porcelli* and *G. ovalis* belong to the family Gyropidae, distinguished by having one or no claws on the second and third pairs of legs.

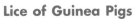 *G. porcelli,* the slender guinea pig louse, is 1 to 1.5 mm × 0.3 to 0.44 mm (Figure 13-16). *G. ovalis,* as its name implies, is more oval than *G. porcelli* and measures 1 to 1.2 mm × 0.5 mm (Figure 13-17). The head of *G. ovalis* is much broader than that of *G. porcelli.* Of these two lice, *G. porcelli* is the more common.

Guinea pig lice can be detected antemortem by careful inspection of the hair coat, either grossly or with a handheld magnifying lens. Postmortem, a method similar to that used to detect lice in other species of animals may be useful; that is, a piece of the pelt from the dead animal may be placed in a covered Petri dish and placed under a mild heat source, such as a small reading lamp. In a short time as the pelt cools, the lice migrate toward the warmth of the lamp and to the tips of the hairs. The lice can be easily observed grossly or with a handheld magnifying lens.

Light infestations of *G. porcelli* and *G. ovalis* usually cause no clinical signs. In heavy infestations, however, alopecia and scablike areas may develop, especially in the areas caudal to the ears of the guinea pig. Excessive scratching may be noticed. Ivermectin can be used to treat *G. porcelli* and *G. ovalis* in guinea pigs.

> *TECHNICIAN'S NOTE* Diagnosis of guinea pig lice is made by finding the living parasites on the animal with a magnifying glass.

Transmission of *G. porcelli* and *G. ovalis* is by direct contact with another host guinea pig or with bedding or other fomites from infested guinea pigs. As with other lice, lice of guinea pigs are species specific and do not cross-infest other species, including humans.

Lice of Rabbits

Parasite: *Hemodipsus ventricosus*
Host: Rabbit

Location of Adult: Within the hair coat
Distribution: Not found
Derivation of Genus: Unknown
Transmission Route: Direct animal-to-animal contact
Common Name: Rabbit louse
Zoonotic: No

Hemodipsus ventricosus is not typically found on domestic rabbits; however, when infestation does occur, it is especially debilitating. *H. ventricosus* is an anopluran louse, with a head narrower than the widest part of the thorax. Its mouthparts are specially designed for sucking blood from the host. It has a small thorax and a large rounded abdomen covered with numerous long hairs. Adult *H. ventricosus* are 1.2 to 2.5 mm long and can be observed antemortem by careful visual examination of the hair coat, especially on the dorsal and lateral aspects of the rabbit. On postmortem examination, hairs may be pulled and placed in a Petri dish under a warm lamp and examined with a dissecting microscope or magnifying glass. Adult lice are drawn by the warmth of the lamp to the tips of the hairs. The oval nits of *H. ventricosus* are 0.5 to 0.7 mm in length and may be found attached to the base of the hair shafts by pulling the fur and examining it microscopically.

> **TECHNICIAN'S NOTE** *Hemodipsus ventricosus* is not commonly found on pet rabbits but can be debilitating if it is found to infest the pet rabbit.

Clinical signs of *H. ventricosus* include alopecia and ruffled fur. Rabbit lice are avid bloodsuckers, so anemia may occur in severe infestations.

H. ventricosus is transmitted from rabbit to rabbit by prolonged direct contact. This mostly occurs between a doe and her litter. Although *H. ventricosus* is not considered zoonotic, it is a vector of *Francisella tularensis,* the etiologic agent that causes tularemia.

DIPTERA (TWO-WINGED FLIES)

The order Diptera is a very large, complex order of insects. As adults all members have one pair of wings (two wings), thus the ordinal name Diptera; *di* means "two," and *ptera* means "wing." The members vary greatly in size, food source preference, and developmental stage or stages that parasitize animals or produce pathology. With regard to their role as ectoparasites, dipterans produce two contrasting pathologic scenarios. As adults, they may feed intermittently on vertebrate blood, saliva, tears, and mucus; as larvae, they may develop in the subcutaneous tissues or internal organs of the host. When adult dipterans make frequent visits to the vertebrate host and intermittently feed on that vertebrate host's blood, they are referred to as **periodic parasites**. When dipteran larvae develop in the tissue or organs of vertebrate hosts, they produce a condition known as myiasis.

> **TECHNICIAN'S NOTE** Dipteran larvae can cause a condition known as *myiasis* (maggot infestation) if they develop in the tissues or organs of vertebrate hosts.

As periodic parasites, blood-feeding dipterans can be classified in several ways according to the way in which the adult male and female dipterans feed on vertebrate blood and their food preference. There are certain dipteran groups in which only the females feed on vertebrate blood; these female flies require vertebrate blood for laying their eggs. Included in this group are biting gnats (*Simulium, Lutzomyia,* and *Culicoides* spp.), the mosquitoes (*Anopheles, Aedes,* and *Culex* spp.), the horseflies (*Tabanus* spp.), and the deerflies (*Chrysops* spp.).

In the second group of blood-feeding dipterans, both male and female adult flies require a vertebrate blood meal. These species include *Stomoxys calcitrans,* the stable fly; *Haematobia irritans,* the horn fly; and *Melophagus ovinus,* the sheep ked.

Another dipteran fly, *Musca autumnalis,* feeds on mucus, tears, and saliva of large animals, particularly cattle.

> **TECHNICIAN'S NOTE** In some types of dipterans the female is the only periodic parasite that feeds on vertebrate blood, whereas in other species of dipterans both males and females feed on vertebrate blood.

Periodic Parasites of Which Only Adult Females Feed on Vertebrate Blood

In the first dipteran group of periodic parasites, only the female dipterans feed on vertebrate blood. The tiniest members of this group are the biting gnats of *Simulium, Lutzomyia,* and *Culicoides* species.

Parasite: *Simulium* species
Host: Domesticated animals, poultry, and humans
Location of Adults: Surface of the skin when feeding; otherwise, in the vicinity of swiftly flowing streams
Distribution: Worldwide, but not in Hawaii or New Zealand
Derivation of Genus: At the same time
Transmission Route: Fly from host to host
Common Name: Black flies or buffalo gnats

Simulium *Species (Black Flies)*

Members of the genus *Simulium* are commonly called **black flies**, although they may vary from gray to yellow, or **buffalo gnats** because their thorax humps over their head, giving the appearance of a buffalo's hump (Figure 13-18). These are tiny flies, ranging from 1 to 6 mm in length. The adults have broad, unspotted wings that have prominent veins along the anterior margins. They have serrated,

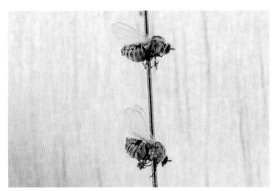

FIGURE 13-18 Members of the genus *Simulium* are commonly called *black flies* (but may be gray to yellow) or *buffalo gnats* (thorax humped over the head gives the appearance of a buffalo's hump). Note the small size compared with the straight pin that is sticking them.

scissorlike mouthparts, and thus their bites are very painful. Because the females lay eggs in well-aerated water, these flies are often found in the vicinity of swiftly flowing streams. They move in great swarms, inflicting painful bites and sucking the host's blood. These flies are voracious feeders (periodic parasites), but only the female flies feed on vertebrate blood. The males feed on nectar and pollen. The females fly great distances to find vertebrate blood. The female needs a vertebrate blood meal to lay her eggs. These flies may keep cattle from grazing or cause them to stampede. The ears, neck, head, and abdomen are favorite feeding sites. Black flies also feed on poultry and can serve as an intermediate host for a protozoan parasite known as *Leucocytozoon* species.

> **TECHNICIAN'S NOTE** The common name *black fly* is a misnomer; not all black flies are black. They can come in a variety of colors from yellow to gray to black.

Black flies prefer the daylight hours and tend to be active in open air. Repellents may offer some relief from these flies. The best method of preventing infestation with black flies is by keeping the equine or bovine hosts in the barn during daylight hours.

Black flies are most often collected in the field (usually in the vicinity of their breeding sites, swiftly flowing streams) and are not found on animals presenting to a veterinary clinic. They are diagnosed by their small size, humped back, and strong venation in the anterior region of the wings. Identification of black flies to the level of genus is probably best left to an entomologist.

> **TECHNICIAN'S NOTE** Black flies are typically found in the field rather than on animals presenting to a veterinary clinic.

Parasite: *Lutzomyia* species and *Phlebotomus* species
Host: Mammals of many species, reptiles, avians, and humans (*Lutzomyia* species); mammals, reptiles, avians, and humans (*Phlebotomus* species)
Location of Adult: On the skin surface when feeding; otherwise in dark, moist, and organic environments

Distribution: Worldwide (*Lutzomyia* species); tropics, subtropics, and Mediterranean regions (*Phlebotomus* species)
Derivation of Genus: *Phlebotomus*, vein cutting; *Lutzomyia*, Frank Eugene Lutz was a renowned entomologist, and *myia* means "fly"
Transmission Route: Fly from host to host
Common Name: New World sand flies (*Lutzomyia* species); sand flies (*Phlebotomus* species)

Lutzomyia *Species (New World Sand Flies)* and Phlebotomus *Species*

Members of the genus *Lutzomyia* are commonly referred to as New World sand flies. *Phlebotomus* species are commonly referred to as *sand flies*. These two genera represent the group of flies called the *phlebotomine sand flies*. They are tiny mothlike flies, rarely more than 5 mm in length. A key feature for identification is that the body (head, thorax, and abdomen) is **hirsute** (covered with fine hairs). *Lutzomyia* and *Phlebotomus* species tend to be active only at night and are weak fliers. These tiny flies transmit a zoonotic protozoan parasite known as *Leishmania* species, and the rodents that reside in the burrows in which the flies live serve as reservoirs for *Leishmania* species.

> **TECHNICIAN'S NOTE** Sand flies and New World sand flies are active only at night and do not fly far to get to a host.

As with black flies, sand flies most often can be collected in the field and are not found on animals presenting to a veterinary clinic. The adult flies are weak fliers and are often collected in rodent burrows, where they breed in moist organic debris. Phlebotomine sand flies can be diagnosed by their small size and hairy wings and bodies. Identification of sand flies is probably best left to an entomologist.

> **TECHNICIAN'S NOTE** Sand flies are diagnosed by their small size and the hairy wings on their bodies.

Parasite: *Culicoides* species
Host: Domestic animals and humans

Location of Adult: On the skin surface when feeding; otherwise in their aquatic or semi-aquatic breeding grounds
Distribution: Worldwide
Derivation of Genus: Mosquito-like
Transmission Route: Fly from host to host
Common Name: No-see-ums, punkies, or sand flies (not to be confused with the phlebotomine sand flies: *Lutzomyia* and *Phlebotomus* species)

Culicoides *Species (No-See-Ums)*

Culicoides gnats are also commonly known as no-see-ums, punkies, or sand flies. They are tiny gnats (1-3 mm in length) and similar to black flies in that they inflict painful bites and suck the blood of their hosts. The adults have a short proboscis and mottled or spotted wings with hairs on the wing margins. They are active at dusk and at dawn, especially during summer months. The adults tend to be found around their aquatic or semiaquatic breeding grounds when not feeding. The developmental stages are primarily aquatic and are seldom observed in a veterinary clinic setting. These female gnats tend to feed on the dorsal or ventral areas of the host during dusk and evening hours; the feeding site preference depends on the species of biting gnat. Horses often become allergic to the bites of *Culicoides* species, scratching and rubbing these areas, causing alopecia, excoriations, and thickening of the skin. This condition has several names, including Queensland itch, sweat itch and sweet itch. Because this condition is often seen during the warmer months of the year, it is also referred to as summer dermatitis. The best prevention for these flies is stabling animals during the hours between dusk and dawn. Repellents may offer some protection against *Culicoides* species. These flies also serve as the intermediate host for *Onchocerca cervicalis,* a nematode whose microfilariae are found in the skin of horses. These flies also transmit the bluetongue virus of sheep.

> **TECHNICIAN'S NOTE** Several of the *Culicoides* species are intermediate hosts for protozoan and helminth parasites and can also transmit viral diseases. They are associated with the transmission of the bluetongue virus.

In contrast to the clear, heavily veined wings of black flies, the wings of *Culicoides* species are mottled. Identification of *Culicoides* species is probably best left to an entomologist.

Parasite: *Anopheles quadrimaculatus, Aedes aegypti,* and *Culex* species
Host: Mammals, reptiles, avians, and humans
Location of Adult: Skin surface when feeding
Distribution: Worldwide
Derivation of Genus: *Anopheles,* hurtful; *Aedes,* unpleasant; *Culex,* gnat
Transmission Route: Fly from host to host
Common Name: Malaria mosquito (*A. quadrimaculatus*), yellow fever mosquito (*A. aegypti*), and mosquito (*Culex* species)

Anopheles quadrimaculatus, Aedes aegypti, *and* Culex *Species (Mosquitoes)*

Although they are tiny, fragile dipterans, mosquitoes are some of the most voracious blood-feeders (Figure 13-19) and strong fliers. Mosquitoes plague livestock, and as with black flies, swarms of mosquitoes have been known to keep cattle from grazing or cause them to stampede. The feeding of large swarms of mosquitoes can cause significant anemias in domestic animals. Because of their aquatic breeding environments, large numbers of mosquitoes can be produced from eggs laid in relatively small bodies of water.

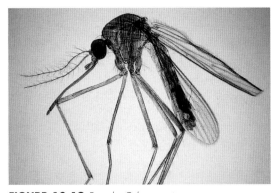

FIGURE 13-19 Female *Culex* species, one genus among several pathogenic genera of mosquitoes. Although mosquitoes are tiny, fragile dipterans, they are some of the most voracious blood-feeders known.

Anopheles quadrimaculatus females lay their eggs on the surface of still water. Each egg possesses two lateral corrugated areas called *floats*. These floats allow the eggs of *A. quadrimaculatus* to float on the water's still surface. At the tip of the *Anopheles* larval abdomen is a breathing pore that lacks a **siphon**. The larva floats parallel to the surface of the water and wriggles in the water if disturbed. The pupa floats right at the surface of the water and if disturbed will tumble down to a lower level within the water and slowly float back to the surface.

> **TECHNICIAN'S NOTE** The female mosquito requires a vertebrate blood meal in order to lay her eggs.

Aedes aegypti females lay their eggs on dry surfaces where water will accumulate. These eggs lack the floats of *A. quadrimaculatus*. The larval *A. aegypti* has three portions: head, thorax, and abdomen. On the tip of the abdomen is a breathing pore at the tip of the siphon. This mosquito larva floats parallel to the surface of the water and wriggles in the water if disturbed. As with *A. quadrimaculatus*, the *A. aegypti* pupa floats right at the surface of the water and if disturbed will tumble down to a lower level within the water and slowly float back to the surface.

> **TECHNICIAN'S NOTE** Mosquito eggs, larvae, and pupae are associated with still water because this is where they carry out the life stages of the mosquito.

Culex species females lay their eggs perpendicular to the surface of water to form a floating "egg raft." The larval mosquito has three portions: head, thorax, and abdomen. In the tip of the abdomen is a breathing pore at the tip of the siphon. This mosquito larva floats parallel to the surface of the water and wriggles in the water if disturbed. The pupa floats right at the surface of the water and if disturbed will tumble down to a lower level within the water and slowly float back to the surface.

Although they are known for spreading malaria (*Plasmodium* spp.), yellow fever, and elephantiasis in humans, mosquitoes are probably best known in veterinary medicine as intermediate hosts for the canine heartworm, *Dirofilaria immitis.*

Many of the repellents on the market are effective against mosquitoes. The repellents must be applied to the entire body at labeled frequencies to provide protection to the animal. In addition, preventing the buildup of small bodies of water on the premises (e.g., water in old tires, small puddles after rain) and cleaning water troughs frequently will help reduce the breeding grounds available to mosquitoes.

The adult and larval body of the mosquito has three portions: head, thorax, and abdomen. Adult mosquitoes have wings and body parts (head, thorax, and abdomen) covered by tiny leaf-shaped scales. The adult female of the *Anopheles* species has a proboscis with long palps. The adult females of the *Aedes* species and *Culex* species have a proboscis with short palps. **Palps** are appendages found near the mouth in invertebrate organisms used for sensation, locomotion, and feeding. All females have a pilose (covered with fine hairs) antenna. Identification of both adult and larval *Anopheles, Aedes,* and *Culex* species is probably best left to an entomologist.

> 📎 *TECHNICIAN'S NOTE* Mosquitoes are capable of transmitting bacteria, viruses, spirochetes, *Chlamydia,* protozoans (e.g., *Plasmodium* species [malaria]), and helminths (e.g., *D. immitis* [heartworm]). Some of these may be zoonotic agents.

Parasite: *Chrysops* species and *Tabanus* species
Host: Large mammals and humans, but small animals and avians can be attacked
Location of Adult: Skin surface when feeding; otherwise around lakes and ponds
Distribution: Worldwide
Derivation of Genus: *Chrysops,* golden eye; *Tabanus,* gadfly
Transmission Route: Fly from host to host
Common Name: Deerflies (*Chrysops* species) and horseflies (*Tabanus* species)

Chrysops *Species (Deerflies) and* Tabanus *Species (Horseflies)*

Tabanus species (horseflies) are **very large** flies (up to 3.5 cm in length), whereas *Chrysops* species are

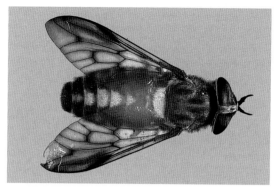

FIGURE 13-20 *Tabanus* species (horseflies) are large (up to 3.5 cm in length), heavy-bodied, robust dipterans with powerful wings. Horseflies are swift, speedy dipterans. These flies have very large eyes. Horseflies are much larger than deerflies.

smaller with banded wings. They both are heavy-bodied, robust, swift dipterans with powerful wings. These flies also have very large eyes. Horseflies and deerflies are the largest flies in this dipteran group in which only the females feed on vertebrate blood (Figure 13-20). Horseflies are much larger than deerflies. Deerflies have a dark band passing from the anterior to the posterior margin of the wings.

> 📎 *TECHNICIAN'S NOTE* Deerflies and horseflies are the largest flies in the dipteran group and are voracious blood-feeders that can consume large amounts of blood.

Adult flies lay eggs in the vicinity of open water such as lakes and ponds. Larval stages of horseflies and deerflies are found in aquatic to semiaquatic environments, often buried deep in mud at the bottom of lakes and ponds. Adults are seen in summer and prefer sunlight. The female flies feed in the vicinity of open water and have reciprocating, scissorlike mouthparts, which they use to lacerate the tissues of vertebrates and lap up the oozing blood. These flies feed primarily on large animals such as cattle and horses. Site preferences include the underside of the abdomen around the navel, the legs, and the neck and withers. Horseflies and deerflies feed several times in multiple sites before becoming filled with blood. When disturbed by the animal's swatting tail or by the panniculus reflex, the flies leave the host, although blood often continues to ooze from the open wound. The bites of these flies are very painful. Cattle and horses become restless in their presence. Stabling cattle and horses during the day will help reduce the annoyance of these parasites. The newer varieties of insect repellents offer a degree of relief to those animals turned out during the day. These flies may act as mechanical transmitters of anthrax, anaplasmosis, and the virus of equine infectious anemia.

The veterinary diagnostician can probably best identify these flies by their large, scissorlike mouthparts. Species identification of intact adult horseflies and deerflies is probably best left to an entomologist.

> **TECHNICIAN'S NOTE** Identification is best made by observation of the large scissorlike mouthparts, whereas species identification is best left to an entomologist.

Periodic Parasites of Which Both Adult Males and Females Feed on Vertebrate Blood

In the second group of blood-feeding dipterans, both male and female adult flies require a vertebrate blood meal. These species include *Glossina* species (tsetse fly); *S. calcitrans*, the stable fly; *H. irritans*, the horn fly; and *M. ovinus*, the wingless sheep ked.

Parasite: *Glossina* species
Host: Mammals, reptiles, avians, and humans
Location of Adult: Skin surface when feeding
Distribution: Continent of Africa
Derivation of Genus: Little tongue
Transmission Route: Fly from host to host
Common Name: Tsetse fly (*tsetse* means "fly destructive to cattle" in Setswana, the language of Botswana and South Africa)

Glossina *Species (Tsetse Fly)*

The tsetse fly, *Glossina* species, is a dipteran biting fly. The adult tsetse fly resembles a wasp or a large honeybee. This biting fly has a bayonet-like proboscis that is designed for piercing the skin and sucking blood. Both male and female flies are avid blood-feeders. There is an onion-shaped bulb at the base of the proboscis. Adult dipterans are identified by their unique wing pattern (**venations**). The tsetse fly has a cleaver or hatchet cell in the middle of each wing.

These flies are unique in that they breed only once during their life cycle. The female retains the larva within her abdomen until she is ready to deposit a single larva at a time. She will produce only four to six eggs during her lifetime. The female deposits individual larvae in loose, sandy soil. The larva develops into a pupa in a short period of time. After pupation, the adults emerge from the pupal case and are on the wing. They copulate only once, and the life cycle begins again.

> **TECHNICIAN'S NOTE** Tsetse flies breed only once in their lifetime, and the female produces only one larva at time.

These flies are found in fly belts (tropical) throughout the continent of Africa. They are periodic parasites; however, they serve as the intermediate host for *Trypanosoma* species, a protozoan parasite that produces both human and animal trypanosomiasis. These flies are not zoonotic because they only transmit animal trypanosomiasis between animals and human trypanosomiasis (African sleeping sickness) between humans. Animal trypanosomiasis is not transmitted to humans. Diagnosis is made by identifying the adult fly.

> **TECHNICIAN'S NOTE** Because tsetse flies breed only once during their lifetime, the flies can be controlled by using the sterile male release technique. Sterile males are released into the wild to compete with the intact males. The sterile male will mate with a female without producing an offspring.

Parasite: *Stomoxys calcitrans*
Host: A variety of animals and humans
Location of Adult: Around large animals, especially areas with large amounts of decaying vegetation
Distribution: Worldwide

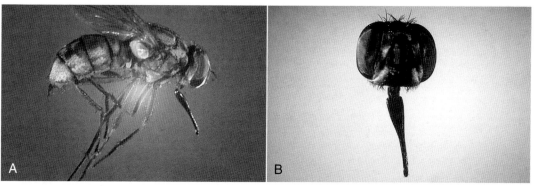

FIGURE 13-21 *Stomoxys calcitrans*, the stable fly or biting housefly, is approximately the size of the housefly, *Musca domestica*. It has a bayonet-like proboscis that protrudes forward from its head.

Derivation of Genus: Mouth sharp
Transmission Route: Fly from host to host
Common Name: Stable fly, biting housefly, or legsticker

Stomoxys calcitrans (Stable Fly)

The stable fly, *S. calcitrans*, is often called the biting housefly. It is approximately the size and coloration of the housefly *Musca domestica,* but instead of having a sponging type of mouthpart, the stable fly has a bayonet-like proboscis that protrudes forward from its head (Figure 13-21). These flies are found worldwide. In the United States they are found in the central and southeastern states, areas known for raising cattle. As mentioned previously both male and female flies are avid blood-feeders, preying on most domestic animals. They usually attack the legs and ventral abdomen but also may bite the ears. These flies tend to feed on the tips of the ears of dogs with pointed or raised ears (commonly called *fly strike*), such as German shepherds. This problem can be resolved by applying topical repellents to the ear tips.

> **TECHNICIAN'S NOTE** These flies prefer to feed on the ear tips of dogs with erect ears, such as German shepherds.

S. calcitrans also feeds on horses and cattle, with horses being the preferred host. The fly usually lands on the host with its head pointed upward. It is a sedentary fly, not moving on the host. The flies inflict painful bites that puncture the skin and bleed freely. Stable flies stay on the host for short periods, during which they obtain their blood meals. This is an outdoor fly; however, in late fall and during rainy weather it may enter barns or other enclosed areas. Topical insect repellents made for large animals work well against *S. calcitrans*. The repellents should be applied as recommended on the label for adequate protection.

Stable flies are mechanical vectors of anthrax in cattle and equine infectious anemia. This fly is the intermediate host for *Habronema muscae*, a nematode found in the stomach of horses, and *Stephanofilaria stilesi*, a nematode found in the skin of cattle, goats, and buffalo. When large numbers of stable flies attack dairy cattle, a decrease in milk production can result. Beef cattle may refuse to graze in the daytime when attacked by large numbers of flies; as a result, these cattle do not gain the usual amount of weight.

Stable flies use decaying organic material for laying eggs. Removing piles of leaves, grass clippings, soiled bedding, and other decaying matter from the premises will reduce the stable fly breeding areas and reduce the *S. calcitrans* population. Eggs hatch and produce larvae. Each larva develops into a pupa in a short period of time. After pupation, the adult emerges from the pupal case and is on the wing.

> **TECHNICIAN'S NOTE**   Control of the stable fly can be accomplished by removing piles of leaves, grass clippings, soiled bedding, and other decaying material from the premises to reduce the breeding areas.

The veterinary diagnostician can easily identify the stable fly by its size (approximately the same size as a housefly) and the bayonet-like proboscis that protrudes forward from the head.

Parasite: *Haematobia irritans*
Host: Cattle and buffalo
Location of Adult: Clustered around the horns but can be around the shoulders, back, sides, and ventral abdomen
Distribution: North America, Europe, and Australia
Derivation of Genus: Bloody life
Transmission Route: Fly from host
Common Name: Horn fly

Haematobia irritans (Horn Fly)

H. irritans is often called the **horn fly**. It is a dark-colored fly, approximately 3 to 6 mm in length, half the size of *S. calcitrans,* the biting housefly. As with the stable fly, the horn fly has a bayonet-like proboscis that protrudes forward from the head (Figure 13-22). These flies are found almost exclusively on cattle throughout North America.

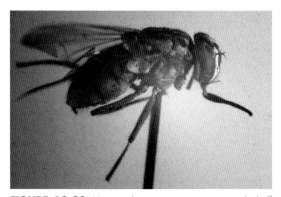

FIGURE 13-22 *Haematobia irritans* is approximately half the size of the stable fly, *Stomoxys calcitrans.* It also possesses a bayonet-like proboscis that protrudes forward from its head.

When the air temperature is below 70° F, horn flies cluster around the base of the horns, thus the common name, *horn fly*. In warmer climates, horn flies often cluster in large numbers on the host's shoulders, back, and sides; these are the areas least disturbed by tail swishing. On hot sunny days, horn flies often accumulate on the host's ventral abdomen. Use of insecticides effective against *H. irritans* will help reduce the horn fly population on the individual cow. This may be accomplished with a fly spray or pour-on solution. A walk-through horn fly trap will cut the individual population in half by mechanically removing the flies from the animal.

Adult horn flies spend most of their life on cattle; females leave the host to deposit their eggs in fresh cow manure. Within the "cow pie," the eggs hatch into larvae. Each larva develops into a pupa in a short period of time. At the end of the larval development, the larvae will crawl from the cow feces and pupate in loose soil. After pupation, the adult flies emerge from the pupal case and are on the wing. The egg, larval, and pupal morphology are significant in a veterinary clinic setting for the ease of control purposes. Disruption of the life cycle can be accomplished by spreading the cow feces so it can dry out.

> **TECHNICIAN'S NOTE**   Although these horn flies can be loosely classified as periodic parasites, they spend most of their adult lives on the animal until they are disrupted. Once disrupted, they fly off the host and either fly back to the same host or fly to a new host.

Using their tiny bayonet-like mouthparts, horn flies feed frequently, sucking blood and other fluids, and cause considerable irritation. Female flies are more aggressive than males. The energy lost in disturbing the feeding flies coupled with the loss of blood often results in reduced weight gain and milk production. Horn flies probably cause greater losses of cattle in the United States than any other blood-feeding fly. Adult horn flies also cause focal midline dermatitis on the ventral abdomen of horses. These flies serve as the intermediate hosts for *S. stilesi,* a filarial parasite that produces ventral plaquelike lesions on the underside of the abdomen of cattle.

The veterinary diagnostician can easily identify *H. irritans* by its dark color and size (approximately half the size of a stable fly). As with the stable fly, the horn fly's bayonet-like proboscis protrudes forward from the head.

> ⬛ *TECHNICIAN'S NOTE* Although horn flies are loosely classified as periodic parasites, they are typically found on the backs of cattle in the pasture in numbers as large as 20,000.

Parasite: *Melophagus ovinus*
Host: Sheep and goats
Location of Adult: Deep within the sheep's wool or the goat's fleece
Distribution: Worldwide
Derivation of Genus: Sheep eater
Transmission Route: Direct contact with infested animals
Common Name: Sheep ked

Melophagus ovinus (Sheep Ked)

M. ovinus is often referred to as the sheep ked. As mentioned earlier, members of the order Diptera usually possess one pair of wings; sheep keds are exceptions to that rule: They are wingless dipterans. Sheep keds have an unusual appearance; they are hairy and appear leathery and measure approximately 4 to 7 mm in length (Figure 13-23). The

head of this dipteran is short and broad and contains piercing (bloodsucking) mouthparts. The thorax is brown, and the abdomen is broad and grayish brown. The legs are strong and armed with stout claws (Figure 13-24). Keds are often described as having a louselike appearance, but they definitely are not lice.

> ⬛ *TECHNICIAN'S NOTE* Although placed in the order Diptera, the sheep ked is a wingless dipteran that has an unusual hairy and leathery appearance.

The female sheep ked does not lay eggs but retains one larva within her abdomen until she is ready to deposit that one larva in the sheep's wool or the goat's fleece. The larvae develop into pupae quickly; the pupae are dark brown and are also found in the wool or fleece. After pupation, the adults emerge from the pupal case and can be found within the wool. The life cycle then begins again with the male and female sheep ked breeding. The entire life cycle of this dipteran takes place on the host.

Keds are permanent ectoparasites of sheep and goats. Their pupal stages are often found attached to the wool or fleece of the host. Keds are avid blood-feeders. Heavy infestations can reduce the condition of the host considerably and even cause significant anemia. The bites of *M. ovinus* cause pruritus over much of the host's body; the infested

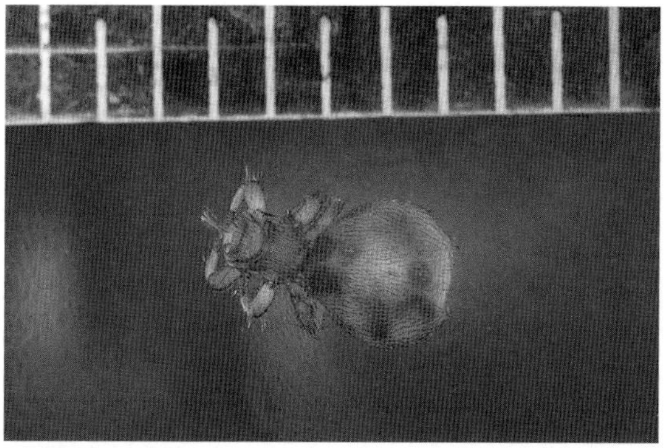

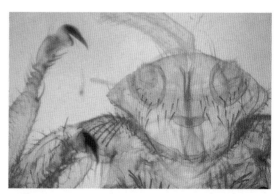

FIGURE 13-23 *Melophagus ovinus*, the sheep ked, is a wingless dipteran that is hairy, leathery, and approximately 4 to 7 mm in length.

FIGURE 13-24 The head of *Melophagus ovinus* is short and broad. The legs are strong and armed with stout claws. Some say keds have a louselike appearance.

sheep often bites, scratches, and rubs itself, thus damaging the wool. Ked feces are dark brown, stain the wool, and do not wash out readily. Keds are most numerous in cold temperatures during fall and winter. Their numbers decline as temperatures rise in spring and summer. Close inspection of the wool and underlying skin reveals infestation by these wingless dipterans. Infested wool often has a dark-brown appearance because of discoloration by ked feces. Control of *M. ovinus* may be accomplished by applying an effective insecticide to the sheep after shearing.

> **TECHNICIAN'S NOTE** There are other species of keds found on other hosts; *Lipoptena cervi* is the deer ked found on deer.

Sheep keds are closely related to the hippoboscid flies, winged dipterans that parasitize wild birds. These flattened, swiftly flying, blood-feeding dipterans are often found among the feathers of wild birds. Two important hippoboscid flies are *Lynchia* and *Pseudolynchia* species (Figure 13-25). They can serve as intermediate hosts for *Haemoproteus* species, a malaria-like parasite of wild birds.

Parasite: *Lynchia* species and *Pseudolynchia* species
Host: Wild birds
Location of Adult: Deep within the feathers
Distribution: Tropical and subtropical regions
Derivation of Genus: Unknown

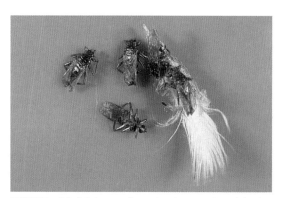

FIGURE 13-25 Louse flies, *Lynchia* or *Pseudolynchia* species, often parasitize wild birds.

Transmission Route: Direct contact with infested bird
Common Name: Bird keds

Lynchia *Species and* Pseudolynchia *Species (Bird Keds)*

The bird keds are winged dipterans in that they possess one pair of wings and are strong and swift fliers. The adults have piercing (bloodsucking) mouthparts. Both males and females are avid blood-feeders. The adults can be found deep within the feathers of the bird. At the end of each of the adult fly's legs is a fierce looking claw designed to grip the feathers.

The female bird ked does not lay eggs but retains a single larva within her abdomen until she is ready to deposit it. The larvae develop into pupae very quickly. The pupae are dark brown. After pupation, adults emerge from the pupal case and can be found among the feathers. The life cycle begins again with the male and female breeding. The entire life cycle usually takes place on the host. Although transmission is usually from infested bird to uninfested bird by direct contact, the adults are strong fliers, so they can fly from host to host; thus they should be considered periodic parasites.

> **TECHNICIAN'S NOTE** If one is handling birds infested with bird keds, the flies may fly off the avian host and try to get in the hair of the veterinarian, technician, or presenting client.

Periodic Parasites That Feed on Mucus, Tears, and Saliva

The final periodic parasites among the dipteran flies discussed here are ones that are not blood-feeders but instead feed on the mucus, tears, saliva, or feces of animals. These flies are known as *M. domestica* (housefly), *M. autumnalis* (face fly), *Calliphora* species, *Lucilia* species, *Phormia* species, *Phaenicia* species, *Sarcophaga* species, and *Hippelates* species.

Parasite: *Musca domestica*
Host: A variety of animals

Location of Adult: Within the house
Distribution: Worldwide
Derivation of Genus: Fly
Transmission Route: Fly from host to host
Common Name: Housefly

Musca domestica (Housefly)

M. domestica, or the houseflies, are medium-sized, mouse-gray flies that have sponging mouthparts. These mouthparts cannot be used for lacerating flesh but are designed for lapping up liquid food, including secretions from animals. These flies are "vomit drop feeders." The adults disgorge their stomach contents, which contain digestive enzymes that liquefy their food. They have a freely movable head and are covered with tiny hairlike bristles called **setae.** Their legs have sticky footpads. These flies are "designed" for spreading pathogens.

> *TECHNICIAN'S NOTE* The larval stage of the housefly life cycle produces a facultative myiasis that is of great veterinary significance.

Egg and pupal morphologies of *M. domestica* are not of great veterinary significance, but larval morphology is very important in the clinic setting. The larval stage is called *facultative myiasis.* In facultative myiasis, the larval stages may be found in tissues or organs of domestic or wild animals and sometimes in humans. This is discussed more in Facultative Myiasis-Producing Flies.

M. domestica are **synanthropic** (living with humans), meaning they are house-invading flies. Houseflies fly freely from feces to food and can transmit a variety of pathogens to animals and humans. The identification of the adult flies is best left to a trained entomologist.

> *TECHNICIAN'S NOTE* Houseflies are efficiently designed for spreading pathogens.

Parasite: *Musca autumnalis*
Host: Cattle predominately
Location of Adult: Feeding around the medial canthus of the eye
Distribution: Worldwide
Derivation of Genus: Fly
Transmission Route: Fly from host to host
Common Name: Face fly

Musca autumnalis (Face Fly)

Face flies, *M. autumnalis,* are so named because they gather around the eyes and muzzle of livestock, particularly cattle. They may also be found on the withers, neck, brisket, and sides. Face flies feed mostly on saliva, tears, and mucus. They usually are not considered blood-feeders because their mouthparts are not piercing or bayonet-like. Instead, their mouthparts are adapted for sponging up saliva, tears, and mucus (Figure 13-26). These flies often follow flies that feed on blood, disturb them during

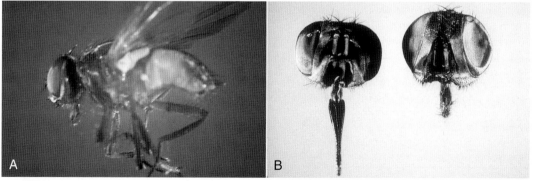

FIGURE 13-26 A, *Musca autumnalis,* the face fly. These flies gather around the eyes and muzzle of livestock, particularly cattle. Their mouthparts are adapted for sponging up saliva, tears, and mucus. **B,** Left, *Stomoxys calcitrans;* right, *Musca autumnalis.*

their feeding process, then lap up the blood and body fluids that ooze and accumulate on the host's skin. Face flies are found on animals that are outdoors; they usually will not follow animals into barns or other enclosures.

Face flies produce considerable pathology because of their annoyance of the host. The irritation around the host's eyes stimulates the flow of tears, which attracts more flies. The flies' activity produces annoyance, which ultimately interferes with the host's productivity. Face flies may be vectors in the transmission of *Moraxella bovis*, a bacterium that causes infectious keratoconjunctivitis, or pinkeye, in cattle. Face flies may be controlled with the application of an insecticide to the animal's body to offer a degree of relief. Spraying potential breeding sites with insecticide will help reduce fly populations. The eggs are laid in fresh cow feces, whereas the larval and pupal stages can be found in the soil surrounding dried cow feces.

> *TECHNICIAN'S NOTE* The face fly is a great annoyance to the host and is a vector for transmitting the etiologic agent for infectious bovine keratoconjunctivitis, *Moraxella bovis*.

Grossly, the face fly is morphologically similar to the housefly, *M. domestica*. These two species in the genus *Musca* can be differentiated only through minor differences in eye position and color of the abdomen. The veterinary diagnostician should probably not attempt to speciate this fly; speciation requires the skills of a trained entomologist. Rather the veterinary diagnostician should remember this rule of thumb: If a fly with sponging mouthparts is found around the face of a cow or horse, it is most probably a face fly.

> *TECHNICIAN'S NOTE* A symbiotic relationship between two organisms of different species in which a smaller organism (*Moraxella bovis*) is carried about by a larger organism (*Musca autumnalis*) is called *phoresis*. The relationship between *M. autumnalis* and *M. bovis* is an excellent example of phoresis.

Parasite: *Calliphora* species, *Lucilia* species, *Phormia* species, and *Phaenicia* species
Host: Domestic animals, wild animals, and humans

Location of Adult: Free-living with humans
Distribution: Australia, England, and North America (*Calliphora*); Worldwide (*Lucilia*, *Phormia*, and *Phaenicia* species)
Derivation of Genus: *Calliphora*, beauty-bearing; *Lucilia*, light
Transmission Route: Fly from feces to food
Common Name: Bottle flies or blowflies

Calliphora *Species*, Lucilia *Species*, Phormia *Species*, and *Phaenicia Species*

These dipteran species are collectively known as the *bottle flies* or *blowflies*. These flies are medium sized, shiny, and iridescent (blue, black, and green resembling the color of glass bottles, hence the name bottle flies) with sponging mouthparts. The mouthparts cannot be used for lacerating flesh but are designed for lapping up liquid food. These flies are vomit drop feeders. The adult flies disgorge their stomach contents, which contain digestive enzymes that liquefy their food. They have a freely movable head and are covered with tiny hairlike bristles called *setae*. Their legs have sticky footpads. These flies are designed for spreading pathogens.

The egg and pupal stages of the life cycle are not of great veterinary significance. However, the morphology of the larval stage is very important in the clinical scenario called *facultative myiasis*. In facultative myiasis, the larval stages of these flies may be found in tissues or organs of domestic or wild animals and sometimes human beings. This is discussed further under the topic *Calliphora*, *Lucilia*, *Phormia*, and *Phaenicia* Species—Larval Stages.

> *TECHNICIAN'S NOTE* Bottle flies or blowflies are important in veterinary parasitology as facultative myiasis–producing flies.

Like the houseflies, the bottle flies or blowflies are synanthropic (living with humans), meaning they are house-invading flies. The bottle flies or blowflies fly freely from feces to food, transmitting a variety of pathogens. These pathogens are spread by the host eating the infected food on which the flies have disgorged their stomach contents. Thus they can spread a variety of zoonotic pathogens.

> **TECHNICIAN'S NOTE** Some of the larvae of some species of bottle flies or blowflies are classified as surgical maggots because their larvae have been purposefully introduced into infected wounds of both animals and humans to facilitate the healing process.

Parasite: *Sarcophaga* species
Host: Domestic animals, wild animals, and humans
Location of Adult: Free-flying in the environment
Distribution: North America and Hawaii
Derivation: Flesh eater
Transmission Route: Fly from feces to food
Common Name: Flesh fly

Sarcophaga *Species (Flesh Fly)*

Sarcophaga species are known as the flesh flies. They are medium- to large-sized flies possessing a striped thorax and a checkerboard abdomen. They possess sponging mouthparts that cannot be used for lacerating flesh but instead are designed for lapping up liquid food. These flies are vomit drop feeders. The adult flies disgorge their stomach contents, which contain digestive enzymes that liquefy their food. They have a freely movable head and are covered with setae. Their legs have sticky footpads. These flies are designed for spreading pathogens.

The female fly retains her eggs within her abdomen. These flies do not lay eggs but instead deposit first-stage larvae in either feces, carrion, or contaminated wounds. The pupal stage is not of great veterinary significance; however, the larval stage is very important in the clinical scenario called *facultative myiasis*. In facultative myiasis, the larval stages of these flies may be found in tissues or organs of domestic and wild animals and sometimes in humans. This is discussed more under the topic *Sarcophaga* Species—Larval Stage.

Adult flesh flies fly freely from feces to food and (like houseflies and bottle flies and blowflies) are efficiently designed for transmitting a variety of pathogens, some of which are zoonotic.

> **TECHNICIAN'S NOTE** Speciation of flesh flies should be left to an entomologist.

Parasite: *Liohippelates* species (formerly *Hippelates*)
Host: Bovines and canines
Location of Adult: On or about mucocutaneous junctions of the eyes, lips, and teats of cattle and the penis of the dog
Distribution: North and South America
Derivation of Genus: Unknown
Transmission Route: Fly from host to host
Common Name: Dog penis gnats

Hippelates *Species*

Liohippelates species of dipterans are known as dog penis gnats because of their proximity to the glans penis of the male dog. These are tiny, nonbiting gnats (not to be confused with the biting gnats *Simulium, Phlebotomus, Lutzomyia,* or *Culicoides* species). Instead of the lacerating mouthparts possessed by the biting gnats, these nonbiting gnats have sponging mouthparts very similar to those of the housefly, *M. domestica.* These flies are found in locations on or about the mucocutaneous junctions around the eyes, lips, and teats of cattle and around the penis of the male dog. These flies are irritating to the host. They feed on moisture associated with the mucocutaneous junctions.

> **TECHNICIAN'S NOTE** Dog penis gnats are often found in the proximity of the glans penis of the male dog, hence the common name, *dog penis gnats.*

Myiasis-Producing Flies

With regard to their roles as ectoparasites, larval dipterans may develop in the subcutaneous tissues of the skin of many domestic animals. When dipteran larvae develop in the tissues or organs of vertebrate hosts, these larvae produce a condition known as *myiasis*. Depending on the degree of host dependence, there are two types of myiases: (1) facultative myiasis, in which the fly larvae are usually **free-living**, and (2) obligatory myiasis. In facultative myiasis, the normally free-living larvae adapt themselves to a parasitic dependence on a host. In obligatory myiasis, the fly larvae are completely parasitic; that is, they are dependent on the host during development through the life cycle. In other words, without the host, the obligatory parasites will die.

> *TECHNICIAN'S NOTE*   Free-living fly larvae can become adapted to being parasitic and being dependent on a host to survive to the next stage of their life cycle.

Dipteran Fly Larvae That Infest the Skin

Facultative Myiasis–Producing Flies. The dipteran larvae capable of producing facultative myiasis in the skin are *M. domestica,* the housefly; *Calliphora, Phaenicia, Lucilia,* and *Phormia* species, the blowflies, or bottle flies; and *Sarcophaga* species, the flesh flies. Larval stages of these flies are usually associated with skin wounds contaminated with bacteria or with a matted hair coat contaminated with feces.

Under normal conditions, adult flies of these genera lay their eggs in decaying animal carcasses or in feces. In facultative myiasis the adult flies are attracted to an animal's moist wound, skin lesion, or soiled hair coat. These sites provide the adult fly with moist media on which to feed. As adult female flies feed in these sites, they lay eggs. The eggs hatch, producing larvae (maggots), which move independently about the wound surface, ingesting dead cells, exudate, secretions, and debris but not live tissue. This condition is known as **fly strike**, or **strike**. These larvae irritate, injure, and kill successive layers of skin and produce exudates. Maggots can tunnel through the thinned epidermis into the subcutis. This process produces tissue cavities in the skin that measure up to several centimeters in diameter (Figure 13-27). Unless the process is halted by appropriate therapy, the infested animal may die of shock, intoxication, histolysis, or infection. A peculiar, distinct, pungent odor permeates the infested tissue and the affected animal. Advanced lesions may contain thousands of maggots. It is important to remember that as adults, these flies can be pestiferous in a veterinary clinical setting. These flies are vomit drop feeders and fly from feces to food, spreading bacteria on their feet and within their disgorged stomach contents.

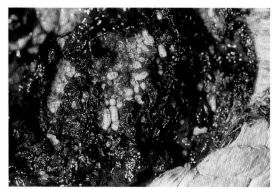

FIGURE 13-27 Fly strike in a Hereford cow. The fly larvae (maggots) move independently about the wound surface, ingesting dead cells, exudate, secretions, and debris but not live tissue. This condition is known as *fly strike,* or *strike.*

> *TECHNICIAN'S NOTE*   A facultative myiasis fly can lay eggs in the moist wound, skin lesion, or soiled hair coat of an animal or human. These eggs then hatch and produce a maggot infestation in that area.

A tentative diagnosis of maggot infestation in any domestic animal can easily be made by a veterinary diagnostician because maggots can be observed in an existing wound or among the soiled, matted hair coat. A specific diagnosis can be made by examining the spiracular plate on the posterior end of the fly maggot. Each species of fly maggot has its own distinctive spiracular plate, much like a fingerprint (Figure 13-28). Dichotomous keys are available for identifying the specific spiracular plate of each species. As soon as a diagnosis of facultative myiasis has been made, the veterinary diagnostician must rule out the possibility of obligatory myiasis caused by *Cochliomyia hominivorax.*

> *TECHNICIAN'S NOTE*   Maggot infestation is easily made by a veterinarian because the maggots can be observed in an existing wound or around the soiled and matted hair coat.

The larval stages of *Calliphora, Lucilia, Phormia, Phaenicia, and Sarcophaga* species are very recognizable by the owner or the veterinarian. The typical larva is fusiform (bullet-shaped). On its anterior

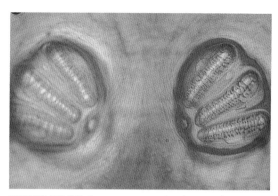

FIGURE 13-28 Diagnostic spiracular plates on the posterior end of a fly maggot. This plate can be used for positive identification of the fly maggot.

end is a pair of hooks that are used to assist the larva in crawling about the contaminated wound surface. *Sarcophaga* species deposit larvae rather than eggs into contaminated wounds (particularly skin wounds) of warm-blooded animals so the larvae can live a "parasitic existence"; thus they are considered facultative parasites. Wounds are not absolutely necessary for the laying of eggs because flies can lay their eggs in the pelage (hair coat) that is contaminated with urine or feces. Bottle fly or blowfly larvae can be differentiated from that of *C. hominivorax* by the absence of the two deeply pigmented (black), parallel tracheal tubes on the dorsal-posterior third of the third-stage larva of *C. hominivorax*.

> **⬚TECHNICIAN'S NOTE** There are some species of bottle flies or blowflies that produce larvae that *only* ingest unhealthy tissues (tissues contaminated with pathogenic species of bacteria). These species are referred to as *surgical maggots*.

Obligatory Myiasis–Producing Flies. The dipteran larvae capable of producing obligatory myiasis in the skin are *C. hominivorax*, *Cuterebra* species, and *Hypoderma* species. In obligatory myiasis the dipteran larvae lead a parasitic existence.

Parasite: *Cochliomyia hominivorax*
Host: Domestic animals

Location of Larva: Fresh, uncontaminated wounds of warm-blooded animals
Distribution: North America
Derivation of Genus: Screw fly
Transmission Route: Fly from host to host
Common Name: Screwworm, primary screwworm, or New World screwworm

Cochliomyia hominivorax. Only one fly in North America, *C. hominivorax*, is a primary invader of fresh, uncontaminated skin wounds of domestic animals. These larvae must not be confused with the larvae of the facultative myiasis–producing flies just described. *C. hominivorax* is often referred to as the screwworm fly. In economic terms, it is the most important of the flies that attack livestock in the southwestern and southern United States. These are nonbiting muscoid flies. Adult female flies are attracted to fresh skin wounds (such as recent surgical sites or recent lacerations) on warm-blooded animals, where they lay batches of 15 to 500 eggs in a shinglelike pattern at the edge of the wounds. The female fly lays several thousand eggs during her lifetime. The cream-colored, elongated eggs hatch within 24 hours. Larvae enter the wound, where they feed for 4 to 7 days before they become third-stage (fully grown) larvae. The veterinarian *must* be able to identify the third-stage larvae of this obligatory myiasis–producing fly. The third-stage larvae are segmented, with each segment being emphasized by the presence of rows of tiny, backward-facing black spines along the segment, giving the larvae the appearance of a spiraling wood screw. These larvae can be as long as 1.5 cm; at this stage they resemble a wood screw, thus the name *screwworm*. The third larval stage is *unique* in its appearance. It possesses two deeply pigmented (black) and parallel tracheal tubes on the dorsal-posterior third of the third-stage larva (Figure 13-29). When fully grown, the larvae drop to the ground, after which the adult flies emerge. The adult male and female flies breed only once during their lifetime, a key fact that is used to control these flies biologically. Adult screwworm flies are shiny, greenish blue with a reddish-orange head and eyes and are 8 to 15 mm long.

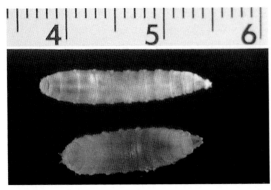

FIGURE 13-29 Larvae of *Cochliomyia hominivorax* can be identified by the wood-screw shape and two deeply pigmented tracheal tubes on the dorsal aspect of the caudal ends of the third larval stage.

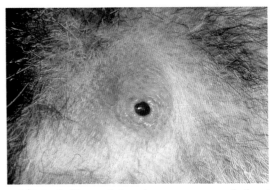

FIGURE 13-30 Larval *Cuterebra* species are usually found in swollen, cystlike subcutaneous sites, with a fistula (pore, or hole) communicating to the outside environment. The larva breathes through the pore.

> **TECHNICIAN'S NOTE** Identification of the distinct third-stage larva is used to diagnose this stage of *Cochliomyia hominivorax*. Unique features include the characteristic wood-screw shape and the presence of two deeply pigmented and parallel tracheal tubes at the dorsal-posterior third of the larva.

Because of the obligatory nature of the screwworm with regard to breeding in the fresh wounds of warm-blooded animals, the veterinary diagnostician must report the parasite to both state and federal authorities. *C. hominivorax* has been eradicated from the United States but occasionally enters the country surreptitiously in imported animals. Although *C. hominivorax* is not a true zoonotic parasite, it can develop in any warm-blooded animal, including humans.

> **TECHNICIAN'S NOTE** *Cochliomyia hominivorax* was once present in most of the United States and Canada; however, it has been eradicated from these portions of North America. Because these flies breed only once in their lifetime, they can be controlled using the sterile male release control technique.

Parasite: *Cuterebra* species
Host: Rabbits, squirrels, mice, rats, chipmunks, occasionally dogs and cats

Location of Larva: Areas around the head and neck
Distribution: North America
Derivation of Genus: Skin borer
Transmission Route: Direct contact with first-stage larvae
Common Name: Warbles or wolves

Cuterebra Species (Wolves, Warbles). Larvae of the genus *Cuterebra* (commonly called wolves or warbles) infest the skin of rabbits, squirrels, mice, rats, chipmunks, and occasionally dogs and cats. The adult flies look almost exactly like bumblebees. Ova are never observed on the animal. A large discrepancy exists concerning the morphologic descriptions of larval *Cuterebra*. Most of the specimens recovered in a clinical setting are of the second-stage or third-stage larvae. Second-stage larvae are grublike, 5 to 10 mm long, and cream to grayish white; this stage is often sparsely covered with tiny, black, toothlike spines. Third-stage larvae are large, robust, and coal black with a heavily spined appearance; they are up to 3 cm in length. Larval stages are usually found in swollen, cystlike subcutaneous sites, with a fistula (pore or hole) communicating to the outside environment (Figure 13-30). It is through this pore that the larval *Cuterebra* breathes.

Adult flies lay eggs near the entrance to rodent burrows. Pets usually contract this parasite while investigating or seeking out rodent prey. As a result, the most frequently affected cutaneous sites in dogs and cats are the subcutaneous tissues of the neck and head. Most cases occur during the late summer and early fall. Among the myiasis-producing flies, this dipteran larva is known for its aberrant or erratic migrations, having been found in a variety of extracutaneous sites such as the cranial vault, the anterior chamber of the eye, the nose, and the pharyngeal regions. Clinical signs vary with the site of infection or infestation. Larval *Cuterebra* species are often discovered in cutaneous sites during physical examination. They are usually removed surgically by enlarging the breathing pore and removing the larva with thumb forceps. Great care must be taken not to crush the larva during the extraction process because anaphylaxis may result.

Cuterebrosis is diagnosed by observing the characteristic swollen, cystlike subcutaneous lesion with its fistula or central pore that communicates to the outside environment. Second-stage or third-stage larvae are usually removed from these cutaneous lesions. These larvae are usually covered with tiny black spines (Figure 13-31).

TECHNICIAN'S NOTE *Cuterebra* species should be removed carefully; great care must be taken not to crush the larva during extraction to avoid a possible anaphylactic reaction in the host.

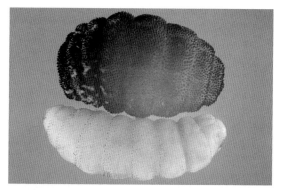

FIGURE 13-31 Different developmental stages of *Cuterebra* species. Larval *Cuterebra* are either sparsely or thickly covered with tiny black spines.

Parasite: *Hypoderma* species
Host: Cattle and in rare instances horses, sheep, and humans
Location of Larva: In large boil-like cysts in the back of the cow
Distribution: Northern and southern United States and Canada
Derivation of Genus: Under the skin
Transmission Route: Adult female flies from host to host
Common Name: Gadflies (adults) and cattle grubs (larvae)

Hypoderma Species (Ox Warbles). Two larval species of *Hypoderma* flies (ox warbles or cattle grubs) infect cattle: *Hypoderma lineatum* and *Hypoderma bovis*. *H. lineatum* is found in the southern United States, and both species are found in the northern United States and Canada. The adult flies are heavy and resemble honeybees; they are often called **heel flies**. These adult flies have very primitive mouthparts, so they are not capable of biting the cow; however, they do produce much annoyance for the cow.

The entire life cycle is almost a year long. Adult flies are bothersome to cattle as they approach to lay eggs. Animals often become apprehensive and disturbed and attempt to escape this pesky fly by running away, an action called gadding. At the end of the adult female's abdomen there is an ovipositor, which she uses to deposit her eggs on the hairs of the cow's leg. The eggs are about 1 mm long and white and are attached to hairs on the legs of cattle. *H. lineatum* deposits a row of six or more eggs on an individual hair shaft; *H. bovis* lays its eggs singly on the hair shaft. The larvae hatch in about 4 days and crawl down the hair shaft to the skin, which they penetrate. The larvae wander through the subcutaneous connective tissues in the leg, migrating through the esophagus (*H. lineatum*) or the region of the spinal canal and epidural fat (*H. bovis*) until they reach the subcutaneous tissues of the back. Here the larvae create breathing holes in the skin of the dorsum; it is through these pores that they later exit and fall to the ground to pupate. The adult flies emerge from the pupae.

> **TECHNICIAN'S NOTE** *Hypoderma* species produces pathology both as an adult (in the form of annoyance and gadding) and as a larval stage (within boil-like cysts in the skin of the back of the cow). If systemic insecticides are used while the larvae are migrating through the spinal cord or esophagus, limb paralysis or bloat may result.

Adult *Hypoderma* species are beelike and are covered with yellow-to-orange hairs. Mature larvae are 25 to 30 mm long, cream to dark brown, and covered with small spines. Lesions consist of large, cystlike swellings on the back, with a central breathing pore (Figure 13-32). As with *Cuterebra* species, great care must be taken not to crush the *Hypoderma* larva during the extraction process because anaphylaxis may result.

Dipteran Fly Larvae That Infect the Gastrointestinal Tract

Parasite: *Gasterophilus* species
Host: Horses and donkeys
Location of Larva: Attached to horse's gastric mucosa
Distribution: Worldwide
Derivation of Genus: Stomach loving
Transmission Route: The adult female lays eggs on the horse's leg, the horse grooms itself, the larvae hatch and penetrate the mucosa
Common Name: Bot flies (adults), horse bots (larvae)

Gasterophilus species (horse bots or stomach bots) have three developmental stages that may be associated with pathology in the horse. Just as adult *Hypoderma* species are annoying to the host, adult *Gasterophilus* species are similarly annoying. These adult flies resemble honeybees. The adult flies have very primitive mouthparts; thus, they are not able to bite the horse. During late summer and early fall, adult females fly around the fetlocks of the forelegs and the chin and shoulders of the horse to oviposit eggs on the hairs in these regions (Figure 13-33). This fly's activity and the accompanying oviposition cause extreme annoyance to the host. Some horses will panic because of the egg-laying activity of these flies. The bot fly eggs are small and white. The female fly "glues" each egg individually to single hairs on the leg of the horse (or appropriate location). Within each egg is a tiny fly larva (first-stage larva), which is ringed by several rows of backward-facing spines. Once the eggs have been laid on the hairs, the horses lick themselves. The abrasive tongue and accompanying saliva are a stimulus for the larvae to hatch from the eggs (Figure 13-34). The larvae penetrate the mucosa of the lips, tongue, and buccal cavity and migrate through the oral mucosa. They eventually emerge and migrate to the cardiac portion of the stomach, where they remain attached for 10 to 12 months. The larvae measure up to 20 mm in length, are red to brown, and possess dense spines on the anterior border of each body segment. There is a pair of

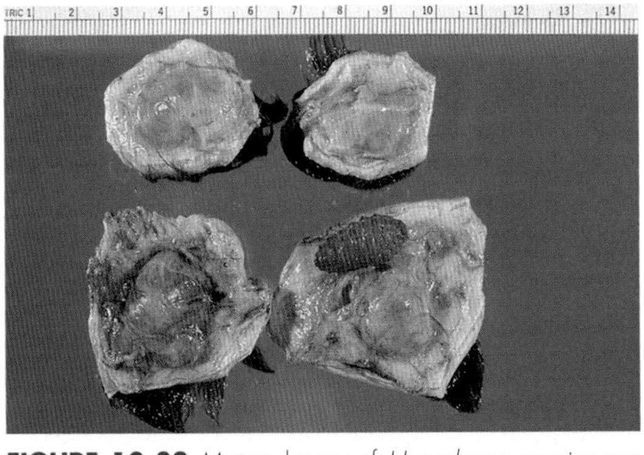

FIGURE 13-32 Mature larvae of *Hypoderma* species are 25 to 30 mm long, cream to dark brown, and covered with small spines. Lesions consist of large cystlike swellings on the back, with a central breathing pore.

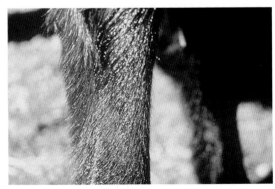

FIGURE 13-33 Numerous eggs cemented to the forelimb of a horse.

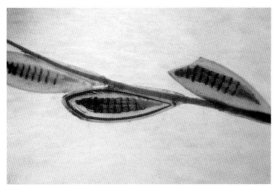

FIGURE 13-34 Individual eggs [?] of *Gasterophilus* species cemented by an adult female fly to the hairs on a horse's leg. Friction and moisture of the horse's licking cause the egg to hatch. Note the emergence of the larval bot.

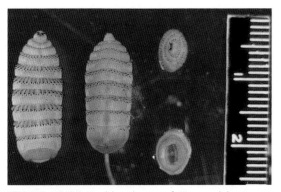

FIGURE 13-35 Final larval stage of *Gasterophilus* species is often found within the feces of the equine host. Note the presence of anterior hooks, with the larva attached to the gastric mucosa.

indistinct mouth hooks (organs of attachment) on the anterior end of the first body segment and a spiracular plate on the posterior end. These larvae usually pass out of the host in the spring (Figure 13-35) and pupate on the ground for 3 to 5 weeks. The adult flies emerge from the pupal case and live during the latter half of the summer. The larval stage of the *Gasterophilus* species can be treated with dichlorvos, trichlorfon, or ivermectin dewormers in the fall and spring seasons. A bot knife may be used on the legs of the animal to remove the eggs before they are able to infect the animal.

> **TECHNICIAN'S NOTE** *Gasterophilus* species produces pathology as both an adult (annoyance) and as a larva (attachment to gastric mucosa).

The veterinary diagnostician should be able to identify the annoying adult female flies seen around the horse in the fall. The telltale egg stages contain tiny larvae, and the dark-brown bots pass out with the feces. It is through the feces that the third larval stage exits the gastrointestinal tract; therefore this parasitic stage may be recovered in horse feces.

Dipteran Fly Larvae That Infect the Respiratory Tract
Parasite: *Oestrus ovis*
Host: Sheep and goats
Location of Larva: Nasal passages
Distribution: Worldwide
Derivation of Genus: Gadfly
Transmission Route: Adult female flies from host to host and lays larvae in the nares
Common Name: Nasal bot fly (adult); grub (larvae)

> **TECHNICIAN'S NOTE** How does a bot fly get a name that sounds like a portion of a female's reproductive cycle? It was once believed that when women were undergoing the estrus phase of their menstrual cycle, they would "act irrationally" or become "hysterical." When sheep are plagued by the adult nasal bot fly, they run about madly, hence the name *Oestrus ovis*.

Oestrus ovis (Nasal Bots). *Oestrus ovis* (nasal bots or nasal bot flies) produce a respiratory myiasis in sheep. The adults are beelike flies and, like both *Hypoderma* and *Gasterophilus* species, are quite annoying to the sheep or goat. The adult female fly flies into the area of the nostrils where she deposits a tiny, first-stage larva. This causes a great deal of annoyance, resulting in the sheep or goat keeping its nostrils very close to the ground as an avoidance mechanism. This tiny white-to-yellow larva crawls upward into the nostrils and sinuses of the sheep or goat, often producing a purulent rhinitis or sinusitis. The larvae grow rapidly into 3-cm,

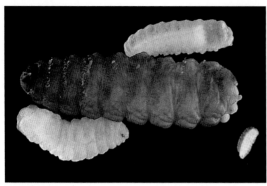

FIGURE 13-36 Several larval stages of *Oestrus ovis* extracted from the nasal passages of sheep.

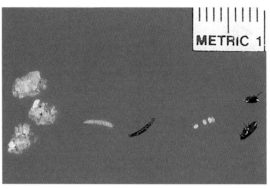

FIGURE 13-37 Life stages of *Ctenocephalides felis*, the cat flea: adult males and females, eggs, larvae, and pupae.

dark-brown larvae with large black oral hooks (Figure 13-36). When fully developed, the larvae drop out of the nostrils and pupate in the ground; the adults then emerge from the pupae. Ivermectin has been shown to be very effective against *O. ovis.*

The veterinary diagnostician should be able to identify the large dark-brown bots as they pass out of the nostrils.

> *TECHNICIAN'S NOTE* Occasionally the larvae of *Oestrus ovis* wander aberrantly and get into the host's cranial vault, producing neurologic abnormalities. This neurologic condition is referred to as *false gid.*

SIPHONAPTERA (FLEAS)

Of all the orders of arthropods discussed thus far, members of the order Siphonaptera, or fleas, are perhaps the most important insect with respect to veterinary economics. Treating for fleas can be a veterinary practice builder. Because of the extreme popularity of dogs and cats and the prolific nature of the flea (and thus its ability to return after populations are exterminated on the animal and within the animal's environment), the veterinarian should pay special attention to diagnosing the various life cycle stages of fleas both on the pet and in the pet's environment (Figure 13-37).

Parasite: *Ctenocephalides felis, Ctenocephalides canis, Cediopsylla simplex, Odontopsylla multispinosus,* and *Echidnophaga gallinacea*

Host: Cats and dogs (*C. felis*), dogs (*C. canis*), rabbits (*C. simplex*), rabbits (*O. multispinosus*), and poultry but will feed on dogs and cats (*E. gallinacea*)
Location of Adult: On the skin
Distribution: Worldwide
Derivation of Genus: Cockle or comblike head (*Ctenocephalides*); monster eater (*Echidnophaga*)
Transmission Route: Host-to-host contact and contact with infested environment
Common Name: Cat flea, dog flea, common eastern rabbit flea, giant eastern rabbit flea, and poultry flea, respectively
Zoonotic: Yes, adults will bite humans for a blood meal but will not infest humans as they do animals

Fleas, or siphonapterans, are small (4-9 mm in length), laterally compressed, wingless insects with powerful hind legs that are used for jumping onto hosts. Their "flatness" allows them to run through the pelage (hair coat). Adult fleas have piercing and sucking (siphonlike) mouthparts that are used to suck the blood of their hosts (Figure 13-38). Adult female fleas are usually larger than male fleas. The adult flea has three body components: the head, the thorax, and the abdomen. They also have three pairs of legs, with the posterior pair being larger than the first two pairs. It is this posterior pair of legs that allows fleas to jump great distances. More than 2000 species of fleas have been identified throughout the world. Adult fleas are always

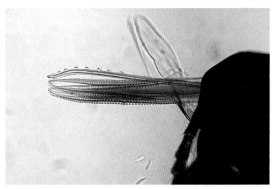

FIGURE 13-38 Mouthparts of *Echidnophaga gallinacea*, the sticktight flea of poultry. Adult fleas are placed in the order Siphonaptera because they possess piercing-sucking (siphonlike) mouthparts used to suck the host's blood.

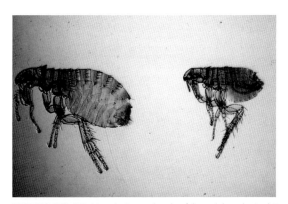

FIGURE 13-39 Morphologic details of the adult male *(right)* and female *Ctenocephalides felis (left)*, cat fleas. Note the penis rods of the male and the spermatheca of the female.

parasitic, feeding on both mammals and birds (Figure 13-39). Dogs and cats are host to comparatively few species of fleas.

> **TECHNICIAN'S NOTE** Adult fleas are able to jump great distances with their very powerful rear legs.

The flea life cycle consists of four stages: (1) adult stage, (2) egg stage, (3) larval stage, and (4) pupal stage. The female flea can lay up to several thousand eggs in her lifetime. The eggs may be laid on the infested animal or in the environment. Eggs laid on the animal will drop to the ground or bedding. The eggs are very tiny and resemble tiny pearls. Typical flea eggs are smooth, white, and oval. They are not sticky, so they will fall off the host and be found in the host's environment. The eggs hatch into larvae within 2 weeks. Flea larvae are maggotlike in appearance and sparsely covered in hairs. The larvae eat organic debris (e.g., dead skin, dead hair, flea feces) from the environment. The larva begins to form a cocoon as it passes into the pupal stage. The pupal stage is carried out entirely within the cocoon and can last for months. The cocoon keeps the pupa from desiccating over long periods (Figure 13-40). The flea pupae are seldom observed by the client or veterinarian. The flea pupa has a loosely spun cocoon that is very sticky—so sticky that environmental debris such as sand and dust adheres to the pupa. Flea eggs, larvae, and pupae are found in the host's environment, from the pet's bedding to the owner's bed—any site to which the infested pet has access. The flea emerges from the pupal stage only if environmental signs (air pressure, vibrations, warmth) indicate a host is present. The adult flea can survive only up to 1 week without a blood meal. Once emerged, the adult flea will find a host, take a blood meal, and begin the life cycle again.

Ctenocephalides felis, the cat flea, is the most common flea found on dogs and cats. The dog flea, *Ctenocephalides canis,* is uncommon and occurs much less frequently on dogs than does the cat flea.

When flea infestation is suspected in domestic rabbits, a complete physical examination of the rabbit hair coat should be performed because different species of fleas prefer different areas of the body surface. *Cediopsylla simplex,* the **common eastern rabbit flea**, is often found around the face and neck of domestic rabbits. *Odontopsylla multispinosus,* the **giant eastern rabbit flea**, is often found over the "tail-head" region at the base of the tail of domestic rabbits (when they curl up in sleep with the head close to the tail).

Echidnophaga gallinacea is also known as the **sticktight flea of poultry** (Figure 13-41; see also Figure 13-38). A common flea of chickens and guinea fowl, *E. gallinacea* also feeds on dogs and cats. This flea has unique feeding habits. The female flea inserts her mouthparts into the skin of the host and remains attached at that site. On first

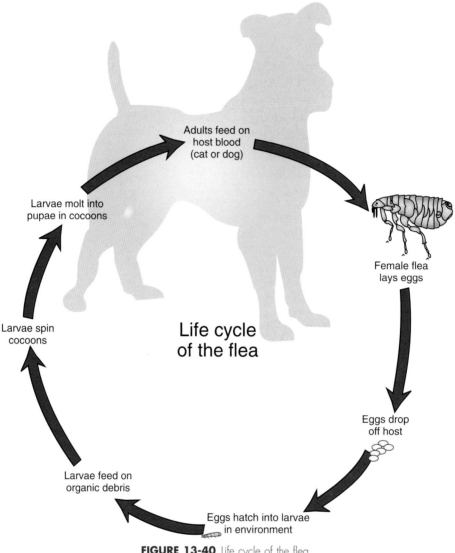

FIGURE 13-40 Life cycle of the flea.

observation, these specimens resemble attached ticks; however, they are indeed fleas. *E. gallinacea* prefer to attach and feed around the eyes and ears of dogs and cats. Because these fleas are usually associated with farm environments, the egg, larval, and pupal stages are rarely observed. However, these stages would be exactly the same as those corresponding to the same stages of *C. felis.*

Fleas are not typically found on either horses or ruminants. In barns where "barn cats" abound and excessive straw is present, large numbers of fleas have been found on calves. Under these conditions, fleas can produce significant anemias in young calves. *Pulex irritans,* the flea of humans, has been recovered from dogs and cats, especially in the southeastern United States.

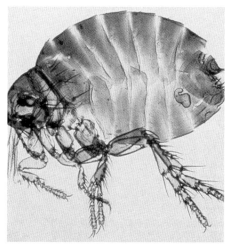

FIGURE 13-41 Adult *Echidnophaga gallinacea*, the stick-tight flea of poultry. Note the angular profile. A common flea of chickens and guinea fowl, it also feeds on dogs and cats.

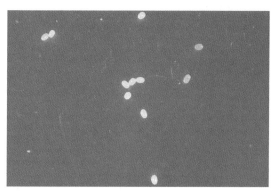

FIGURE 13-42 Eggs of *Ctenocephalides felis*, the cat flea. Flea eggs resemble tiny pearls; they are nonsticky, 0.5 mm long, white, oval, and rounded at both ends.

> *TECHNICIAN'S NOTE* Cat and dog fleas will get on human hosts and bite them. Certain species of fleas are also capable of transmitting zoonotic disease (e.g., *Yersinia pestis*, the bacterium that causes bubonic plague, is transmitted from rats to humans by fleas).

Although the adult flea is the life cycle stage most often encountered, the veterinary diagnostician may also be presented with flea eggs or with larval fleas from the pet's environment. Flea eggs and larvae are frequently found in the owner's bedclothes, the pet's bedding, travel carriers, doghouses, and clinic cages. Flea eggs resemble tiny pearls; they are nonsticky, 0.5 mm long, white, oval, and rounded at both ends (Figure 13-42). Flea larvae resemble tiny fly maggots; they are 2 to 5 mm long, white (after feeding they become brown), and sparsely covered with hairs (Figures 13-43 and 13-44).

Adult fleas are usually encountered on the animal but may also be collected in the pet's environment. Observed on recovery from the pet, the larger fleas with an orange-to-light brown abdomen are females; the smaller, darker specimens are males.

Because adult fleas spend most of their time on the host, diagnosis of flea infestation or siphonapterosis is usually obvious. However, in animals with flea

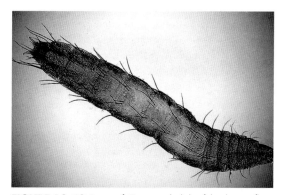

FIGURE 13-43 Larva of *Ctenocephalides felis*, the cat flea. Flea larvae resemble tiny fly maggots; they are 2 to 5 mm long, white (after feeding they become brown), and sparsely covered with hairs.

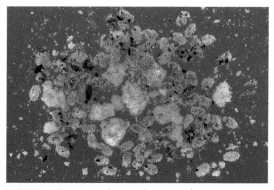

FIGURE 13-44 Sand-covered pupae of *Ctenocephalides felis*, the cat flea.

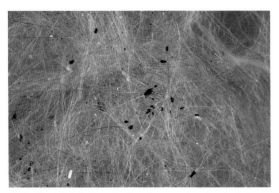

FIGURE 13-45 Flea dirt (flea feces or flea frass) of *Ctenocephalides felis*, the cat flea. Flea dirt can be used to diagnose current or recent infestations by fleas. If water is slowly dropped onto flea dirt on a gauze sponge, the flea dirt will reconstitute to the host's blood.

allergy dermatitis, fleas may be so few on the pet that the diagnosis of flea infestation is quite difficult.

Definitive diagnosis of a flea infestation requires demonstration of the adult fleas and/or their droppings (flea dirt, flea feces, or flea frass) (Figure 13-45). Flea dirt can be used to diagnose current or recent infestations of fleas. Fleas can be easily collected by spraying the pet with an insecticide. After a few minutes, dead fleas drop off the animal. Alternatively, fleas may be collected using a fine-toothed flea comb, available from any veterinary supply company or pet store.

> **TECHNICIAN'S NOTE** Flea infestation on a dog with flea allergy dermatitis can be difficult to diagnose because there may be only a few fleas on this type of allergic dog.

Adult fleas defecate large quantities of partially digested blood, commonly called flea dirt or flea frass. These feces are reddish black and can appear as fine pepperlike specks, comma-shaped columns, or long coils. To collect a sample of flea dirt, the diagnostician must comb the pet with a flea comb and place the collected debris on a white paper towel moistened with water. Rubbing the flea dirt with a fingertip causes the flea dirt to dissolve, producing a characteristic blood-red or rust-red color.

Flea control is important because fleas not only cause discomfort and irritation to the pet but also serve as intermediate hosts to certain helminth parasites. Fleas serve as intermediate host for *Dipylidium caninum,* the double-pored tapeworm of dogs and cats, and for *Acanthocheilonema reconditum,* the filarial parasite that resides in the subcutaneous tissues of dogs. Some types of fleas can also transmit diseases such as bubonic plague and endemic typhus to humans.

> **TECHNICIAN'S NOTE** The sale of flea control products for dogs and cats can be a practice builder in a veterinary clinic; however, many of these products are sold over the counter in pet stores.

Flea control makes up a large part of pet care costs in the United States. There are many different types and styles of flea prevention products on the market. Flea prevention should encompass three different areas to ensure proper control: (1) the yard, (2) the house, and (3) the animal. The yard is the major source of initial flea infestation. A good-quality yard spray approved for fleas will reduce the flea population in the outside environment, thus reducing the chances of the pet bringing new adult fleas into the home. The house is a major source of animal reinfestation. Once the adult fleas breed and the female lays eggs, the eggs are present in the house. The pupae that result from the life cycle of the flea remain in the house and hatch as adults to reinfest the pet. Several types of products are available for use in the house, including foggers, sprays, and powders. Each of these products may incorporate an **adulticide** to kill the adult fleas and an **insect growth regulator** (IGR) to prevent the other life stages from developing to maturity. Although many products can be used to treat the yard and home, great improvements have been made in products for animal application. There are daily or weekly sprays and powders available. However, the greatest advancements include once-a-month applications. Topical products such as Frontline Top Spot™, Advantage™, Advantix™, and Advantage Multi™ can be applied once a month, are resistant to water, and contain an adulticide or an adulticide and IGR. Other products such as Program™ and Sentinel™ (also contains heartworm prevention) contain IGR and are given monthly in pill form to dogs. Program™ can also be given as a 6-month injection to cats. Capstar™ can be given to dogs and cats orally for the treatment of adult fleas over a 24-hour period; however, there is no residual activity after 36 hours. Regardless of the product used, all three forms of flea prevention (yard, house, animal) should be used for proper control of the flea population.

> **TECHNICIAN'S NOTE** Once-a-month flea preventatives have undergone great advances and make client compliance with flea preventative use much higher than it was in the past.

MITES AND TICKS

Kingdom: Animalia
    Phylum: Arthropoda (arthropods)
        Subphylum: Chelicerata (possess chelicerate mouthparts)
            Class: Acarina (mites and ticks)

Because mites and ticks belong to the class Acarina, any infestation of domestic animals by either mites or ticks is referred to as acariasis. The four developmental stages in the typical life cycle of the mite or tick are (1) the egg stage, (2) the six-legged larval stage, (3) the eight-legged nymphal stage, and (4) the eight-legged adult stage.

MITES OF VETERINARY IMPORTANCE

The first group of parasitic mites can be classified as **sarcoptiform mites**. As sarcoptiform mites, they have the following key features in common:

1. These mites can produce severe dermatologic problems in a variety of domestic animals. This dermatitis is usually accompanied by a severe pruritus, or itching.
2. Typically, sarcoptiform mites are tiny mites barely visible to the naked eye, approximately the size of a grain of salt.
3. In silhouette the bodies of sarcoptiform mites have a round-to-oval shape.

CASE PRESENTATION 13-1

Setting Up the Scenario

Ms. Leonard brought in her 10-year-old, female-spayed bichon frise, Betsy, for hair loss and scratching. The technician got Betsy's weight, temperature, and flea comb analysis. The technician found live adult fleas on the flea comb and noted the finding in the patient record. After the examination, the technician was asked to discuss fleas with Ms. Leonard.

What Information Must the Veterinary Technician Convey to Ms. Leonard?

"Ms. Leonard, Betsy has fleas. Fleas will make Betsy itch so she scratches, and the more she scratches the more likely it is that she will scratch out her hair. Because Betsy has fleas, it means there are fleas in your house. Betsy most likely picked up the fleas outside, where the eggs were dropped by wild animals such as raccoons. The eggs developed through several stages (larva and pupa) to become adults that then jumped on Betsy. Once Betsy was infected, she brought the adult fleas into your house. The fleas mated and produced eggs that have fallen off Betsy and onto the carpets, bedding, and furniture in your house.

Fleas can be difficult to control once they infest the house, so we need to get a handle on this problem. I see you have another dog and two cats. Part of flea control will be using a flea prevention product on all of your pets. We have several very good options that we recommend." The technician then discussed the products recommended by the clinic.

"In addition to treating all of your pets, you will also need to treat your house. The best way is to vacuum each room and then throw the used vacuum cleaner bag into the outdoor garbage after spraying with a flea spray to kill the adults in the bag. This will reduce the eggs, larvae, and pupae in the carpets. You will then need to treat each room (carpets and furniture) with a flea product."

The technician explained the products recommended by the clinic.

"Finally, because wild animals tend to spread the eggs as they pass through your yard, you should also treat it with a yard and kennel spray. The areas to concentrate on are the shaded areas of the yard. Do you have any questions?"

The technician noted the discussion in the patient record.

4. Sarcoptiform mites have legs that have pedicels, or stalks, at the tips. The pedicels may be long or short. If the pedicel is long, it may be straight (unjointed) or jointed. At the tip of each pedicel there may be a tiny sucker. Veterinary diagnosticians should use the description of the pedicel (long or short, jointed or unjointed) to identify sarcoptiform mites.

> **TECHNICIAN'S NOTE** Sarcoptiform mites can cause severe dermatologic problems in a variety of domestic animals and even humans.

Sarcoptiform mites can be broken down into two basic families: the Sarcoptidae family, sarcoptiform mites that burrow or tunnel within the epidermis, and the Psoroptidae family, sarcoptiform mites that reside on the surface of the skin or within the external ear canal. Sarcoptidae includes *Sarcoptes, Notoedres, Cnemidocoptes,* and *Trixacarus* species. Psoroptidae includes *Psoroptes, Chorioptes,* and *Otodectes* species.

> **TECHNICIAN'S NOTE** Sarcoptiform mites are broken down into two families: Sarcoptidae mites that burrow or tunnel within the epidermis and Psoroptidae mites that reside on the surface of the skin or within the external ear canal.

Family Sarcoptidae (Mites)

Members of the family Sarcoptidae burrow or tunnel within the epidermis of the infested definitive host. The entire four-stage life cycle is spent on the host. Male and female mites breed on the skin surface. The female mite penetrates the keratinized layers of the skin and burrows or tunnels through the epidermis. Over a 10- to 15-day period, she deposits 40 to 50 eggs within the tunnel. After egg deposition, the female dies. Six-legged larvae emerge from the eggs in 3 to 10 days and exit the tunnel to wander on the skin surface. These larvae molt to the eight-legged nymphal stage within tiny pockets in the epidermis. Nymphs become sexually active adults in 12 to 17 days, and the life cycle begins again.

Sarcoptes scabei (Scabies Mite)

The disease caused by *Sarcoptes scabiei* is called scabies, or **sarcoptic acariasis**. Sarcoptic acariasis is extremely pruritic. *Sarcoptes* species exhibit host specificity. For example, *S. scabiei* variety *canis* affects only dogs, and *S. scabiei* variety *suis* affects only pigs. Almost every domestic animal has its own distinct variety of this mite, which does not infest other hosts.

> **TECHNICIAN'S NOTE** *Sarcoptes scabiei* species are species specific; however, *S. scabiei* variety *canis* can cause a self-limiting infestation in humans, so it is considered zoonotic. *S. scabiei* variety *hominis* is the human sarcoptic mite that causes scabies in humans.

Parasite: 🅩 *Sarcoptes scabiei* variety *canis*
Host: Canines
Location of Adult: Tunneling in the superficial layers of the epidermis for the majority of their life cycle; for a short period of their life cycle, can be found on the skin surface
Distribution: Worldwide
Derivation of Genus: Flesh cutters
Transmission Route: Direct contact from host to host
Common Name: Scabies mite of the dog
Zoonotic: Yes

Canine scabies is caused by *S. scabiei* variety *canis,* which produces lesions consisting of an erythematous, papular rash. Scaling, crusting, and excoriations are common. The ears, lateral elbows, and ventral abdomen are sites that are likely to harbor mites. The animal's entire body, however, may be infested. The eight-legged adult mite has a unique silhouette—an oval shape. Each leg possesses a sucker (much like the "cup" of a plumber's plunger) on the ends of some of its legs. If present, the sucker is connected to the legs by a pedicel. The condition of the pedicel (long or short; jointed or unjointed) assists in speciating or identifying the Sarcoptiform mites. *S. scabei* has long, unjointed pedicels. The anus of the adult *S. scabiei* is terminal, not dorsal. These mites are spread by direct contact or by combs and brushes containing mites and/or their eggs and can affect all dogs in the household. For only a short period of their life cycle these mites are found on the skin surface. For most of their life cycle, however, they may be found tunneling in the superficial layers of the epidermis. *S. scabiei* variety *canis* is extremely contagious. The dog owner can become infested with this mite, but the disease is self-limiting. The mites burrow into the skin of humans, producing a papulelike lesion; however, the mites will not establish a full-blown infestation in humans. Therefore *S. scabiei* variety *canis* is considered to be zoonotic. Some dogs may be asymptomatic carriers of *S. scabiei* variety *canis*.

> **TECHNICIAN'S NOTE** *Sarcoptes scabiei* variety *canis* is extremely contagious, and dogs can be asymptomatic carriers of the mite.

Superficial skin scrapings (to the extent that a bit of capillary blood is drawn) are used to diagnose this mite. Impression smears on glass slides can also be used. The skin scrapings or impression smears are viewed microscopically for the developmental stages of mites (egg, larva, nymph, adult).

Parasite: 🄳 *Sarcoptes scabiei* variety *felis*
Parasite: *S. scabiei* variety *suis, bovis, equi,* and *ovis*
Host: Feline (*felis*), pigs (*suis*), cattle (*bovis*), horses (*equi*), and sheep and goats (*ovis*)
Location of Adult: For most of its life cycle, it is found tunneling in the superficial layers of the epidermis. For a short period of its life cycle, it is found on the surface of the skin.
Distribution: Worldwide
Derivation of Genus: Flesh cutters
Transmission Route: Direct contact from host to host
Common Name: Scabies mite of cats, scabies mite of pigs, scabies mite of cattle, scabies mite of horses, and scabies mite of sheep and goats, respectively
Zoonotic: Yes for *S. scabiei* variety *felis*

Cats also are parasitized by a variety of this mite, *S. scabiei* variety *felis*. Feline scabies caused by this variety is an extremely rare condition.

Among large animals, pigs are most often affected by scabies. Lesions caused by *S. scabiei*

variety *suis* include small red papules, alopecia, and crusts, most frequently on the trunk and ears. Scabies in cattle (*S. scabiei* variety *bovis*) is rare. The main areas of infestation are the head, neck, and shoulders. Scabies in horses (*S. scabiei* variety *equi*) is an even rarer entity. The main area of infestation is the neck. *S. scabiei* variety *ovis* affects the face of sheep and goats rather than the fleece.

Areas with an erythematous, papular rash and crust should be scraped, especially the areas most associated with sarcoptic infestation in dogs, that is, the ears, lateral elbows, and ventral abdomen. Adult sarcoptic mites are oval and approximately 200 to 400 μm in diameter, with eight legs. The key morphologic feature used to identify this species is the long, unjointed pedicel with a sucker on the end of some of the legs. The anus is located on the caudal end of the body (Figure 13-46). The eggs of *Sarcoptes* mites are oval (Figure 13-47).

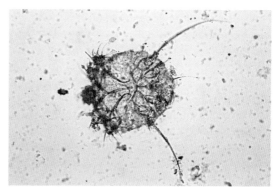

FIGURE 13-46 Adult *Sarcoptes scabei* mite. The anus is located on the caudal end of the body.

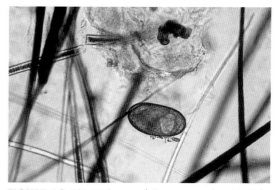

FIGURE 13-47 Oval eggs of *Sarcoptes scabei*. Note the emergence of the six-legged larval mite.

S. scabei can be treated with ivermectin, lime sulfur dips, or amitraz (not used for horses).

Parasite: ⬢**Z** *Notoedres cati*
Host: Felines and occasionally rabbits
Location of Adult: Most of its life cycle, the adult is found tunneling in the superficial layers of the epidermis, but for a short period of its life cycle, it can be found on the surface of the skin around the ear pinna, face, neck, and feet of the cat
Distribution: Worldwide
Derivation of Genus: Back (referring to the dorsal anus)
Transmission Route: Direct contact from host to host
Common Name: Notoedric mange mite of cats or feline scabies mite
Zoonotic: Yes (per American Association of Veterinary Parasitologists)

Notoedres cati (Feline Scabies Mite) and Notoedres muris

Although cats may be parasitized by *S. scabiei* variety *felis,* the mite most often associated with feline scabies is *Notoedres cati.* This mite infests mainly cats but occasionally parasitizes rabbits. This sarcoptiform mite is found chiefly on the ears, back of the neck, face, and feet; in extreme cases, however, the entire body may be affected. This mite is almost identical to the mite *S. scabiei* except for the position of the anus. The anus in *S. scabiei* is terminal, whereas the anus in *N. cati* is dorsal. Like *S. scabiei, N. cati* has long, unjointed pedicels. The life cycle is similar to that of *S. scabei,* with the mite burrowing or tunneling in the superficial layers of the epidermis and with only a short period of the life cycle being spent on the surface of the skin. The characteristic lesion of notoedric acariasis is a yellowing crust in the region of the ears, face, or neck.

> **TECHNICIAN'S NOTE** *Notoedres cati* parasitize the cat but can occasionally infest the rabbit. It is found mainly around the ear pinna, back of the neck, face, and feet but can affect the entire body in extreme cases.

Superficial skin scrapings (with a bit of capillary blood being drawn) and impression smears can be used to microscopically diagnose this mite of the cat. Diagnosis is made by identifying the developmental stages of the mite life cycle (egg, larva, nymph, and adult). Notoedric mites are easier to demonstrate in cats than are sarcoptic mites in dogs. Again, likely infestation sites should be scraped. As with *Sarcoptes* species, *Notoedres* mites have a long, unjointed pedicel with a sucker on the end of some of the legs. Adult notoedric mites are similar to sarcoptic mites but are smaller, with a dorsal subterminal anus. The eggs of notoedric mites are oval. *N. cati* can be transmitted to humans where it causes pruritic papules. Therefore it is a zoonotic parasite.

> **TECHNICIAN'S NOTE** *Notoedres cati* is easier to demonstrate on cats with a skin scraping or impression smears than *Sarcoptes scabiei* is in the dog.

N. cati mites are treated with ivermectin. The best prevention is avoiding contact between infected cats and uninfected cats.

Parasite: *Notoedres muris*
Host: Rats
Location of Adult: Most of the life cycle is spent tunneling in the superficial epidermis, with only a short period being spent on the skin surface
Distribution: Worldwide
Derivation of Genus: Back (referring to the dorsal anus)
Transmission Route: Direct contact from host to host
Common Name: Scabies mite of rats
Zoonotic: No

A related species, *Notoedres muris,* produces otic acariasis in rats (Figure 13-48). This mite resembles *S. scabiei,* with a rounded body and suckers on the first two pairs of legs of female mites and on the first, second, and fourth pairs of legs of male mites. Female *N. muris* can be distinguished from female *S. scabiei* by the dorsal subterminal anal opening of *N. muris.* The anal opening of *S. scabiei* is terminal (Figure 13-49).

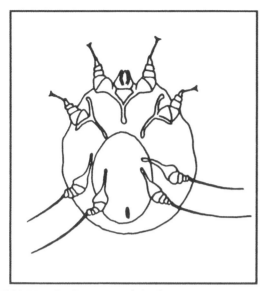

FIGURE 13-48 Drawing of the female *Notoedres muris* showing the dorsal subterminal anal opening.

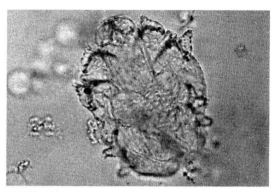

FIGURE 13-50 *Trixacarus caviae,* typical sarcoptiform mite of guinea pigs.

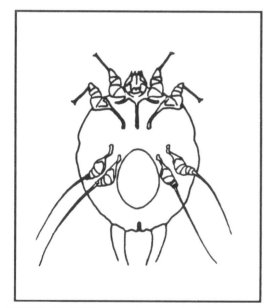

FIGURE 13-49 Drawing of the female *Sarcoptes scabei* showing the terminal anal opening.

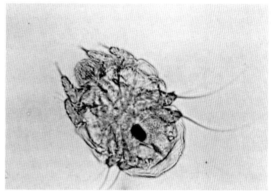

FIGURE 13-51 Adults of *Psoroptes cuniculi,* occurring most often in the external ear canal of rabbits but also collected from horses, goats, and sheep. Mites exhibit characteristic long, jointed pedicels with suckers on ends of some legs.

The burrowing mite *N. muris* usually can be detected and diagnosed before and after death by collecting deep skin scrapings from the edges of suspected lesions. Lesions are usually on the unfurred parts of the body, such as the ear pinnae, tail, nose, and extremities. Lesions appear as crusted areas with reddened vesicles. *N. muris* is quite common in wild rodents. Transmission is by direct contact, so owners should be cautioned to keep pet rats safely away from wild rodent contact. This mite is also known to infest guinea pigs, but it does not infest humans.

Rabbits can be infested by notoedric and sarcoptic acarines. These mites cause similar lesions, usually on the head, neck, and legs. Lesions may also appear on the pinnae, making it necessary to distinguish *N. cati* and *S. scabiei* (see Figure 13-49) from the guinea pig mite *Trixacarus caviae* (Figure 13-50) and the rabbit ear mite *Psoroptes cuniculi* (Figure 13-51).

In general notoedric mites are smaller than sarcoptic mites, and *P. cuniculi* is larger than both.

Except for size the major distinguishing characteristic of *N. cati* and *S. scabiei* is the location of the mite's anus. The anus is dorsal and subterminal in *N. cati* and terminal in *S. scabiei*. In both *N. cati* and *S. scabiei*, suckers are found at the end of long, unjointed stalks on the first two pairs of legs in adult females and on the first, second, and fourth pairs of legs in adult males. Psoroptic mites are distinguished by suckers at the end of long, jointed stalks on the first, second, and fourth pairs of legs in adult females and on the first, second, and third pairs of legs in adult males.

Diagnosis of infestation by *N. cati* and *S. scabiei* is by identification of larval, nymphal, or adult mites or the eggs from deep skin scrapings. Deep skin scrapings from the edges of lesions are necessary to detect the burrowing mites. Lesions normally begin near the nose or lips, spread over the face, and may eventually involve the external or lateral pinnae, extremities, and genital region. Both *N. cati* and *S. scabiei* cause intense pruritus that may result in self-mutilation. A crust or scale may develop over infested areas, and the skin may become thick and wrinkled. Secondary bacterial infection may occur.

> **TECHNICIAN'S NOTE** *Notoedres muris* can be diagnosed with deep skin scrapings at the edges of suspected lesions, usually found at the ear pinnae, tail, nose, and extremities.

Transmission of notoedric and sarcoptic mites is by direct contact. *S. scabiei* is extremely contagious from rabbit to rabbit and from rabbit to human. The pet owner can become infested with this mite, but the disease is self-limiting. The mites burrow into the skin of humans, producing a papulelike lesion; however, the mites will not establish a full-blown infestation. Both *N. cati* and *S. scabiei* are considered to be zoonotic.

> **TECHNICIAN'S NOTE** *Sarcoptes scabiei* and *Notoedres cati* cause an intense pruritus that can result in self-mutilation of the host. Lesions are characterized by crusting and scaling, whereas the skin may become thick and wrinkled.

Parasite: *Cnemidocoptes pilae* and *Cnemidocoptes mutans*
Host: Budgerigars and parakeets (*C. pilae*) and poultry (*C. mutans*)
Location of Adult: *C. pilae* spends most of its life cycle tunneling under the superficial epidermis of the feet, cere, and beak, whereas *C. mutans* tunnels under the superficial epidermis of the feet. They both spend a short period on the surface of the skin.
Distribution: Worldwide
Derivation of Genus: *Koptein* means "to cut" in Greek
Transmission Route: Direct contact from host to host
Common Name: Scaly leg mite of parakeets and scaly leg mite of chickens, respectively
Zoonotic: No

Cnemidocoptes pilae (Scaly Leg Mite of Budgerigars)

Cnemidocoptes pilae is the sarcoptiform mite that causes scaly leg or scaly face in budgerigars and parakeets. This mite tunnels in the superficial layers of the epidermis, affecting the pads and shanks of the feet; in severe cases, it may also affect the beak and the cere, the junction of the feathers and the beak. The mite characteristically produces a yellow-to-gray white mass resembling a honeycomb. This condition can be quite disfiguring to the parakeet. The parasites pierce the skin underneath the scales, causing an inflammation with exudate that hardens on the surface and displaces the scales upward. This process causes the thickened scaly nature of the skin. In canaries, *Cnemidocoptes* species produces a syndrome called **tasselfoot**, a proliferation of the toes and feet. A related species, *Cnemidocoptes mutans*, produces a condition called scaly leg in chickens, turkeys, and wild birds. These mites are extremely pruritic, producing a severe disfigurement of the beak, cere, and feet of parakeets and the legs of chickens.

> **TECHNICIAN'S NOTE** *Cnemidocoptes pilae* cause an extreme pruritus on the feet of parakeets but can also affect the beak and cere (the junction of the feathers and the beak).

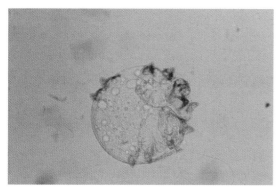

FIGURE 13-52 Adult *Cnemidocoptes pilae*, a sarcoptiform mite that causes scaly leg or scaly face in budgerigars and parakeets. Adults are eight-legged, round to oval in silhouette, and about 500 μm in diameter. Adult females have very short legs and lack suckers. Adult males have longer legs and long, unjointed pedicels with a sucker on the end of some legs.

Infestation sites should be scraped. Great care should be taken in handling the infested birds because parakeets and canaries are fragile creatures. The adult mites are eight-legged, round to oval in silhouette, and about 500 μm in diameter (Figure 13-52). The adult female mites have very short legs and lack suckers. The adult male has longer legs and possesses the long, unjointed pedicel with a sucker on the end of some of the legs.

C. pilae is treated with ivermectin.

> **TECHNICIAN'S NOTE** *Cnemidocoptes* species have very short, stubby legs, very similar in appearance to the legs of a tortoise.

Parasite: *Trixacarus caviae*
Host: Guinea pigs
Location of Adult: Most of its life cycle, the adult can be found tunneling into the superficial epidermis, whereas a short period is spent on the surface of the skin
Distribution: Europe and North America
Derivation of Genus: Unknown
Transmission Route: Direct contact from host to host
Common Name: Burrowing mite of guinea pigs
Zoonotic: No

Trixacarus Caviae

A burrowing or tunneling mite that infests guinea pigs is *T. caviae* (see Figure 13-50). *T. caviae* is a typical sarcoptiform mite with a rounded body and suckers on long, unjointed stalks on the first two pairs of legs of females and on the first, second, and fourth pairs of legs of males.

Deep skin scrapings from the edges of suspected lesions around the back, neck, and shoulders are necessary to detect this mite both antemortem and postmortem. Lesions include dry, scaly skin with pruritus, alopecia, and dermatitis.

> **TECHNICIAN'S NOTE** *Trixacarus caviae* mites cause lesions with dry, scaly skin, pruritus, alopecia, and dermatitis.

Other burrowing mites that may infest guinea pigs are *S. scabei* (see Figure 13-49) and *N. muris* (see Figure 13-48). *S. scabiei* can be transmitted from rabbits to guinea pigs, in which they produce scabby lesions on the nose and lips. Young guinea pigs are particularly susceptible and may become anorectic to the point of death if not treated. (See previous discussion on identification, detection, and transmission of *S. scabiei* in rabbits.) *N. muris* is generally associated with rats but has also been reported in guinea pigs. This mite produces red, crusty lesions on the face of guinea pigs. (See previous discussion on identification, detection, and transmission of *N. muris* in rats.)

Psoroptidae

Members of the family Psoroptidae reside on the surface of the skin or within the external ear canal. The entire five-stage life cycle (egg, larva, protonymph, deutonymph or pubescent female, and adult ovigerous female) is spent on the host. Adult male and female mites breed on the skin surface. The female produces 14 to 24 elliptic, opaque, shiny white eggs that hatch within 1 to 3 days. The six-legged mites are small, oval, soft, and grayish brown. Eight-legged nymphs are slightly larger than larvae. Larval and nymphal stages may last 7 to 10 days. The life cycle is completed in about

10 to 18 days. Under favorable conditions, mites can live off the host for 2 to 3 weeks or longer. Under optimum conditions, mite eggs may remain viable for 2 to 4 weeks.

Parasite: *Psoroptes cuniculi*
Host: Rabbits (most common), horses, goats, and sheep
Location of Adult: External ear canal
Distribution: Worldwide
Derivation of Genus: Scabby
Transmission Route: Direct contact from host to host
Common Name: Rabbit ear mite or rabbit ear canker mite
Zoonotic: No

> **TECHNICIAN'S NOTE** *Psoroptes cuniculi* mites are commonly seen in the ears of rabbits but have also been reported in horses, goats, and sheep.

Psoroptes cuniculi *(Ear Canker Mite of Rabbits)*

P. cuniculi occurs most often in the external ear canal of rabbits but has also been collected from horses, goats, and sheep. These nonburrowing mites reside on the surface of the skin and feed on the rabbit host by puncturing the epidermis to obtain tissue fluids. Within the external ear canal of the infested host are the characteristic dried crusts of coagulated serum. (In chronic cases, the rabbit's ears appear to be packed with dried cornflakes cereal.) Affected animals shake their head and scratch their ears. Although usually associated with otitis media produced by secondary infection with *Pasteurella multocida*, the ear mites themselves are not responsible for this condition. Lesions sometimes occur on the head and legs. *P. cuniculi* are extremely pruritic, and severely infested animals may become debilitated. Loss of equilibrium may occur with torticollis, abnormal contraction of neck muscles.

Diagnosis can be made by superficial skin scrapings or the removal of the scablike lesions. The samples are viewed microscopically for the developmental stages of the mite (egg, larva, nymph, and adult). The *P. cuniculi* mites within the

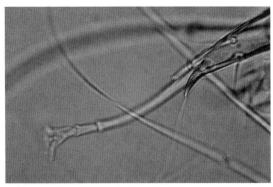

FIGURE 13-53 Detail of long, jointed pedicel on the leg of *Psoroptes cuniculi*.

cornflakelike crusty debris inside the ear can be easily isolated. The brownish-white female mite is large, 409 to 749 μm × 351 to 499 μm; males are 431 to 547 μm × 322 to 462 μm (see Figure 13-51). The mites exhibit characteristic long, jointed pedicels with suckers on the ends of some of the legs (Figure 13-53). The anus is in a terminal slit. In addition, mites can be observed with the unaided eye or with a handheld magnifying glass.

Transmission of *P. cuniculi* is by direct contact. This parasite has no zoonotic potential. Treatment may be accomplished with the use of ivermectin otic (not approved for rabbits), milbemycin otic, or thiabendazole-dexamethasone–neomycin sulfate solution.

> **TECHNICIAN'S NOTE** *Psoroptes cuniculi* mites are easily diagnosed with an ear cytology specimen viewed under the microscope for the eggs, larval, nymphal, and adult stages of the parasite. Adult mites can also be seen with the aid of a magnifying glass or with an otoscope.

Parasite: *Psoroptes ovis, Psoroptes bovis,* and *Psoroptes equi*
Host: Sheep, cattle, and horses, respectively
Location of Adult: Skin surface on the body (*P. ovis*); withers, neck, and rump (*P. bovis*); and mane and tail (*P. equi*)
Distribution: Worldwide
Derivation of Genus: Scabby

Transmission Route: Direct contact from host to host
Common Name: Scabies mites of sheep, cattle, and horses, respectively
Zoonotic: No

Psoroptes of Large Animals

Psoroptes ovis, Psoroptes bovis, and *Psoroptes equi* are the scab mites of large animals residing on sheep, cattle, and horses, respectively. These mites are host specific and reside within the thick-haired or long-wooled areas of the animal. The adults are eight-legged with an oval shape. Each mite possesses a sucker on the ends of some of its legs. If present, the sucker is connected to the legs by a pedicel. The mites are surface dwellers and feed by puncturing the host's epidermis to feed on lymphatic fluid. Serum exudes through the puncture site; after the serum coagulates and forms a crust, wool is lost. The feeding site is extremely pruritic, and the animal excoriates itself, producing further wool loss. Mites migrate to undamaged skin. As *Psoroptes* mites proliferate, tags of wool are pulled out and the fleece becomes matted. Finally patches of skin are exposed, and the skin becomes parchmentlike, thickened, and cracked and may bleed easily. Infested sheep constantly rub against fences, posts, farm equipment, and any object that might serve as a scratching post. The disease is spread by direct contact or infested premises.

> **TECHNICIAN'S NOTE** *Psoroptes* species of large animals are extremely pruritic and cause the host to rub the affected area against fences, posts, equipment, or any object it can use as a scratching post. This can lead to areas of alopecia (hair loss) and excoriations.

P. bovis produces lesions on the withers, neck, and rump that consist of papules, crusts, and wrinkled, thickened skin. *P. equi* in horses is rare and affects the base of the mane and tail.

Because of the intense pruritus and the highly contagious nature of this infestation, the occurrence of *Psoroptes* species in large animals should be reported to both state and federal authorities.

This disease is reportable to the United States Department of Agriculture.

Mites of *Psoroptes* species that infest large animals are host specific. Adults are up to 600 μm in length. The mites exhibit characteristic long, jointed pedicels with suckers on the ends of some of the legs.

Large-animal *Psoroptes* species can be treated with lime sulfur dips or ivermectin.

> **TECHNICIAN'S NOTE** The species of *Psoroptes* that are found on large animals produce a highly pruritic, highly transmissible dermatologic condition known as *scabies*. These species of *Psoroptes* mites in large animals are reportable parasites to both state and federal authorities, whereas *Psoroptes cuniculi* is not a reportable parasite.

Parasite: *Chorioptes equi, Chorioptes bovis, Chorioptes caprae,* and *Chorioptes ovis*
Host: Horses, cattle, goats, and sheep, respectively
Location of Adult: Surface of skin, particularly lower hind legs, flanks and shoulders, and on dairy cattle in the region of the escutcheon
Distribution: Worldwide
Derivation of Genus: Membrane visible
Transmission Route: Direct contact from host to host
Common Name: Foot and tail mites or itchy leg mite
Zoonotic: No

Chorioptes Species (Foot and Tail Mite, Itchy Leg Mite)

Chorioptes equi, Chorioptes bovis, Chorioptes caprae, and *Chorioptes ovis* are the foot and tail mites of large animals, residing on horses, cattle, goats, and sheep, respectively. As with *Psoroptes,* these mites are found on the skin surface. Their predilection sites are on the lower part of the hind legs, but they may spread to the flank and shoulder areas. On cattle, they are frequently found in the tail region, especially in the area of the escutcheon. These mites do not spread rapidly or extensively. They puncture the skin, causing serum to exude. Thin crusts of

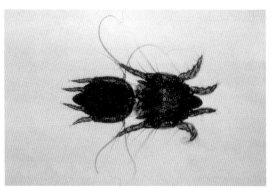

FIGURE 13-54 Female and male *Chorioptes* species. Note the short, unjointed pedicels.

coagulated serum form on the skin surface. The skin eventually wrinkles and thickens, although pruritus is not severe. The presence of these mites on the lower limbs may cause intense pruritus, although the pruritus is not normally severe, with much scratching and licking of the area.

Infested horses stamp, bite, and kick, especially at night. Mites typically infest the pasterns, especially those of the hind legs.

Characteristic mites of the genus *Chorioptes* can be identified from skin scrapings of infested areas. The mites have characteristic short, unjointed pedicels with suckers on the ends of some of the legs. The female mites are about 400 μm long (Figure 13-54). Because these mites can be licked by the infected animal, developmental stages of these mites may be found on fecal flotation.

Ivermectin and lime sulfur dips are used to treat *C. equi, C. bovis, C. caprae,* and *C. ovis.*

> **TECHNICIAN'S NOTE** On superficial inspection, *Chorioptes* species have been found to have the same configuration of pedicels as *Otodectes cynotis.* The "pedicel formula" (position of suckers and pedicels on the mite's limbs) may be similar, but the *Chorioptes* species are found on the legs of large animals while *Otodectes cynotis* is found in the ears of small animals.

Parasite: 🅉 *Otodectes cynotis*
Host: Canines, felines, and ferrets
Location of Adult: External ear canal
Distribution: Worldwide

Derivation of Genus: Ear biter or ear receiver
Transmission Route: Direct contact from host to host
Common Name: Ear mites
Zoonotic: Yes, but extremely rare (per American Association of Veterinary Parasitologists and Companion Animal Parasite Council)

Otodectes cynotis *(Ear Mites)*

Ear mites, *Otodectes cynotis,* are a common cause of otitis externa in dogs, cats, and ferrets. Although they occur primarily in the external ear canal, ear mites may be found on any area of the body. A common infestation site is the tail-head region, because as dogs and cats curl up to sleep, their head (and ears) are often close to the base of the tail. These mites are spread by direct contact and are highly transmissible both among and between dogs, cats, and ferrets.

> **TECHNICIAN'S NOTE** *Otodectes cynotis* mites are highly transmissible from host to host and can be found at the tail-head region because of the way dogs, cats, and ferrets tend to sleep curled up.

Mites are found within the external ear canal, where they feed on epidermal debris and produce intense irritation. Infestation is usually in both ears. The host responds to the mite infestation by shaking its head and scratching its ears. In cases of infestation with these mites, the "massaging" or petting of the external ear canal elicits a scratching response by the animal called the *pedalpinnal response* (foot-ear response). In severe infestations, otitis media with head tilt, circling, and convulsions may occur. Auricular hematomas may develop.

Ear mites are usually identified with an otoscope, through which the mites appear as white motile objects. Exudate collected by swabbing the ear may be placed in mineral oil on a glass slide and the mites observed under a compound microscope using the 10× objective. These mites are fairly large, approximately 400 μm (Figure 13-55); they can also be easily seen with the unaided eye. The mites exhibit characteristic short, unjointed pedicels with

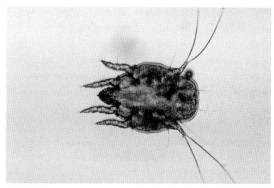

FIGURE 13-55 Adult male ear mite *Otodectes cynotis*.

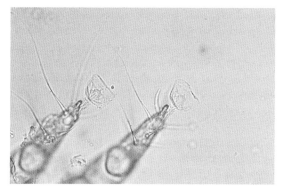

FIGURE 13-56 Detail of the leg of *Otodectes cynotis* with a short, unjointed pedicel.

suckers on the ends of some of the legs (Figure 13-56). The anus of *O. cynotis* is terminal.

Ivermectin otic, milbemycin otic, and thiabendazole-dexamethasone–neomycin sulfate solution are used to treat *O. cynotis*. In addition to use of medication, the ears should be cleaned to remove the debris and mites.

> **TECHNICIAN'S NOTE** If *Otodectes cynotis* is found in one pet of the household, all pets (hosts) in the household should be treated.

Nonsarcoptiform Mites

The following group of parasitic mites are discussed together because they are not sarcoptiform mites. They can, however, produce severe dermatologic problems in a variety of domestic animals. These

mites lack the pedicels, or stalks, on their legs that are so important in diagnosing the sarcoptiform mites.

Parasite: *Demodex* species
Host: Domestic animals and humans (host specific)
Location of Adult: Hair follicles and sebaceous glands of the skin
Distribution: Worldwide
Derivation of Genus: Fat worm or tallow receiver
Transmission Route: Direct contact, especially intimate contact between dam and neonates
Common Name: Red mange mite, follicular mite, canine follicular mite, or demodectic mange mite
Zoonotic: No

Demodex *Species*

Mites of the genus *Demodex* reside in the hair follicles and sebaceous glands of humans and of most domesticated animals. In many species, mites of the genus *Demodex* are considered normal, nonpathogenic fauna of the skin. These mites are host specific and are not transmissible from one species of host to another. The clinical disease caused by many of these mites is called demodicosis.

Demodex mites resemble eight-legged alligators or cigars, and some even say they have a carrot shape—elongated with very short, stubby legs. No other mite looks like this mite. Adult and nymphal stages have eight legs, and larvae have six. Adult *Demodex* mites are approximately 250 μm long (Figure 13-57). The eggs are spindle-shaped or tapered at each end (Figure 13-58).

> **TECHNICIAN'S NOTE** The *Demodex* mite has a characteristic carrot-, cigar-, or alligator-shaped body with very short and stubby legs. The nymphal and adult stages have eight legs, whereas the larval stage has six legs.

Of all the domestic animals infested with *Demodex* species, the dog is the most often and the most seriously infested. These mites are considered part of the normal skin flora of all dogs; in some dogs with immunodeficiencies, however, they proliferate to

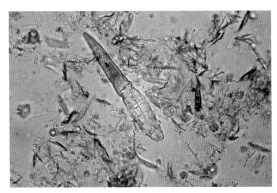

FIGURE 13-57 Adult *Demodex canis*. *Demodex* mites resemble eight-legged alligators; they are elongated, with very short, stubby legs. Adult and nymphal stages have eight legs; larvae have six legs.

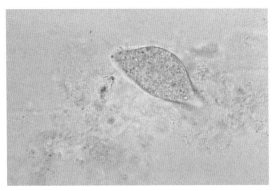

FIGURE 13-58 Egg of *Demodex canis* is either spindle-shaped or tapered at each end.

the point that they produce pathology. The clinical syndromes relative to the form of demodicosis present in dogs are localized demodicosis and generalized demodicosis.

The predominant clinical sign of the localized form of demodicosis is a patchy alopecia, especially of the muzzle, face, and forelimbs. It is thought that *Demodex* mites are acquired during the close, intimate contact that develops as the dam nurses the puppy. As a result of that contact, localized demodicosis often develops in the region of the face or forelimbs.

Generalized demodicosis is characterized by diffuse alopecia, erythema, and secondary bacterial contamination over the entire body surface of the dog. An inherited defect in the dog's immune system is thought to be an important factor in the development and the pathogenesis of generalized demodicosis. Generalized demodicosis can affect the entire skin surface, and on occasion demodectic mites have been known to infect internal organs.

> **TECHNICIAN'S NOTE** *Demodex* mites can produce three syndromes in animals—the asymptomatic carrier, localized demodecosis, and generalized demodecosis.

Cats are infested by two species of demodectic mites, *Demodex cati* and an unnamed species of *Demodex*. *D. cati* is an elongated mite similar to *Demodex canis*. The unnamed species has a broad, blunted abdomen, unlike the elongated abdomen of *D. cati*. The presence of either species in the skin of cats is rare. In localized feline demodicosis, patchy areas of alopecia, erythema, and occasionally crusting occur on the head (especially around the eyes), ears, and neck. In generalized feline demodicosis the alopecia, erythema, and crusting usually involve the entire body. Demodicosis also has been associated with ceruminous otitis externa.

Demodectic mites reside in the hair follicles of other species of domestic animals but rarely produce clinical disease. Cattle and goats are most often infested, and then only rarely.

> **TECHNICIAN'S NOTE** *Demodex* mites live within the hair follicles and sebaceous glands of the skin, but dogs are the hosts most commonly seen with clinical signs of infestation.

In cattle, *Demodex bovis* causes large nodules or abscesses on the shoulders, trunk, and lateral aspects of the neck. In goats, *Demodex caprae* occurs in small, papular, or nodular lesions on the shoulders, trunk, and lateral aspects of the neck. Rarely in sheep, *Demodex ovis* causes pustules and crusting around the coronet, nose, ear tips, and periorbital areas. Rarely in pigs, *Demodex phylloides* produces pustules and nodules on the face, abdomen, and ventral neck. In horses, *Demodex equi* occurs around the face and eyes and rarely produces clinical disease.

Demodex aurati (Figure 13-59) and *Demodex criceti* (Figure 13-60) infest hamsters. As with other *Demodex* species, they live in hair follicles and adjacent sebaceous glands. Deep skin scrapings at the edges of the lesions are necessary to detect the mites. Lesions are most often seen on the dorsum of the hamster near the rump.

Clinical signs that may indicate demodicosis in the hamster include alopecia and dry scaly skin or scabby dermatitis, particularly over the rump and on the back of the hamster. Demodicosis is most often observed in aged or otherwise stressed hamsters. The mite population in hamsters is usually greater in males than in females. As with *D. canis* in dogs, *D. aurati* and *D. criceti* may be present without producing clinical signs.

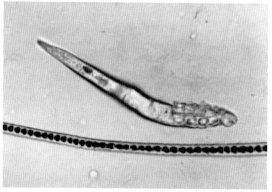

FIGURE 13-59 *Demodex aurati*, a burrowing mite of hamsters.

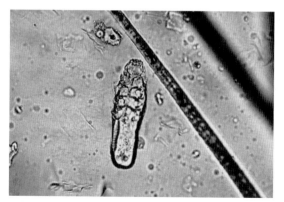

FIGURE 13-60 *Demodex criceti*, a hamster mite, is distinguishable from *Demodex aurati* by its blunt body shape.

Gerbils have been reported to carry two species of *Demodex*, *D. aurati* and *D. criceti* (see Figures 13-59 and 13-60). These mites are similar in size and shape to the demodectic mites of hamsters. Demodectic mites also have been recovered from gerbils with facial dermatitis. As in other species with demodectic acariasis, infested gerbils have other concomitant disease. Lesions are similar to those described in the hamster.

Demodicosis may be detected on postmortem examination by histopathologic examination of skin sections. Transmission is by direct contact, with the primary route thought to be from mother to suckling young. *Demodex* species of hamsters are considered to be species specific, with the possible exception of the gerbil, and thus are not likely to cross-contaminate other species or pose a zoonotic problem to humans.

> **TECHNICIAN'S NOTE** *Demodex* infestation in animals showing clinical symptoms is diagnosed by deep skin scrapings to find the developmental stages of the mite (egg, larva, nymph, and adult).

Skin with altered pigmentation, obstructed hair follicles, erythema, or alopecia should always be scraped with a deep skin scraping to the extent of drawing capillary blood. In localized demodicosis, the areas most often affected are the forelegs, the perioral region, and the periorbital regions. In generalized demodicosis of dogs, the entire body may be affected; however, the face and feet usually are the most severely involved. In dogs, normal skin should also be scraped to determine whether the disease is generalized. The areas should be clipped and a fold of skin gently squeezed to express any mites from the hair follicles. Scraping should be continued until capillary blood is observed oozing because these mites live deep in the hair follicles and sebaceous glands (Figure 13-61).

Nodular lesions in large animals should be incised with a scalpel and the caseous material within smeared on a microscope slide with mineral oil, covered with a coverslip, and examined for mites.

The veterinary diagnostician should count the mites on the glass slide and determine the live:dead ratio. The presence of larval or nymphal stages or eggs should be noted. Treatment for demodicosis involves dipping the affected animal in an amitraz (not used on horses) or trichlorfon dip. During therapy for *Demodex* species a decrease in the number of eggs and the number of live or moving mites is a good prognostic indicator.

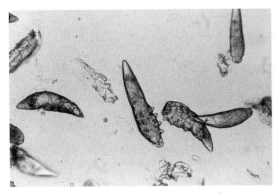

FIGURE 13-61 Results of a thorough, deep skin scraping revealing numerous mites of *Demodex canis.*

> **TECHNICIAN'S NOTE** The veterinarian or technician should count the live versus dead mites for a live:dead ratio to determine the prognosis of treating the infection during therapy.

Parasite: *Trombicula* species
Host: Domestic animals, wild animals, and humans
Location of Larva: The larval stage is the only stage that parasitizes animals and humans. It is found attached to the skin of the host.
Distribution: Worldwide
Derivation of Genus: Unknown
Transmission Route: Direct contact of host and larval mites within forest environments with underbrush
Common Name: Chiggers or red bugs
Zoonotic: No

Trombicula *Species (Chiggers)*

The **chigger,** *Trombicula* species, is yellow to red, has six legs, and ranges in size from 200 to 400 μm in diameter (Figure 13-62). The larval stage is the only developmental stage that parasitizes humans,

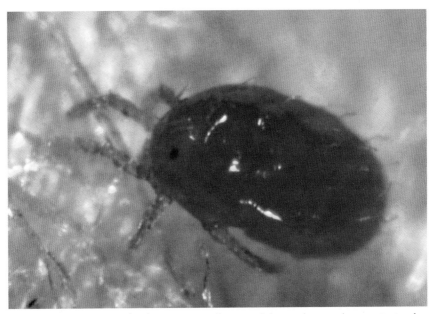

FIGURE 13-62 The chigger, *Trombicula* species, is yellow to red, has six legs, and ranges in size from 200 to 400 μm in diameter. (From Bowman: *Georgis' Parasitology for Veterinarians,* ed 10, 2013, Elsevier.)

domestic animals, and wild animals. The larvae are most common during the late summer and early fall and are transmitted by direct contact of the host with the ground or by brushing against foliage in fields or heavy underbrush. The nymphal and adult stages of chiggers are nonparasitic and are free-living in nature.

Larval chiggers do *not* burrow into the skin, as commonly believed, nor do they feed primarily on host blood. Their food consists of the serous components of tissues. Chiggers attach firmly to the host a..d inject a digestive fluid that produces liquefaction of host cells. The host's skin becomes hardened, and a tube called a **stylostome** forms at the chigger's attachment site. Chiggers suck up liquefied host tissues. When the mite has finished feeding, it loosens its grip and falls to the ground. The injected digestive fluid causes the attachment site to itch intensely. In animals, cutaneous lesions tend to be restricted to areas of the body that come in contact with the ground or underbrush, that is, the head, ears, limbs, interdigital areas, and ventrum.

The most common chigger mite affecting animals and humans is *Trombicula alfreddugesi,* the **North American chigger**. Lesions caused by *T. alfreddugesi* consist of an erythematous, often pruritic, papular rash on the ventrum, face, feet, and legs.

The diagnosis of chiggers is based on the presence of an orange crusting dermatosis, a history of exposure (roaming outdoors), and identification of the typical six-legged larval stage on skin scraping or on collection from the host. The larval chigger remains attached to the skin only for several hours. Consequently, **trombiculosis** may be difficult to diagnose because the pruritus persists after the larva has dropped off the host.

> TECHNICIAN'S NOTE Diagnosis of chiggers is made by finding the six-legged larval stage of the parasite on the affected skin of the host on skin scraping.

Parasite: *Pneumonyssus (Pneumonyssoides) caninum*
Host: Canines
Location of Adult: Nasal turbinates and nasal sinuses
Distribution: Worldwide

Derivation: Lung piercer
Transmission Route: Direct contact from host to host
Common Name: Nasal mites
Zoonotic: No

Pneumonyssus (Formerly, Pneumonyssoides) Caninum (Nasal Mites of Dogs)

Pneumonyssus (Pneumonyssoides) caninum is a rare species of mite that lives in the nasal turbinates and associated paranasal sinuses of dogs. Generally nasal mites are considered to be nonpathogenic; however, reddening of the nasal mucosa, sneezing, shaking of the head, and rubbing of the nose often accompany infestation. Fainting, labored breathing, asthmalike attacks, and orbital disease have been associated with this mite. Sinusitis caused by these mites may lead to disorders of the central nervous system. Owners will observe these mites exiting the nostrils.

The life cycle of *P. caninum* is unknown, but it apparently takes place entirely within the host. Adult males, females, and larvae have been identified, but no nymphal stages have been observed. Transmission probably occurs through direct contact with an infested animal.

> TECHNICIAN'S NOTE Diagnosis of *Pneumonyssus (Pneumonyssoides) caninum* infestation can be made from the owner's observation of mites exiting the dog's nostrils.

Nasal mites are oval and pale yellow. They are 1 to 1.5 mm × 0.6 to 0.9 mm and possess a smooth cuticle with very few hairs. The abdomen lacks setae (fine hairs). Larvae have six legs, and adults have eight legs. All legs are located on the anterior half of the body (Figure 13-63). Diagnosis is usually made at necropsy on asymptomatic animals by finding the characteristic adult mites.

> TECHNICIAN'S NOTE When dogs infested with *Pneumonyssus (Pneumonyssoides) caninum* lie down in front of a fireplace with a roaring fire, the mites may be seen temporarily exiting the nares of the dog as they are attracted to the warmth of the fire.

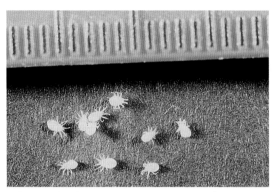

FIGURE 13-63 *Pneumonyssus (Pneumonyssoides) caninum,* a rare mite that lives in the nasal passages and associated paranasal sinuses of dogs.

Parasite: *Ornithonyssus sylviarum* and *Dermanyssus gallinae*

Host: Poultry

Location of Adult: On the skin of poultry (*O. sylviarum*); in the environment of poultry (*D. gallinae*)

Distribution: Worldwide in temperate zones (*O. sylviarum*); worldwide (*D. gallinae*)

Derivation of Genus: Bird piercer (*Ornithonyssus*); skin piercer (*Dermanyssus*)

Transmission Route: Direct contact from host to host (*O. sylviarum*); direct contact with infested environment (*D. gallinae*)

Common Name: Northern fowl mite (*O. sylviarum*); red fowl mite (*D. gallinae*)

Zoonotic: No

Ornithonyssus sylviarum (Northern Mite of Poultry) and Dermanyssus gallinae (Red Mite of Poultry)

Ornithonyssus sylviarum and *Dermanyssus gallinae* both parasitize poultry but differ in the sites where they are collected. *O. sylviarum* is a 1-mm, elongate-to-oval mite with eight legs usually found on birds; it also may be found on nests or within poultry houses. The adults are sparsely covered with setae. In specimens that have been cleared in lactophenol, on the ventral surface of the mite there is an anal plate. The anus of this mite is on the posterior half of that anal plate. This species, the northern mite of poultry, feeds intermittently on birds, producing

irritation, weight loss, decreased egg production, anemia, and even death. These mites have been known to bite humans. The adult is the only life stage that feeds on the host. The larval and nymphal stages do not feed on the host.

D. gallinae is similar in appearance to *O. sylviarum* except the anus is on the anterior surface of the anal plate and is approximately 1 mm in length; elongate to oval; whitish, grayish, or black; and feeds on birds. This mite has a distinct red color when it has recently fed on its host's blood, thus its common name the **red fowl mite**. *D. gallinae* lays its eggs in the cracks in the walls of poultry houses. Both the nymphal stage and the adults are periodic parasites, hiding in the cracks and crevices of poultry houses and making frequent visits to the host to feed. Because of their blood-feeding activity, these mites may produce significant anemia and much irritation to the host. Birds are listless, and egg production may decrease. Loss of blood may result in death. These mites also occur in bird nests in the eaves of houses or in air conditioners. They migrate into homes and attack humans. *D. gallinae* can be treated with pyrethrin sprays or ivermectin. If a flock is infected with *D. gallinae*, dichlorvos strips may be used to treat the flock.

TECHNICIAN'S NOTE Because *Ornithonyssus sylviarum* and *Dermanyssus gallinae* are similar in appearance, it is important to determine the location of the anus on the anal plate for identification of these mites.

Because of their similar morphology, these mites are difficult to differentiate. *O. sylviarum* is usually found on the avian host, whereas *D. gallinae* is a periodic parasite usually found in the host's environment. If specimens are recovered, they should be cleared in lactophenol and the ventral anal plates examined under a compound microscope. The anus of *O. sylviarum* is on the anterior half of the ventral anal plate, whereas that of *D. gallinae* is on the posterior half of the ventral anal plate.

Parasite: *Ornithonyssus bacoti*

Host: Rats and mice; can infect hamsters and guinea pigs

Location of Adult: In host environment most of life cycle; on skin surface when feeding
Distribution: Tropical and subtropical climates
Derivation of Genus: Bird piercer
Transmission Route: Direct contact with contaminated environment
Common Name: Tropical rat mite
Zoonotic: No

Ornithonyssus (Liponyssus) bacoti

Ornithonyssus (Liponyssus) bacoti is commonly called the tropical rat mite. This bloodsucking mite can cause severe problems in rats and mice and can also infect hamsters and guinea pigs. It is especially common in tropical and subtropical climates. *O. bacoti* has a wide host range beyond rodents and can also infect hamsters and guinea pigs.

Oddly, even though *O. bacoti* is a bloodsucking mite, it is more closely related to ticks than mites. This mite is unusual in that it spends most of its life cycle off the host animal, in the host's environment. Both male and female mites are bloodsuckers. The females are larger than the males. These mites may be filled with blood, which produces a reddish-brown color, or if they have not fed, they may be white. The mites can measure up to 750 μm in length (Figure 13-64).

> **TECHNICIAN'S NOTE** The tropical rat mites can cause anemia in rats and mice; however, they can also infect hamsters and guinea pigs. They are bloodsucking mites that are found on the host only when they feed.

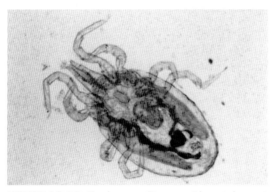

FIGURE 13-64 *Ornithonyssus (Liponyssus) bacoti,* the tropical rat mite.

O. bacoti mites intermittently feed on rodent blood, dropping into nests or surrounding cracks and crevices between feedings. These mites can gain access to other pet animals by dropping from wild or feral animals; days later, when the original host is no longer in the area, they may attack a pet animal for a blood meal.

Infestation with *O. bacoti* is usually diagnosed by observing the blood-filled mites in the bedding, nests, or cracks and crevices near the cages of pet animals. Animals in an environment infested with *O. bacoti* may be anemic and may exhibit a marked reproductive decline. The mite can transmit rickettsial organisms and cause allergic dermatitis in humans. In the absence of a suitable rodent host, *O. bacoti* readily attacks humans for a blood meal.

O. bacoti has a wide host range beyond rodents and is especially common in tropical and subtropical climates.

> **TECHNICIAN'S NOTE** *Ornithonyssus bacoti* can carry rickettsial organisms that can be transmitted to humans and cause allergic dermatitis in humans.

Fur Mites
Parasite: ⓩ *Cheyletiella parasitivorax*
Host: Dogs, cats, and rabbits
Location of Adult: Surface of the skin and hair coat
Distribution: Worldwide
Derivation of Genus: Small lip
Transmission Route: Direct contact from host to host
Common Name: Walking dandruff
Zoonotic: Yes (per the American Association of Veterinary Parasitologists)

Cheyletiella *Species (Walking Dandruff)*

Mites of the genus *Cheyletiella* are surface-dwelling (nonburrowing) mites that reside in the keratin layer of the skin and in the hair coat of various definitive hosts, which may be dogs, cats, or rabbits. These mites ingest keratin debris and tissue fluids and are often referred to as walking dandruff because the motile mites resemble large, moving flakes of dandruff. Cheylettid mites have unique morphologic features. They are large mites (386 × 266 µm), visible to the naked eye. The compound microscope allows easy visualization of this mite's most characteristic morphologic feature, enormous hooklike accessory mouthparts (**palpi**) on the anterior end. These palpi assist the mite in attaching to the host as it feeds on tissue fluids. The mite also has comblike structures at the tip of each of its legs. Members of the genus are also known for their characteristic body shape, a silhouette that has been reported as resembling a shield, a bell pepper, the acorn of an oak tree, or a western horse saddle when viewed from above (Figure 13-65). Eggs are 235 to 245 µm long × 115 to 135 µm wide (smaller than louse nits) and supported by cocoonlike structures bound to the hair shaft by strands of fibers. Two or three eggs may be bound together on one hair shaft or found in the keratin debris of pet dander.

> **TECHNICIAN'S NOTE** Walking dandruff has been reported to look like a bell pepper from the lateral view or an acorn from an oak tree.

The key feature of active infestation by *Cheyletiella parasitivorax* is often the moving, white, dandrufflike flakes along the dorsal midline and head of the host. A handheld magnifying lens or a binocular headband magnifier (e.g., OptiVISOR) may be used to view questionable dandruff flakes or hairs;

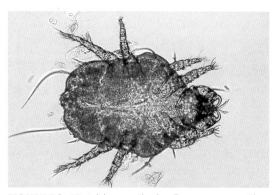

FIGURE 13-65 Adult mite, *Cheyletiella parasitivorax*. *Cheyletiella* species have hooklike accessory mouthparts (palpi) on the anterior end and comblike structures at the tip of the legs. These mites have a characteristic body shape variously described as a shield, bell pepper, acorn, or western horse saddle when viewed from above.

these are perhaps the quickest methods of diagnosing **cheyletiellosis**. A fine-toothed flea comb may be used to collect mites; combing dandrufflike debris onto black paper often facilitates visualization of these highly motile mites. Using clear cellophane tape to entrap mites collected from the hair coat often simplifies localization and viewing under the compound microscope.

C. parasitivorax can be treated with ivermectin (not approved for rabbits) and malathion dips.

> **TECHNICIAN'S NOTE** Superficial combing with a flea comb onto black paper, examination of the dorsal midline and head of the host, and the cellophane tape technique are used to diagnose *Cheyletiella parasitivorax*.

Parasite: *Lynxacarus radovskyi*
Host: Cats
Location of Adult: Hair shafts on the back, neck, thorax, and hind limbs
Distribution: Tropical or warm regions of the United States and Puerto Rico, Australia, and Fiji
Derivation of Genus: Lynx mite
Transmission Route: Direct contact from host to host
Common Name: Feline fur mite
Zoonotic: No

Lynxacarus radovskyi (Feline Fur Mite)

Lynxacarus radovskyi, the feline fur mite, is found attached to the shafts of individual hairs on the back, neck, thorax, and hind limbs of cats residing in tropical or warm areas of the United States such as Florida, Puerto Rico, and Hawaii. These fur mites are laterally compressed. The adults are approximately 500 µm long (Figure 13-66). Pruritus is not always associated with infestations of *L. radovskyi* in cats. These mites are diagnosed by observing the mites attached to hair shafts and examining the dander and other debris after combing. This mite may also affect humans who handle infested cats, producing a papular dermatitis.

> **TECHNICIAN'S NOTE** The feline fur mite can be diagnosed by seeing the adult mites attached to the hair shafts and examining the dander and debris after combing.

Parasite: *Myobia musculi*, *Myocoptes musculinus*, and *Radfordia affinis*

Host: Mice

Location of Adult: Hair shafts

Distribution: Worldwide

Derivation of Genus: Unknown

Transmission Route: Direct contact from host to host

Common Name: Mouse fur mites

Zoonotic: No

Myobia musculi, Myocoptes musculinus, *and* Radfordia affinis *(Mouse Fur Mites)*

The three most common fur mites of the mouse are *Myobia musculi*, *Myocoptes musculinus*, and *Radfordia affinis*. Mice housed in close association with rats may become infested with *Radfordia ensifera*, a fur mite of rats (see next discussion). Rodent mites have life cycles similar to those of mites of other animal species, with larval and nymphal stages. Larval mites have only six legs, whereas nymphal stages (Figure 13-67, *A*) and adult specimens have eight legs (Figure 13-67, *B*).

The first pair of legs of *M. musculi*, *R. affinis*, and *M. musculinus* are distinctly short and adapted for clasping the hair of the host, with the first two pairs of legs being somewhat clublike at the ends (Figure 13-67, *C*).

The second pair of legs of *M. musculi* and *R. affinis* end with clawlike features referred to as empodia. The empodia of *M. musculi* and *M. musculinus* are long and single (Figure 13-68, *A*), whereas *R. affinis* has a shorter pair of empodia of unequal length on the second set of legs (Figure 13-68, *B*). This feature distinguishes *R. affinis* from both *M. musculi* and *M. musculinus*.

Adult females of *M. musculi* are about 400 to 500 μm long and 200 μm wide. Males are similarly

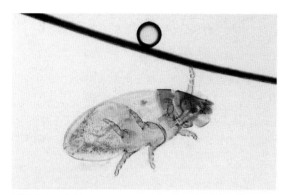

FIGURE 13-66 *Lynxacarus radovskyi,* the feline fur mite, attaches to hair shafts on the back, neck, thorax, and hind limbs of cats.

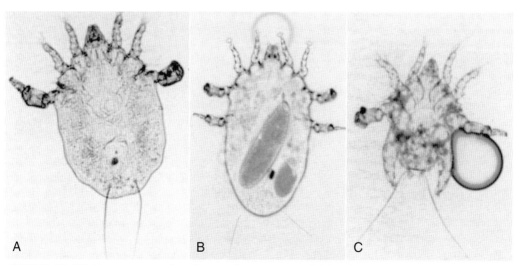

A   B   C

FIGURE 13-67 *Myocoptes musculinus,* fur mite of mice. **A,** Nymphal female. Note the absence of adult's hind legs. **B,** Adult female. The oval shape within is an egg. **C,** Adult male with an air bubble artifact.

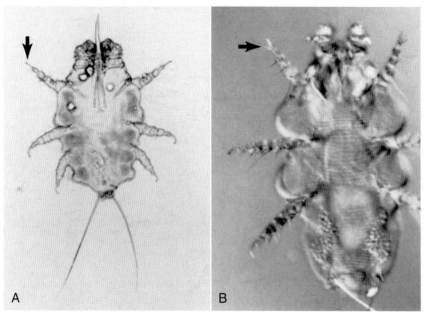

FIGURE 13-68 A, Eight-legged nymphal form of *Myobia musculi* showing a single long empodial claw on the second pair of legs (arrow). The extended mouthpart is typical of the nymphal form. **B,** *Radfordia affinis* showing paired empodial claws on the second leg pair (arrows).

shaped but proportionately smaller. *R. affinis* is similar in size and shape to *M. musculi*. Adult females of *M. musculinus* are smaller than those of other fur mites of mice, measuring 300 × 130 μm. The male is 190 × 135 μm.

> **TECHNICIAN'S NOTE** The second pair of legs end with clawlike features referred to as *empodia*. Empodia of *M. musculi* and *M. musculinus* are longer than those of *R. affinis*.

Fur mite eggs can be found attached near the base of the host's hairs. The eggs are oval and about 200 μm long (Figure 13-69).

To detect fur mites on a live mouse, fur can be obtained by plucking with forceps or by pressing the adhesive side of cellophane tape on the pelt of the mouse. The plucked fur can be placed in a drop of mineral oil on a glass slide and examined microscopically for mites or eggs. The cellophane tape can be placed adhesive side down on a drop of mineral oil on a glass slide and similarly examined.

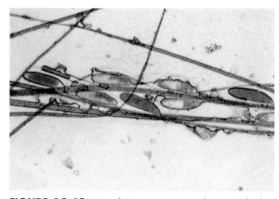

FIGURE 13-69 Nits of *Myocoptes musculinus* attached to the hair shafts of a mouse.

Fur samples should be taken from the neck or shoulder area because that is where the mites most often reside and produce lesions.

Postmortem detection of fur-inhabiting mites of mice may be approached as with the antemortem method, or the dead mouse may be placed under a warm lamp for a few minutes. The heat attracts the mites in the pelt, causing them to migrate to the tips of the hairs. A handheld magnifying glass, a head loupe, or a dissecting microscope aids in the detection of the mites. The mites may be collected on the tip of a metal probe or similar instrument that has been dipped in mineral oil, then placed in a drop of mineral oil on a glass slide and under a coverslip and examined microscopically.

> **TECHNICIAN'S NOTE** Diagnosis of the mouse fur mites can be made by plucking the fur or using the cellophane tape technique to find the mites under a microscope. Samples should be taken from the neck or shoulder areas.

The pathogenicity of mouse fur mites varies greatly with the host and the degree of infestation, similar to demodectic acariasis in dogs. Clinical signs may be absent or may include alopecia, pruritus, and ulceration. More severe lesions may be the result of host sensitivity to the mites, in which case few if any mites are observed.

Transmission of mouse fur mites is by direct contact. Although mites are generally host specific, the owner of multiple species of rodents should be advised that *M. musculi* and *R. affinis* may infest rats and guinea pigs housed in the same area with mice infested with *M. musculi* and *R. affinis*. The three species of mouse fur mites are not known to infest humans.

M. musculi and *M. musculinus* are treated with ivermectin.

Parasite: *Radfordia ensifera*
Host: Rats
Location of Adult: Hair shafts
Distribution: Worldwide
Derivation of Genus: Unknown
Transmission Route: Direct contact from host to host
Common Name: Rat fur mite
Zoonotic: No

Radfordia ensifera (Rat Fur Mite)

R. ensifera, a fur mite of rats, is similar to *M. musculi* and *R. affinis* (see Figure 13-68). *R. ensifera* is distinguished from *M. musculi* and *R. affinis* by the

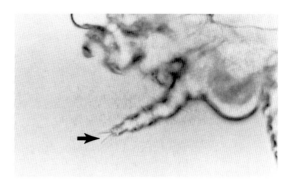

FIGURE 13-70 Second leg of *Radfordia ensifera* showing equal length of the empodial claws *(arrow)*.

empodial claws of the second pair of legs. *M. musculi* has a single, long empodial claw (see Figure 13-68, *A*), whereas *R. ensifera* and *R. affinis* both have a pair of short claws. The two empodial claws of *R. ensifera* are of equal length (Figure 13-70), whereas those of *R. affinis* are of unequal length (see Figure 13-68, *B*).

Antemortem or postmortem, *R. ensifera* is detected using methods described for mouse fur mites. Light infestation of *R. ensifera* usually causes no clinical signs; however, self-inflicted trauma may be seen in heavy infestations. Transmission is by direct contact. *R. ensifera* is not known to infest humans.

> **TECHNICIAN'S NOTE** The rat fur mite can be diagnosed by plucking fur or with use of the cellophane tape method to identify adult mites under the microscope.

Parasite: *Chirodiscoides caviae*
Host: Guinea pig
Location of Adult: Within the pelt
Distribution: Worldwide
Derivation of Genus: Disklike hand
Transmission Route: Direct contact from host to host
Common Name: Guinea pig fur mite
Zoonotic: No

Chirodiscoides caviae (Guinea Pig Fur Mite)

The fur mite that typically infests guinea pigs is *Chirodiscoides caviae*. *C. caviae* is an elongated mite, with a triangular cranial portion that appears similar to the head of the mite. All eight legs are adapted for grasping onto hair. There are no empodial claws on the first two pairs of legs. The male is about 363 × 138 µm (Figure 13-71), and the female is 515 by 164 µm (Figure 13-72).

C. caviae is somewhat difficult to observe antemortem with the unaided eye. It may be detected by pulling hairs, either with forceps or by the cellophane tape method, then examining the specimen microscopically. *C. caviae* is found in the pelt and occurs in the greatest numbers in the area over

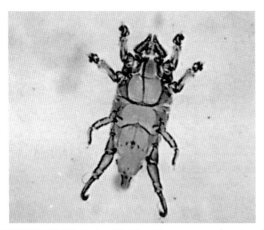

FIGURE 13-71 Male *Chirodiscoides caviae*, a fur mite of the guinea pig.

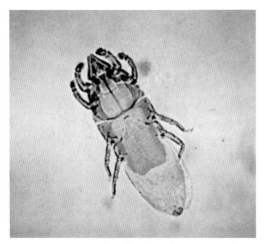

FIGURE 13-72 Female *Chirodiscoides caviae*, a fur mite of the guinea pig.

the rump. Postmortem a piece of the pelt from the rump of the dead animal may be placed in a Petri dish to cool and then examined with a handheld magnifying glass or dissecting microscope for mites at the tip of the hairs.

> **TECHNICIAN'S NOTE**   Diagnosis of the guinea pig fur mite can be made by plucking hairs or using the cellophane tape technique and observing the adult mites under the microscope.

Usually there are no clinical signs unless infestation is severe, when alopecia and pruritus may be seen. Although *C. caviae* is not considered transmissible to humans, transient infestation causing a pruritic, papular urticarial skin condition has been reported.

M. musculinus and *R. affinis* are also transmissible to guinea pigs (see previous discussion).

Parasite: *Listrophorus gibbus*
Host: Rabbits
Location of Adult: Hair shafts
Distribution: Worldwide
Derivation of Genus: Not found
Transmission Route: Direct contact from host to host
Common Name: Rabbit fur mite
Zoonotic: No

Listrophorus gibbus (Rabbit Fur Mite)

Similar to *C. parasitivorax* (see Figure 13-65), *Listrophorus gibbus* is a small, nonburrowing fur mite of rabbits. *L. gibbus* females are about 435 µm long, and males are 340 µm long. Both species have a dorsal hoodlike projection covering the mouthparts. Males are further characterized by the clasping organs at their caudal end.

In the same manner as for *C. parasitivorax*, *L. gibbus* may be detected by pulling fur with forceps or cellophane tape and then examining the hairs under a dissecting microscope. Combing or brushing of the fur may also be used to obtain mites for identification. *L. gibbus* mites are most likely located on the back and abdomen of rabbits. This mite appears to produce no clinical signs, even in heavy infestations.

L. gibbus is transmitted by direct contact. Infestation with *L. gibbus* is treated with malathion dips or ivermectin (not approved for rabbits). This mite is more often associated with wild rabbits than with domestic species, so owners should be aware that control of this parasite depends on controlling the rabbit's environment. *L. gibbus* is not a known vector of disease and has no zoonotic significance in humans.

> **TECHNICIAN'S NOTE** The rabbit fur mite is more commonly associated with wild rabbits than with pet rabbits.

TICKS OF VETERINARY IMPORTANCE

Ticks are small to medium-sized acarines with dorsoventrally flattened, leathery bodies. The tick's head, the capitulum, has two cutting, or lacerating, organs called chelicerae; a penetrating, anchorlike sucking organ, the hypostome; and two leglike accessory appendages, the pedipalps, that act as sensors or supports when the tick fastens to the host's body. The tick's body may be partially or entirely covered by a hard, chitinous plate, the scutum. Mouthparts may be concealed under the tick's body or may extend from the anterior border of the body. Most ticks are inornate, meaning solid-colored (reddish or mahogany) and unpatterned.

Some species are ornate; that is, they demonstrate distinctive white patterns on the dark reddish or mahogany background of the scutum. Larval ticks have six legs, and nymphal and adult ticks have eight legs with strong claws on the ends.

> **TECHNICIAN'S NOTE** The tick's body has a capitulum (head) with chelicerae (two cutting or lacerating organs); a hypostome (penetrating and anchorlike sucking organ); and pedipalps (two leglike accessory appendages) that act as sensors or supports when the tick fastens to the host's body.

Ticks are important parasites because of their voracious blood-feeding activity. They are also important because they are capable of transmitting many parasitic, bacterial, viral, rickettsial, and other pathogenic diseases, such as borreliosis (Lyme disease), among animals and from animals to humans. These pathogenic organisms may be transmitted passively, or the tick may serve as an obligatory intermediate host for certain protozoan parasites.

Ticks are also important because the salivary secretions of some female ticks are toxic and can produce a syndrome known as tick paralysis in humans and domestic and wild animals. Tick species associated with tick paralysis are *Dermacentor andersoni*, the Rocky Mountain spotted fever (RMSF) tick; *Dermacentor occidentalis*, the Pacific Coast tick; *Ixodes holocyclus*, the paralysis tick of Australia; and *Dermacentor variabilis*, the wood tick.

> **TECHNICIAN'S NOTE** Ticks are important veterinary parasites because they are voracious blood-feeders and act as vectors for transmitting various parasitic, bacterial, viral, rickettsial, and other pathogenic diseases, as well as causing tick paralysis.

The ticks of veterinary importance can be divided into two families, the argasid, or soft ticks and the ixodid, or hard ticks. Argasid ticks lack a scutum, the hard, chitinous plate that covers the body of the tick. The mouthparts of the adult soft tick cannot be seen when viewed from the dorsal aspect. Ixodid ticks, on the other hand, have a hard, chitinous scutum that covers all the male tick's dorsum and about a third or less of the female tick's dorsum, depending on the degree of engorgement. As a rule of thumb, male ticks are much smaller than female ticks.

Among the argasid ticks, two species are important: *Otobius megnini*, the spinose ear tick, and *Argas persicus*, the fowl tick. In the ixodid tick family, there are 13 economically important tick species. These include *Rhipicephalus sanguineus*, *Ixodes scapularis*, *Dermacentor* species, and *Amblyomma* species. Of these species, *R. sanguineus* infests buildings such as dwellings and kennels; the other ticks attack their hosts in outdoor environments.

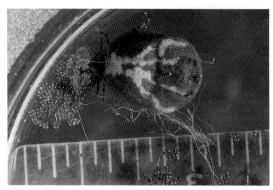

FIGURE 13-73 Adult female *Dermacentor variabilis* laying hundreds of eggs.

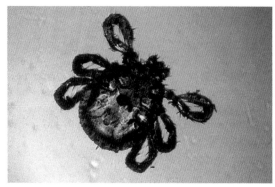

FIGURE 13-74 Six-legged larva, or seed tick, of *Rhipicephalus sanguineus* hatches from the egg and feeds on the host.

> **TECHNICIAN'S NOTE** There are two families of ticks: the argasid ticks (ticks with soft bodies) and the ixodid ticks (ticks with hard bodies).

Specific identification of ticks is difficult and should be performed by a veterinary parasitologist or trained acarologist or arthropodologist. Ticks are usually identified by the shape and length of the capitulum or mouthparts, the shape and color of the body, and the shape and markings on the scutum. Male and unengorged female ticks are easier to identify than engorged female ticks. It is most difficult to speciate larval or nymphal ticks. The common species can be identified by their size, shape, color, body markings, host, and location on the host.

There are four major stages in the life cycle of ticks: egg, larva, nymph, and adult. After their engorgement on the host, female ticks drop off the host and seek protected places, such as cracks and crevices or under leaves and branches, to lay their eggs (Figure 13-73). The six-legged larvae, or seed ticks, hatch from the eggs and feed on the host (Figure 13-74). The larva molts to the eight-legged nymphal stage, which resembles the adult stage but lacks the functioning reproductive organs of adult ticks. After one or two blood meals, the nymph becomes mature and molts to the adult stage.

During the larval, nymphal, and adult stages, ticks may infest one, two, three, or even many different host species (Figure 13-75). This ability to feed on several hosts during the life cycle plays an important role in the transmission of disease pathogens among hosts. It is important to remember that any infestation of domestic animals by either mites or ticks is referred to as *acariasis*.

> **TECHNICIAN'S NOTE** There are four stages to the tick life cycle: egg, larval, nymphal, and adult. In addition, ticks can be one-, two-, three-, or many-host ticks—meaning the tick uses one host for its entire life cycle, one host for a particular life stage, and another host for the other life stages, etc. A three-host tick uses a different host for each life stage.

Most ticks do not tolerate direct sunlight, dryness, or excessive rainfall. They can survive as long as 2 to 3 years without a blood meal, but female ticks require a blood meal before fertilization and subsequent egg deposition. Tick activity is restricted during the cold winter months but increases dramatically during the spring, summer, and fall seasons.

Tick prevention is the best way to avoid acariasis by ticks. Prevention includes inspecting the animal for ticks each time the animal is outside and

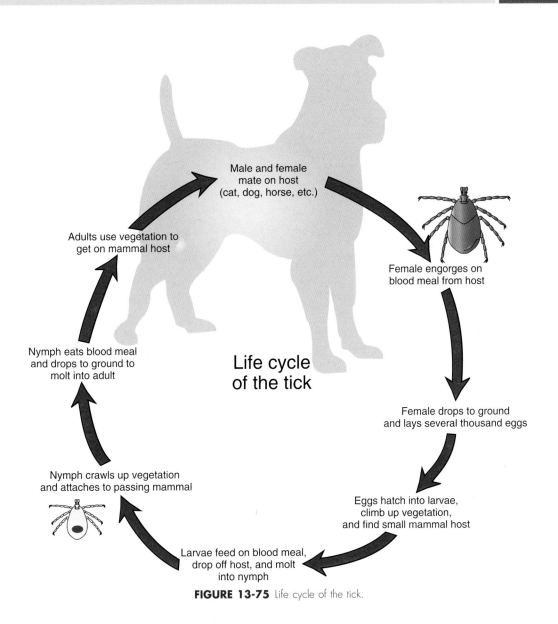

FIGURE 13-75 Life cycle of the tick.

removing the ticks as soon as possible. Tick products, such as Frontline™ or Frontline Plus™ and Advantix™ will kill some species of ticks and are applied once a month. Amitraz is an effective dip for ticks, although there is no long-term residual benefit. Amitraz may also be purchased as a tick collar and is effective against ticks. New monthly preventatives and collars are being developed constantly.

Argasid (Soft) Ticks

Parasite: *Otobius megnini*

Host: Horses, cattle, sheep, goats, and dogs

Location of Adult: Environment of the animal; only larval and nymphal stages feed on the external ear canal of the animal

Distribution: Associated with arid and semiarid regions of the southwestern United States but can be found throughout North America

Derivation of Genus: Ear way of life
Transmission Route: Direct contact with infested environment
Common Name: Spinose ear tick

> **TECHNICIAN'S NOTE** *Otobius megnini* can attach to humans and cause tick paralysis. (NOTE: Every tick has the potential to cause tick paralysis.)

Otobius megnini *(Spinose Ear Tick)*

O. megnini, the spinose ear tick, is an unusual soft tick in that only the larval and nymphal stages are parasitic. The eight-legged adult stages are not parasitic but instead are free-living and are found in the environment of the definitive host, usually in dry protected places, in cracks and crevices, and under logs and fence posts. The larval and nymphal stages feed on horses, cattle, sheep, goats, and dogs. These ticks are associated with the semiarid or arid areas of the southwestern United States; with widespread interstate transportation of animals, however, this soft tick may occur throughout North America. As with most soft ticks, the mouthparts may not be visible when viewed from the dorsal aspect (Figure 13-76). The nymphal stage of *O. megnini* is widest in the middle and is almost

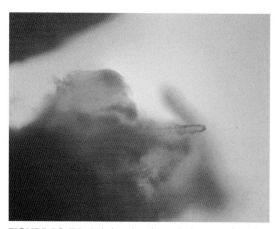

FIGURE 13-76 Only larval and nymphal stages of *Otobius megnini*, the spinose ear tick, are parasitic. Mouthparts of this soft tick may not be visible when viewed from the dorsal aspect.

violin-shaped. It is covered with tiny backward-projecting spines, thus the name **spinose**. The larval and nymphal forms are usually found within the ears of the definitive host, thus the name **ear tick**. The body of the larval stage is covered with stout, tiny spines, whereas the nymphal stage resembles the adult tick on a smaller scale.

> **TECHNICIAN'S NOTE** Only the larval and nymphal stages of *Otobius megnini* feed on the animal host, where they can consume large amounts of blood without engorging or swelling.

Spinose ear ticks are extremely irritating to the definitive host. They often occur in large numbers deep within the external ear canal. These ticks imbibe large amounts of host blood; however, because they are soft ticks, they do not engorge or swell. Large numbers of these ticks may produce ulcerations deep within the external ear. The ears become highly sensitive, and the animals may shake their heads. The pinnae may become excoriated by the constant shaking and rubbing of the animal's head.

The ticks may be visualized in situ with an otoscope. Any waxy exudate should be examined for the presence of larval (six-legged) and nymphal (eight-legged) stages of the spinose ear tick.

Parasite: *Argas persicus*
Host: Chickens, turkeys, and wild birds
Location of Adult: Attached to the skin of the bird when feeding and in the bird's environment when not actively feeding
Distribution: Worldwide
Derivation of Genus: Named for the 100-eyed monster that Hermes slayed in Greek mythology
Transmission Route: Direct contact with infested environment
Common Name: Fowl tick

Argas persicus *(Fowl Tick)*

Argas persicus, the fowl tick, is a soft tick of chickens, turkeys, and wild birds. These ticks are periodic parasites, hiding in cracks and crevices during the day and becoming active during the evening hours when they feed intermittently on the avian host. The adults are 7 mm long and 5 mm wide. In the unengorged state, they are reddish brown, but after engorgement, they take on a slate-blue color. These ticks are flat and leathery, and the tegument is covered with tiny bumps. Because they are soft ticks, they lack a scutum. The mouthparts are not visible when the adult tick is viewed from the dorsal aspect.

Birds heavily infested with *A. persicus* may develop significant anemias. These ticks are worrisome to birds, particularly during the evening hours. The feeding activity of these ticks may cause the birds' egg laying to decrease or even cease.

All stages of *A. persicus* may be collected from infested birds, but it is most often found in cracks, crevices, and contaminated bedding in poultry houses.

> **TECHNICIAN'S NOTE** *Argas persicus* adults are reddish brown before feeding, but after feeding, they turn slate blue.

Ixodid (Hard) Ticks

Parasite: *Ixodes scapularis*
Host: Larval and nymphal stages: mice and voles; adult stage: horses, dogs, deer, and humans
Location of Adult: Attached to host for feeding, environment when not feeding, and can be found on tips of vegetation waiting for a host
Distribution: United States east of the Ohio River Valley
Derivation of Genus: Sticky, like bird-lime
Transmission Route: Direct contact with life stage on tip of vegetation
Common Name: Deer tick

Ixodes scapularis (Deer Tick)
I. scapularis, the deer tick, is a hard-bodied three-host tick. The deer tick is found in regions east of the Ohio River Valley in the eastern United States. The adult ticks have eight legs that lack **festoons** (indentations or folds along the margin of an external body part such as the scutum, the posterior edge of the body, or the legs). The palps (mouthparts)

are long, and the anal groove surrounds the anus anteriorly. The adult females have a small scutum, whereas the males have a large scutum. Adult females engorge or swell up when they take a blood meal. The eggs laid by the female are tiny and round. The larvae have six legs, whereas the nymphs have eight legs like the adult tick.

> **TECHNICIAN'S NOTE** Deer ticks can be found from the Atlantic Ocean to the Ohio River Valley and can be vectors in transmitting several bacteria and parasites.

I. scapularis is a bloodsucking tick that requires a blood meal before developing to the next life stage or laying eggs. These ticks are vectors for bacterial diseases such as tularemia, *Babesia microti*, *Borrelia burgdorferi* (Lyme disease), and granulocytic ehrlichiosis (in humans). All developmental stages can be collected from the tips of vegetation where they await the opportunity for a host to pass by so they can attach themselves to the host. The adults can attach to humans and transmit Lyme disease, tularemia, and babesiosis to the human host. The tick does not cause disease itself, although it can cause tick paralysis, but serves as a vector and intermediate host for the bacteria and parasites that do cause disease.

> **TECHNICIAN'S NOTE** *Ixodes scapularis* is the vector for spreading Lyme disease to dogs, horses, and humans.

Parasite: *Rhipicephalus sanguineus*
Host: Dogs
Location of Adult: Attached below the hair coat on the body but especially the external ear canal and between the toes
Distribution: North America
Derivation of Genus: Fan head
Transmission Route: Direct contact with infested environment
Common Name: Brown dog tick

Rhipicephalus sanguineus (Brown Dog Tick)
R. sanguineus, the brown dog tick, is an unusual hard tick in that it invades both kennel and

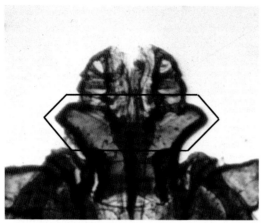

FIGURE 13-77 The area including the basis capitulum of *Rhipicephalus sanguineus* has a unique hexagonal shape. (From Bowman: *Georgis' Parasitology for Veterinarians*, ed 10, 2013, Elsevier.)

household environments. This tick is widely distributed throughout North America. It has an inornate, uniformly reddish-brown scutum and feeds almost exclusively on dogs, thus the common name, brown dog tick. The adult can be found in the hair coat all over the dog's body but is especially fond of the external ear canal and the area between the toes. *R. sanguineus* also has a distinguishing key morphologic feature: Its basis capitulum (or head) has prominent lateral extensions that give the structure a decidedly hexagonal appearance (Figure 13-77). The engorged female is often slate gray. In southern climates the tick is found outdoors, but in northern climates it becomes a serious household pest, breeding indoors in both home and kennel environments.

The bites of this tick can be very irritating to the dog. In severe infestations, heavy blood loss may occur. This tick is also an intermediate host for *Babesia canis,* the etiologic agent that causes canine piroplasmosis.

> **TECHNICIAN'S NOTE** *Rhipicephalus sanguineus* ticks do not transmit any zoonotic diseases but can cause tick paralysis in humans.

R. sanguineus can be identified (with dichotomous keys) by its inornate brown color and characteristic lateral projections of the basis capitulum. These ticks are unique in that they can be found in an indoor or a kennel environment. Treatment can be accomplished by foggers that kill ticks or a house spray labeled for use against ticks. This treatment kills ticks indoors or in the kennel.

Parasite: *Dermacentor variabilis*
Host: Small mammals, dogs, and humans
Location of Adult: Attached to skin when feeding
Distribution: Primarily the eastern two thirds of the United States but can be found throughout the United States
Derivation of Genus: Skin stabber or skin puncturer
Transmission Route: Direct contact with life stage at tip of infested vegetation
Common Name: American dog tick or wood tick

Dermacentor variabilis (American Dog Tick, Wood Tick)

D. variabilis, the American dog tick or wood tick, is found primarily in the eastern two thirds of the United States; however, with the increased mobility of American households, the tick may become distributed throughout the country. Unlike *R. sanguineus,* the *D. variabilis* tick inhabits only grassy, scrub-brush areas, especially roadsides and pathways. This three-host tick initially feeds on small mammals such as field mice and other rodents. However, dogs and humans can serve as preferred hosts for this ubiquitous tick. *D. variabilis* can serve as a vector of RMSF, tularemia, and other microbes. It has also been associated with tick paralysis in domestic and wild animals and in humans. This tick has an ornate scutum that is dark brown with white striping. The adults have eight festooned legs, and the hypostome and palps are somewhat shortened. Unfed adult ticks are approximately 6 mm long; the adult engorged female is about 12 mm and is blue gray (Figure 13-78). *D. variabilis* is a seasonal annoyance to humans and domestic animals.

> **TECHNICIAN'S NOTE** The American dog tick is commonly found on dogs in the United States. *Dermacentor variabilis* can transmit RMSF, tularemia, and other microbes. It is a source for tick paralysis.

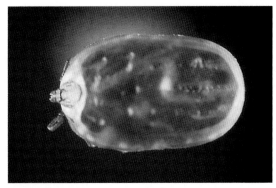

FIGURE 13-78 Engorged, adult female *Dermacentor varia-bilis*. Unfed adults are approximately 6 mm long; engorged adult females are about 12 mm long and blue gray.

D. variabilis can be diagnosed by its key morphologic features (with a dichotomous key) and the rectangular base of the capitulum and characteristic white markings on the dorsal shield.

Parasite: *Dermacentor andersoni*
Host: Larval and nymphal stages: small rodents; adult stage: dogs, horses, cattle, goats, sheep, and humans
Location of Adult: Attached to the skin surface
Distribution: Rocky Mountain regions but can travel on host to other parts of the United States and North America
Derivation of Genus: Skin sticker or skin puncturer
Transmission Route: Direct contact with infested vegetation
Common Name: Rocky Mountain wood tick

Dermacentor andersoni (Rocky Mountain Wood Tick)

D. andersoni, or the **Rocky Mountain wood tick**, is typically seen in the Rocky Mountain regions, but with the ease of travel, the host is able to carry it to other regions in the United States and North America. This is an ornate tick, and the adult has eight festooned legs. The hypostome and palps are short, with the female having a small scutum and the male having a large scutum. The eggs tend to be tiny and round. The female tick can lay as many as 4000 eggs in her lifetime. The larval stage has six legs, whereas the nymph has eight legs.

> **TECHNICIAN'S NOTE** *Dermacentor andersoni* is the Rocky Mountain wood tick that is considered the primary vector for the spread of RMSF.

The larval (seed ticks) and nymphal stages are found on many small mammals, especially rodents. The adult stages are found on large mammals that include horses, dogs, cattle, sheep, goats, and humans. The male and female ticks are blood-feeders that can serve as vectors for a variety of animal and human pathogens. All life stages can be collected from the tips of vegetation where they await a host to pass by.

These ticks can be identified by matching their short palps and hypostome, festooned legs, and ornate scutum with a dichotomous key. These ticks are capable of transmitting RMSF to animals and humans and are considered the primary vector for the transmission of RMSF.

> **TECHNICIAN'S NOTE** *Dermacentor andersoni*, being a three-host tick, is an excellent vector for spreading diseases of animals and humans.

Parasite: *Dermacentor occidentalis*
Host: Larval and nymphal stages: small mammals; adult stage: large mammals such as dogs, deer, cattle, horses, sheep, rabbits, and humans
Location of Adult: Attached to the skin of the host when feeding
Distribution: Sierra Nevada Mountains to the Pacific Ocean
Derivation of Genus: Skin stabber or skin puncturer
Transmission Route: Direct contact with infested vegetation
Common Name: Pacific Coast dog tick

Dermacentor occidentalis (Pacific Coast Dog Tick)

D. occidentalis, or the Pacific Coast dog tick, is a brown tick with eight festooned legs. The adult has short palps and a hypostome. The female has a small scutum, whereas the male possesses a large scutum. This tick is found in the United States between the

Sierra Nevada Mountains and the Pacific Ocean from Oregon to Southern California.

The eggs are tiny and round, whereas the larvae have six legs. The nymphal stage resembles a smaller version of the adult tick with eight legs. The larval and nymphal stages can be found feeding on small mammals, especially rodents. The adults are typically found feeding on large mammals including horses, deer, cattle, donkeys, rabbits, sheep, and humans. All developmental stages can be collected from the tips of infested vegetation where they await a host to pass by so they can attach to it.

All developmental stages are blood-feeders and can act as vectors or intermediate hosts for a variety of animal and human pathogens including tularemia. In addition, the tick can serve as a cause for tick paralysis in animals and humans.

> **TECHNICIAN'S NOTE** *Dermacentor occidentalis,* or the Pacific Coast dog tick, is typically found between the Sierra Nevada Mountains and the Pacific Ocean. However, with the ease of travel, the host can carry it to other regions of the United States and North America.

Parasite: *Amblyomma americanum*
Host: Larval and nymphal stages: small mammals; adult stage: wide range of mammal hosts including humans
Location of Adult: Attached to the skin of the host, particularly the ear
Distribution: Southern United States, Midwest, and Atlantic Coast of the United States
Derivation of Genus: Dull eye
Transmission Route: Direct contact with infested vegetation
Common Name: Lone star tick

Amblyomma americanum *(Lone Star Tick)*

Amblyomma americanum demonstrates a characteristic white spot on the apex of its scutum, thus its common name, the lone star tick. The spot is more conspicuous on male than female ticks. This tick is distributed throughout the southern United States but is also found in the Midwest and on the Atlantic Coast. All developmental stages can be collected from infested vegetation where they await a host to pass by to which to attach.

This three-host tick is found most often in spring and summer, parasitizing the head, belly, and flanks (the ear is the favored site) of wild and domestic animal hosts. It also will feed on humans and is said to have a painful bite. It can produce anemia and has been incriminated as a vector of tularemia and RMSF.

A. americanum is easily diagnosed by the white spot on its scutum.

> **TECHNICIAN'S NOTE** *Amblyomma americanum* is a vector for the transmission of tularemia and RMSF in animals and humans. It can be identified by a single white spot on its scutum.

Parasite: *Amblyomma maculatum*
Host: Larval and nymphal stages: ground birds; adult stage: cattle, horses, sheep, dogs, and humans
Location of Adult: Attached to the skin of the host when feeding
Distribution: Regions of high humidity such as the Atlantic Coast and Gulf Coast of the United States
Derivation of Genus: Dull eye
Transmission Route: Direct contact with infested vegetation
Common Name: Gulf Coast tick

Amblyomma maculatum *(Gulf Coast Tick)*

Amblyomma maculatum, the Gulf Coast tick, is a three-host tick found in the ears of cattle, horses, sheep, dogs, and humans. It occurs in areas of high humidity on the Atlantic and Gulf Coast seaboards. It produces severe bites and painful swellings and is associated with tick paralysis. This tick has silvery markings on its scutum. Larval and nymphal stages occur on ground birds throughout the year. The numbers of adult ticks on cattle decreases during winter and spring and increases in summer and fall. When the ear canals of cattle and horses are infested, the pinnae may droop and become deformed.

A. maculatum is easily diagnosed by the silvery markings on its ornate scutum (Figure 13-79).

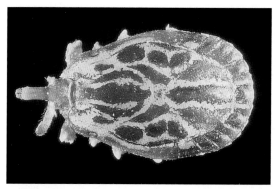

FIGURE 13-79 Ornate adult male, *Amblyomma maculatum*. *A. maculatum* is easily diagnosed by the silvery markings on its scutum.

> **TECHNICIAN'S NOTE** Although *Amblyomma maculatum* is not associated with the transmission of any diseases in humans, it can cause tick paralysis.

Parasite: *Boophilus annulatus*
Host: Cattle
Location of Adult: Attached to the skin of host while feeding
Distribution: Mexico or enzootic areas of the United States
Derivation of Genus: Cattle lover
Transmission Route: Direct contact from host to host; all stages are found on the host
Common Name: Texas cattle fever tick or North American tick

Boophilus annulatus (Texas Cattle Fever Tick)

Boophilus annulatus, the Texas cattle fever tick or North American tick, uses only one host. This tick has historical significance in that it was the first arthropod shown to serve as an intermediate host for *Babesia bigemina,* a protozoan parasite of cattle. This tick therefore marks a milestone in veterinary parasitology. *B. annulatus* has been completely eradicated from the United States; however, if it is ever diagnosed by a veterinary diagnostician, that fact *must* be reported to the proper regulatory agencies. The tick should be identified by a specialist and the appropriate control methods applied. *B. annulatus* frequently enters the United States from Mexico.

The engorged *B. annulatus* female is 10 to 12 mm in length, and the male is 3 to 4 mm. The mouthparts are very short, and there are no festoons on the posterior aspect of the abdomen. It is an inornate tick.

> **TECHNICIAN'S NOTE** In 1892, Theobald Smith and the veterinarian F.L. Kilbourne found that *Boophilus annulatus* was the first arthropod to be shown to serve as an intermediate host for a protozoan parasite (*Babesia bigemina*).

Because this is a one-host tick, larvae, nymphs, and adult ticks may be found on cattle. They do not leave the host to complete the life cycle. Animals with heavy infestations are restless and irritated. To rid themselves of ticks, they rub, lick, bite, and scratch. Irritated areas may become raw and secondarily infested. If ticks are numerous, anemia may occur.

The veterinary diagnostician must use a key to identify adults of *B. annulatus*. Again, ticks identified as such must be reported to both state and federal authorities. Determining the origin of suspect ticks is of paramount importance. Most often these ticks may be collected from within an enzootic area in the United States or from animals originating from Mexico.

Parasite: *Haemaphysalis leporispalustris*
Host: Larval and nymphal stages: rabbits, birds, and occasionally dogs, cats, and humans; adult stage: rabbits
Location of Adult: Attached to the skin of the host when feeding
Distribution: Worldwide
Derivation of Genus: Blood bladder or blood bubble
Transmission Route: Direct contact with infested vegetation
Common Name: Continental rabbit tick

Haemaphysalis leporispalustris (Continental Rabbit Tick)

Although numerous kinds of ticks may infest rabbits, most have a limited geographic distribution and are generally recognized by veterinarians in each geographic area. This discussion centers on

Haemaphysalis leporispalustris, the continental rabbit tick. This tick has the widest geographic distribution of rabbit ticks in the Western Hemisphere. *H. leporispalustris* is a three-host tick, meaning that each developmental stage (larva, nymph, and adult) requires a separate host for a blood meal. Although rabbits may serve as the host for each stage, they seem to be the definitive host for only the adult stage. Larval and nymphal stages also feed on birds, occasionally on dogs and cats, and rarely on humans. Feeding on birds is thought to account for much of the wide geographic distribution of *H. leporispalustris,* because these birds are often migratory.

> **TECHNICIAN'S NOTE** *Haemaphysalis leporispalustris* is a three-host tick that may use the rabbit in all developmental stages, but the rabbit is the definitive host for the adult stage of the tick.

H. leporispalustris is a small, eyeless tick and is distinguished in all stages of the life cycle by the laterally pointed angles formed at the base of the mouthparts, the basis capitulum. The basis capitulum causes the mouthparts to resemble a triangular head. Males are 2.2 mm long, and females are 2.6 to 10 mm long, depending on whether they are engorged with blood. The ticks may be found in the external ear canal and on the pinnae but are more frequently seen on the head and neck.

In extreme cases large numbers of these ticks may produce emaciation and death. These rabbit ticks may spread diseases such as RMSF, Q fever, and tularemia. In general *H. leporispalustris* occurs more frequently on wild than domestic rabbits, so owners should be warned of the disease potential for domestic rabbits that are not kept safely away from wild rabbits and birds.

> **TECHNICIAN'S NOTE** The continental rabbit tick is known to harbor and spread Q fever, RMSF, and tularemia to humans and can also cause tick paralysis.

CHAPTER THIRTEEN TEST

MATCHING 1—Match the term with the correct phrase or term.

A. Arthropodology
B. Crustaceans
C. Centipedes and millipedes
D. Blister beetles (Spanish fly)
E. Caterpillars
F. Kissing bugs

G. *Cimex lectularius*
H. Mallophagans (chewing lice)
I. Anoplurans (sucking lice)
J. Dictyopterans
K. Nit
L. Pediculosis
M. *Simulium* species
N. *Lutzomyia* species
O. *Culicoides* species

1. Egg of either an anopluran or a mallophagan
2. Bedbug
3. No-see-ums
4. Cockroaches and grasshoppers
5. Black flies
6. Importance: first intermediate host for *Paragonimus kellicoti,* *Diphyllobothrium latum, Spirometra mansonoides,* and *Dracunculus insignis*
7. Head wider than widest part of thorax
8. Cantharidin
9. Sand flies capable of transmitting *Leishmania* species
10. The study of arthropods, creatures with jointed appendages
11. Head more narrow than widest part of thorax
12. Intermediate host for *Trypanosoma cruzi* (Chagas disease)
13. Infestation with lice, either mallophagan or anopluran
14. Urticating or stinging hairs
15. Produce venomous substances

MATCHING 2—Match the term with the correct phrase or term.

AA. *Chrysops* species, *Tabanus* species
BB. *Stomoxys calcitrans*
CC. *Haematobia irritans*
DD. *Melophagus ovinus*
EE. *Musca autumnalis*
FF. Myiasis
GG. Facultative myiasis
HH. Obligatory myiasis
II. *Calliphora, Phaenicia, Lucilia,* and *Phormia* species
JJ. *Musca domestica*
KK. Strike or fly strike
LL. Posterior spiracular plate
MM. *Cochliomyia hominivorax*
NN. *Cuterebra* species
OO. *Hypoderma* species

1. Free-living dipteran fly larvae developing a parasitic dependence
2. Heel flies or ox warbles
3. Dipteran fly larvae or maggots within contaminated wounds
4. Stable fly or biting housefly
5. Wolves or warbles in the skin of dogs and cats
6. Housefly
7. Horn flies
8. Blowflies or bottle flies
9. Primary screwworm; dipteran larvae reportable to U.S. Department of Agriculture
10. Sheep ked
11. Face fly
12. Morphologic feature used to identify or speciate dipteran fly larvae
13. Infestation or infection with dipteran larvae or "maggots"
14. Completely parasitic dipteran fly larvae
15. Deerflies, horseflies

MATCHING 3—Match the term with the correct phrase or term.

AAA. Gadding

BBB. *Gasterophilus* species
CCC. *Oestrus ovis*

DDD. *Ctenocephalides felis*
EEE. *Echidnophaga gallinacea*
FFF. Larval siphonapterans
GGG. Flea eggs
HHH. Flea frass
III. Pedicel
JJJ. Acariasis
KKK. Scabies

LLL. *Notoedres cati*
MMM. *Cnemidocoptes pilae*
NNN. *Trixacarus caviae*
OOO. *Psoroptes cuniculi*

1. Resemble tiny pearls; nonsticky, 0.5 mm long, white, oval, and rounded at both ends
2. Ear canker mite of rabbits
3. Colloquial term used to describe cattle running or evading adult heel flies
4. Feline scabies mite
5. Guinea pig mite

6. Horse bots
7. Cat flea
8. Infestation with either mites or ticks
9. Scaly leg mite of budgerigars (parakeets)
10. Sticktight flea of poultry
11. Stalk at the tip of a sarcoptiform mite's leg: They can be long or short, jointed or unjointed
12. Infection with *Sarcoptes scabei*
13. Resemble tiny fly maggots, sparsely covered with tiny hairs
14. Nasal bot fly of sheep and goats
15. Reddish-black, pepperlike specks found with dog or cat's hair coat; actually dried flea feces

MATCHING 4—Match the term with the correct phrase or term.

aa. *Psoroptes* species of large animals
bb. *Chorioptes* species
cc. *Otodectes cynotis*
dd. *Demodex canis*
ee. *Trombicula* species
ff. *Pneumonyssoides caninum*
gg. *Ornithonyssus bacoti*

hh. *Cheyletiella* species
ii. *Lynxacarus radovskyi*
jj. Argasid ticks
kk. Ixodid ticks
ll. *Otobius megnini*
mm. *Argas persicus*
nn. *Rhipicephalus sanguineus*
oo. *Dermacentor variabilis*
pp. *Amblyomma americanum*
qq. *Boophilus annulatus*
rr. *Haemaphysalis leporispalustris*
ss. Ornate ticks
tt. Inornate ticks

1. Tick reportable to the U.S. Department of Agriculture (USDA); Texas cattle fever tick
2. Spinose ear tick
3. Mite reportable to the USDA
4. American dog tick
5. Feline fur mite
6. Foot and tail mite; itchy leg mite
7. Hard ticks with scutum with a pattern of white on a dark background
8. Follicular mite of dogs
9. Lone star tick
10. Hard ticks with a dark-colored scutum
11. Tropical rat mite
12. Canine and feline ear mite
13. Soft ticks
14. Rabbit tick
15. Walking dandruff of dogs, cats, and rabbits
16. Hard ticks
17. Fowl tick
18. Nasal mite of dogs

19. Brown dog tick
20. Chiggers

QUESTIONS FOR THOUGHT AND DISCUSSION

1. Of all the arthropods in this chapter, which do you think is the best practice builder in a small animal veterinary clinic?

2. Of all the arthropods in this chapter, which do you think is the most important parasite to be able to successfully identify with respect to your reputation or standing with your state veterinarian or with the U.S. Department of Agriculture?

3. One of the major ways in which arthropods are important is that they are capable of serving as intermediate hosts for both protozoan and helminth parasites. List 10 arthropods and link them to the protozoans or parasites with which they are associated.

4. What morphologic features or characteristics can be used to identify the following:
   - Adult dipteran flies
   - Larval dipterans (maggots)
   - Sarcoptiform mites
   - Ticks

Introduction to the Phylum Arthropoda, Subphylum Pentastomida

OUTLINE

LEARNING OBJECTIVES

After studying this chapter, the reader should be able to do the following:
- Describe the life cycle of the pentastomes.
- Understand the zoonotic potential for reptilian pentastomes and the importance of thorough handwashing after contact with snake feces.

KEY TERMS

Larval pentastome

Linguatuliasis

Linguatulids

Linguatulosis

Nymphal pentastome

Pentastome

Pentastomiasis

Pleomorphic

Tongue worms

PENTASTOMES (PARASITES OF REPTILES)

Reptiles have served as hosts to protozoan and metazoan parasites for eons. One of the oldest continuing host-parasite relationships is that between snakes and pentastomes. Pentastomes are almost exclusively parasites of the reptilian respiratory system. According to theory, the pentastomes' ancestors were once land animals that invaded the respiratory passages of reptiles. These rare parasites hold serious zoonotic consequences for humans, who can unwittingly serve as incidental hosts.

Pentastomes have lost most of their morphologic similarity to other major phyla; they are a taxonomist's dilemma. During their life cycle, pentastomes are pleomorphic (demonstrating a variety of morphologic forms). They resemble acarines (mites) during their larval stage but look like annelids (earthworms) during their nymphal and adult stages. It is difficult to assign them to either phylum, which probably means that they possess a common ancestor with annelids and arthropods. Therefore these creatures have been assigned to the subphylum Pentastomida.

> **TECHNICIAN'S NOTE** Pentastomes resemble mites during their larval stage and annelids during their nymphal and adult stages; therefore they have been assigned to the subphylum Pentastomida.

MORPHOLOGY

The name pentastome (*penta* meaning "five" and *stome* meaning "mouth," thus five mouths) was chosen because, as adults, these parasites have a mouth on the anterior end that is surrounded by four hooked claws. Early investigators erroneously believed these claws to be four additional mouths; one mouth plus four mouths equals five mouths. Pentastomes have also been called tongue worms and linguatulids because of their distinct tongue-shaped appearance, being wider anteriorly than posteriorly (Figure 14-1). Infection with pentastomes is referred to as pentastomiasis, linguatuliasis, linguatulosis, or rarely porocephalosis or porocephaliasis (after Porocephalida, one of two orders composing the subphylum Pentastomida).

Grossly, pentastomes resemble helminths; however, they are often grouped with the phylum Arthropoda because of the mitelike larval stage that appears during their life cycle.

Pentastomes are almost always parasites of reptiles; the exceptions to this rule are species of *Linguatula serrata* (which parasitize carnivores) and *Reighardia sternae* (a parasite of seagulls and terns). Within the phylum are nine genera that parasitize snakes, three that parasitize lizards, four that parasitize crocodiles, and two that favor turtles. Among snakes, the most common genera are *Armillifer* species that parasitize pythons and vipers, *Kiricephalus* that parasitize cobras, and *Porocephalus* that parasitize boas and rattlesnakes (Figure 14-2).

TECHNICIAN'S NOTE With the exception of two species of pentastomes, almost all pentastomes parasitize reptiles.

LIFE CYCLE

Adult reptilian pentastomes are dioecious parasites; they have separate sexes, and there are both male and female pentastomes. Pentastomes are parasites that occur almost exclusively within the lungs, trachea, and nasal passages of the reptilian definitive host, feeding on tissue fluids and blood cells. Female pentastomes produce several million fully embryonated eggs, each containing a single larva with two or three pairs of rudimentary clawed legs. Eggs are "coughed up," swallowed, and passed to the outside environment within the host feces. The oval, tailed larval pentastome with four to six stumpy legs, each with one or two retractable, pincerlike claws, hatches from the egg and is infective for the intermediate host. Figure 14-3 shows the life cycle of a reptilian pentastome.

Intermediate hosts include rodents, herbivores, carnivores, nonhuman primates, and humans. The larval pentastome bores through the intestinal wall of the intermediate host and passes with the blood to the mesenteric lymph nodes, the liver, the lungs, the omentum, or other internal organs where it becomes encysted. The larva becomes "quiescent"

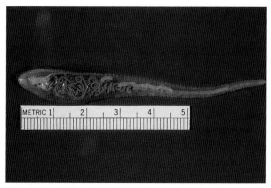

FIGURE 14-1 Distinctive tongue-shaped appearance of a pentastome. Because these strange parasites are flattened and wider anteriorly than posteriorly, they are often referred to as tongue worms. The canine pentastome, *Linguatula serrata*, has a transversely striated cuticle. The female is 8 to 13 cm long, and the male is 1.8 × 2 cm.

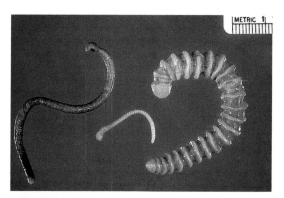

FIGURE 14-2 Assorted adult reptilian pentastomes from the respiratory tracts of snakes. *Left to right,* mature *Kiricephalus* species, immature *Kiricephalus* species, and mature *Armillifer* species.

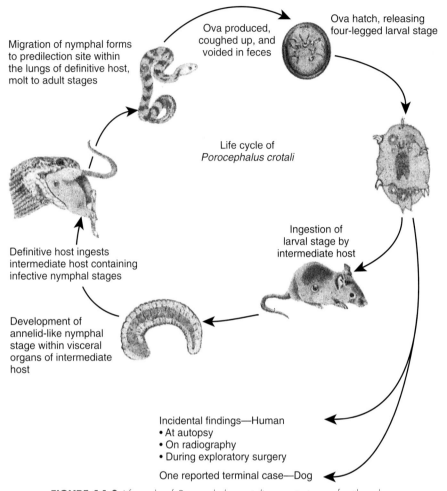

Ova produced, coughed up, and voided in feces

Ova hatch, releasing four-legged larval stage

Migration of nymphal forms to predilection site within the lungs of definitive host, molt to adult stages

Life cycle of *Porocephalus crotali*

Ingestion of larval stage by intermediate host

Definitive host ingests intermediate host containing infective nymphal stages

Development of annelid-like nymphal stage within visceral organs of intermediate host

Incidental findings—Human
• At autopsy
• On radiography
• During exploratory surgery

One reported terminal case—Dog

FIGURE 14-3 Life cycle of *Porocephalus crotali*, a pentastome of rattlesnakes.

and changes into the annelid (wormlike) nymphal stage, which can pass through as many as five molts. The reptilian definitive host becomes infected by ingesting the intermediate host with its encysted nymphal pentastomes. The infective nymphs penetrate the host's intestine and bore into the lungs, where they become sexually mature adult parasites. The life cycle of the typical pentastome is an oddity in that the organism serving as the intermediate host (e.g., a mammal) is *higher* in the phylogenetic classification scheme than the definitive host (the reptile); this situation is uncommon among the life cycles of parasites. With most parasites, the organism serving as the intermediate host is *lower* in the phylogenetic classification scheme than the host that serves as definitive host.

> **TECHNICIAN'S NOTE** The intermediate hosts for reptilian pentastomes include rodents, herbivores, carnivores, nonhuman primates, and humans.

DIAGNOSIS

Definitive Host

Clinical signs of reptilian pentastomiasis include lethargy, anorexia, dyspnea, and production of blood-tinged sputum or mucus within the pharynx or the trachea. The sputum can contain eggs that microscopically appear to contain four-legged to six-legged larvae with retractable claws. These pentastome eggs also can be found in the feces of the definitive host. Hematologic studies might demonstrate leukocytosis and eosinophilia. Radiographic examination might reveal adult worms or remnants of calcified cysts.

Adult reptilian pentastomes are not confined to the lungs. Adult and juvenile pentastomes might attempt to exit the host through the reptile's nostrils or mouth or through the body wall and skin whenever the reptile is stressed. Reptilian pentastomiasis also can be diagnosed by biopsy of infected tissues or recovery of the parasite at necropsy.

> **TECHNICIAN'S NOTE** Pentastome eggs can be found on standard fecal flotation procedures on the feces of the definitive host.

Incidental Host

In contrast to pentastomid infections in natural intermediate hosts, infections in incidental hosts are striking. An incidental host is usually asymptomatic to nymphal invasion; nymphs are often found during radiographic examination, during surgery, or at necropsy. Nymphs can affect vital structures and produce pathology that leads to demonstration of related clinical signs. Death can result.

A case of incidental nymphal pentastomiasis has been reported in dogs. Eosinophilic inflammatory responses were noted in thoracic and abdominal cavities. These responses were presumably caused by the extensive migratory paths of the pentastomes. During exploratory surgery, it was noted that all peritoneal and visceral surfaces were covered with 3- to 5-mm, C-shaped, cystic structures, each of which contained an elongated, coiled nymph. The nymphs were identified as those of *Porocephalus crotali*, a pentastome of rattlesnakes.

Humans also are incidental mammalian hosts of pentastomids. The fact that humans can serve as intermediate hosts for reptilian pentastomes is sufficient reason for veterinarians to recognize the zoonotic potential of these parasites. Human infections with reptilian pentastomes have been reported from all continents but are most common in Africa and Malaysia. Almost all recorded infections in humans have been incidental findings during radiographic examination (pentastomes often die in tissue locations and become calcified), exploratory surgery, or autopsy. Those pentastomes recovered during autopsy are usually not related to the cause of death; however, under certain circumstances, nymphs may cause significant pathology because of the organ location, the large number of nymphs involved, or their extensive tissue migrations.

> **TECHNICIAN'S NOTE** With the exception of humans, incidental infection with pentastomes can cause death to the incidental host related to the migration of larval and nymphal stages and the damage to organs that these migrations produce.

On histopathologic examination of tissue, the characteristic C shape of the nymph can be seen. Pentastomid nymphs have a pseudosegmented body with a prominent body cavity, a striated musculature, a digestive tract with numerous villi, and acidophilic glands surrounding the intestine. The nymphal pentastome's cuticle may be spiny, smooth, or annulated and may possess numerous acidophilic skin glands that communicate with the cuticle through sclerotized openings. Most of these morphologic features can be identified by either a trained pathologist or a parasitologist.

Antemortem diagnosis of pentastomiasis in the intermediate host can be accomplished by radiographic examination. In these hosts, pentastomes may die in their tissue sites and become calcified; these calcified pentastomes may be visible on radiography.

> **TECHNICIAN'S NOTE** Diagnosis of pentastomiasis in the intermediate host can be made by radiographic examination for calcified pentastomes.

ADULT PENTASTOME THAT INFECTS NASAL PASSAGES AND TURBINATES OF A MAMMALIAN HOST

Parasite: *Linguatula serrata*
Host: Dogs

Location of Adult: Nasal passages and sinuses
Distribution: Worldwide
Intermediate Host: Cats, rats, porcupines, guinea pigs, rabbits, hedgehogs, pigs, and ruminants
Derivation of Genus: Small tongue
Transmission Route: Ingestion of infective intermediate host
Common Name: Canine pentastome
Zoonotic: No

L. serrata, the canine pentastome, is found in the nasal passages and sinuses of dogs and other canids. Intermediate hosts are cats, rats, porcupines, guinea pigs, rabbits, hedgehogs, pigs, and wild and domestic ruminants. In North America, rabbits are the most common intermediate hosts. Both adult and nymphal stages of this parasite may infect humans. Humans harbor nymphal stages after ingesting eggs from contaminated feces. Nymphs may be found in a variety of organs—the spleen, liver, and mesenteric lymph nodes. Humans become definitive hosts by eating raw or undercooked meat or meat by-products that contain the nymphal stages.

> **TECHNICIAN'S NOTE** In North America, the rabbit is the common intermediate host for *Linguatula serrata*; humans can harbor nymphal stages after ingesting eggs from contaminated feces.

DIAGNOSIS

Definitive Host

Usually there are no signs of infection; however, dogs may exhibit catarrhal or suppurative rhinitis and bleeding of the nose usually related to inflammatory damage. Restlessness, sneezing, difficulty breathing, and a reduced sense of smell have been observed. The adult parasite may be observed in its predilection site or may be sneezed out or coughed up. The adult parasite resembles a helminth (worm), but as with all pentastomes, it is an arthropod. The parasite is tongue-shaped and flattened and has a transversely striated cuticle. The female is 8 to 13 cm long, and the male is 1.8 × 2 cm in size (see Figure 14-1).

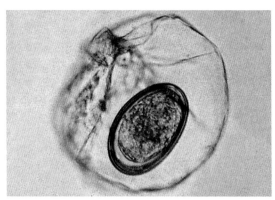

FIGURE 14-4 Eggs of *Linguatula serrata* are yellow brown, oval, and 70 × 90 μm and have a thick chitinous shell. An embryo with two pairs of irregularly arranged chitinous claws may be observed on the inside of the egg. Each egg is initially enclosed in a thin, bladderlike envelope containing clear fluid. This envelope is usually removed during passage through the gastrointestinal tract.

Eggs may be observed on fecal flotation or nasal swabs. Eggs are yellow brown, oval, and 70 × 90 μm and have a thick chitinous shell. An embryo with two pairs of irregularly arranged, chitinous claws may be observed on the inside of the egg. Each egg is initially enclosed in a thin, bladderlike envelope containing a clear fluid. This envelope is usually removed during passage through the gastrointestinal tract (Figure 14-4).

Intermediate Host

Nymphs of *L. serrata* in the intermediate host are detected by biopsy, exploratory laparotomy, postmortem examination, and subsequent histopathology.

The veterinarian must remember that pentastomes are rare, unusual parasites of snakes and dogs. It is important to note that the hands should *always* be washed after handling snake feces. Humans can serve as an intermediate host for this strange parasite.

> **TECHNICIAN'S NOTE** Although pentastome infections are rare, hands should always be washed after handling snake feces as a precautionary measure.

CHAPTER FOURTEEN TEST

MATCHING—Match the term with the correct phrase or term.

A. Pentastomes

B. Pentastome's larval stage

C. Pentastome's nymphal or adult stage

D. Reptiles

E. *Porocephalus crotali*

F. *Linguatula serrata*

G. Prevention of human pentastomiasis

H. Acidophilic glands around the intestine

I. Nasal passages and sinuses

J. Five mouths

1. Derivation of the term *pentastome*

2. Thorough handwashing after handling of snakes or snake feces

3. Tongue worms or linguatulids

4. Rattlesnake pentastome

5. Very similar to an annelid; they are very wormlike in appearance

6. Site of infection for canine pentastomes

7. Characteristic trait of pentastome nymph in histopathologic section

8. Very similar to a mite; it has jointed appendages

9. Principal definitive hosts for pentastomes

10. Canine pentastome

QUESTIONS FOR THOUGHT AND DISCUSSION

1. Snakes are becoming increasingly popular with the public at large. From a public health view, how might one counsel a client with regard to maintaining a snake in the home?

2. What should a veterinarian tell the owner of a dog infected with adult *Linguatula serrata*?

The Phylum Annelida

OUTLINE

LEARNING OBJECTIVES

After studying this chapter, the reader should be able to do the following:

- Describe the morphology of leeches.
- Describe the pathology associated with hirudiniasis.
- Describe the beneficial use of leeches in both human and veterinary medicine.

KEY TERMS

Annelids	Hirudineans	*Hirudo medicinalis*	Stepping
Hirudin	Hirudiniasis	Pseudosucker	Swimming

Kingdom: Animalia
   Phylum: Annelida
      Class: Hirudinea

Leeches and earthworms are annelids. Leeches are not considered to be true helminths but are often described as parasitic worms. As external parasites of humans and domesticated and wild animals, leeches are members of the phylum Annelida and the class Hirudinea.

> **TECHNICIAN'S NOTE** Although leeches are considered ectoparasites, one species is used for medicinal purposes.

HIRUDINEA (LEECHES)

Leeches or hirudineans can be predatory or scavenging. Most often they are parasitic on a wide variety of vertebrates and invertebrates. The ectoparasitic leeches feed on blood from fish, crustaceans, frogs, turtles, mollusks, birds, and land animals such as cattle, horses, assorted primates, and humans. These ectoparasites range in size from tiny species that are 5 mm long to varieties such as *Haemopis sanguisuga,* the horse leech, which has been reported to be as long as 45 cm when extended and swimming.

MORPHOLOGY

Leeches have slender, leaf-shaped bodies that lack bristles. The typical leech has two suckers, a large, adhesive posterior sucker and a smaller anterior sucker. The anterior sucker is actually a pseudosucker and surrounds the mouth. As a member of the phylum Annelida, the leech is segmented and lacks a hard exoskeleton; in its place the leech has a thin, flexible cuticle. Because of this thin cuticle, leeches dry out quickly and must always be closely associated with water. A few leeches are found in saltwater; a few terrestrial (land) leeches are found in moist, damp locations. For the most part, leeches should be considered aquatic animals.

> **TECHNICIAN'S NOTE** The leech has a segmented body that lacks a hard exoskeleton. Instead, it has a thin, flexible cuticle.

As a result of these different habitats, leeches have developed two widely different locomotory habits, swimming and stepping. Swimming is the method of locomotion used when the leech is in water. The leech's body becomes flattened dorsoventrally as waves of muscular contraction pass down its length. The result is an undulating motion that propels the leech forward.

Stepping is the method of locomotion used when the leech is on solid ground. While in this mode, the leech moves in an "inchwormlike" manner, using its cranial and caudal suckers as organs of attachment to move along the substrate (surface). The layer of circular muscle just beneath the epidermis contracts, and the leech becomes long and thin. The cranial sucker then attaches to the substrate, the caudal sucker releases, and the longitudinal muscle layer beneath the circular muscle brings the caudal sucker up to the vicinity of the cranial sucker, where it attaches. The overall effect is "stepping."

> **TECHNICIAN'S NOTE** When on land, the leech moves using an inchwormlike motion called *stepping*. It alternates using its cranial and caudal suckers to attach to and move along surfaces.

While the leech is attached to the host with its caudal sucker, it uses the cranial sucker to explore the host's skin to locate a suitable feeding site and to attach tightly. Three rows of jaws with approximately 100 teeth are found in the cranial sucker. These teeth operate similar to a circular saw, penetrating through the skin to a depth of 1.5 mm. The wound produced by the leech bite is a characteristic Y-shaped skin incision. When the incision is made, the host feels very little pain.

In the past, analgesia was thought to be caused by the release of an anesthetic in the leech saliva, but it is now believed that leech saliva does *not* contain an anesthetic. The ability of a leech to feed is made easier by the secretion of powerful anticoagulants into the site of attachment. A histamine-like substance is added to the wound to prevent the collapse of adjacent capillaries. As blood passes through the mouth, the anticoagulant hirudin is added to it. Hirudin is a 64–amino acid peptide with a function similar to that of antithrombokinase. It has been described as the most powerful anticoagulant known. Active agents in the saliva of various species of leeches include a hyaluronidase, a collagenase, and two fibrinases.

> **TECHNICIAN'S NOTE** Hirudin, one of the most powerful anticoagulants known, is secreted into the bite wound of the leech to keep the host bleeding as the leech feeds.

When engorged with blood, the leech is dark and bloated; some leeches can ingest blood meals that are 900% of their body weight. True bloodsucking leeches require a blood meal only occasionally; consumed blood is used very slowly, so slowly that some leeches have been kept in captivity for more than 2 years without being fed. The mouth leads to a pharynx with salivary glands that secrete hirudin, a crop where ingested blood is stored, a stomach, an intestine, a rectum, and an anal pore near the caudal sucker.

LIFE CYCLE OF THE LEECH

As with the flatworms (flukes and tapeworms), leeches are hermaphroditic. Because male and female organs are located on adjacent body segments, self-fertilization is impossible, and cross-fertilization must take place. After copulation, both partners are fertilized. Eggs are laid in cocoons. The cocoon of each species of leech has a characteristic shape and design. *Hirudo medicinalis*, the medicinal leech, produces from one to seven cocoons, each of which may contain 5 to 15 eggs. Depending on the species of leech, cocoons may be attached to the parent's body or adhere to solid surfaces within the aquatic environment. Young leeches hatch from the eggs, feed for a few days on the yolk, and develop to the adult bloodsucking mode. Adult leeches can live for as long as 18 to 27 years.

The term hirudiniasis is derived from the classic Linnaean nomenclature and can be defined as invasion of the nose, mouth, pharynx, or larynx by leeches or the attachment of leeches to the skin. The terrestrial, or land, varieties of leeches are primarily found in the tropical regions of the world, particularly Southeast Asia, the Pacific islands, the Indian subcontinent, and South America. Land leeches are found on the surface of trees and grasses and under stones in damp places. One terrestrial leech, *Haemopis terrestris*, has been plowed up in fields in the Midwestern United States.

> **TECHNICIAN'S NOTE** Land leeches are found on the surface of trees and grasses or under stones in damp places. They mostly occur in tropical regions of the world.

Punctures made in the skin by land leeches are painless, remain open, and continue to bleed long after the leech has detached. Land leeches in Southeast Asia and India congregate in such large numbers on the legs of cattle, horses, and other native animals that they interfere with the ambulation of the host. Because leeches can ingest so much blood, further complications for the host include anemia and even death from blood loss.

Terrestrial leeches that attach to the skin should never be pulled off but instead must be induced to detach. If pulled off, these leeches may leave their jaws embedded in the skin; such remnants can induce ulceration and serve as a site of infection. Drops of concentrated salt solution, alcohol, or strong vinegar applied around the mouth of the leech or heat with a lighted match or cigarette applied to the leech's body will cause land leeches to release their hold. The open wound should be treated with a styptic and an antiseptic.

> **TECHNICIAN'S NOTE** Never pull an attached leech off of a host; instead, the leech must be induced to detach on its own. Pulling the leech off can result in leaving mouthparts in the skin, resulting in ulceration of the site and possibly infection.

Aquatic leeches can be external or internal parasites. Two genera of aquatic leeches (*Limnatis* and *Dinobdella*) have veterinary significance because they parasitize monkeys and domestic animals. *Theromyzon tessulatum* parasitizes wild and domestic aquatic birds. These genera reside in freshwater, where they come in contact with the vertebrate host.

Leeches entering the mouth or nostrils of the host can pass to the nasopharynx, epiglottis, esophagus, trachea, and bronchi. After attaching itself to the mucous membranes, the leech secretes its anticoagulant and engorges. Depending on the site of attachment, leeches may cause the host to exhibit nosebleeds, cough up blood, or vomit blood. A leech attached in the laryngeal region may produce a cough with a bloody discharge, difficulty in breathing, pain, and even suffocation. A leech localized in the region of the epiglottis may cause difficulty in swallowing. In severe breathing disturbances, the host's neck may be extended, and the animal may exhibit open-mouthed breathing.

> **TECHNICIAN'S NOTE** Aquatic leeches can attach to the nasopharynx, epiglottis, esophagus, trachea, and bronchi causing nosebleeds and the coughing up and vomiting of blood.

Parasite: *Hirudo medicinalis*
Host: Humans
Location of Adult: On the skin
Distribution: Worldwide for medicinal use but native to Europe, Asia, and South America
Derivation of Genus: Leech
Transmission Route: Intentional placement for medicinal purposes
Common Name: Medicinal leech
Zoonotic: No

Several species of leeches have proved to be beneficial to humans. Perhaps the best-known leech used for bloodletting is *H. medicinalis,* the European medicinal leech. This leech is a native of Europe, parts of Asia, and (after its introduction) South America. It possesses a distinct green pattern of pigmentation with brown stripes and ranges in size from less than 1 cm to more than 20 cm in length (Figures 15-1 and 15-2). On its anterior end is a

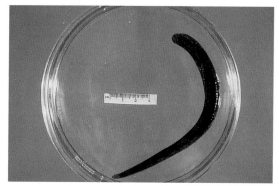

FIGURE 15-1 Extended *Hirudo medicinalis* in a Petri dish. Note that the narrow end is the cranial end and has an oral sucker. The wide end is the caudal end with a sucker.

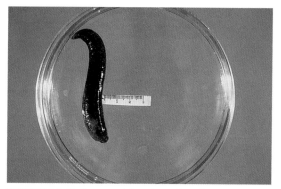

FIGURE 15-2 Contracted *Hirudo medicinalis* in a Petri dish. Note the external segmentation on the body.

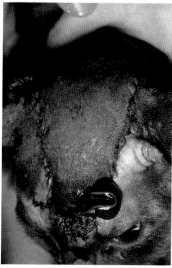

FIGURE 15-3 *Hirudo medicinalis* feeding on a full-thickness skin graft in a cat 24 hours after surgery. Surgical techniques used were a single-pedicle advancement flap and full-thickness mesh with graft bed. Note the congested area in the rostral portion of the pedicle flap.

muscular sucker that contains three sharp chitinous jaws armed with saw-shaped teeth; its caudal end has a characteristic suckerlike disk. This species can ingest an amount of blood up to five times its own weight. When the leech has taken a blood meal from the host, it may take as long as 200 days for digestion. This leech is reported to have gone without food for as long as 18 months.

TECHNICIAN'S NOTE Medicinal leeches can consume blood up to five times their own weight.

H. medicinalis has been the leech used most often for bloodletting purposes throughout history. Its present use in reconstructive and microvascular surgery in humans is gaining impetus. Medicinal leeches have also been used in applications in both veterinary surgery and medicine. Recently there has been revived interest in these unique ectoparasites.

TECHNICIAN'S NOTE Medicinal leeches are most often thought of in conjunction with bloodletting throughout history.

H. medicinalis serves as an important medical tool because it can produce a small bleeding wound that mimics venous outflow in tissues with impaired venous circulation (Figure 15-3). Leeches are indicated only for tissues with such impairment. The leech's main benefit is not the average 5 mL of blood removed during attachment but rather the volume of blood (reportedly as much as 50 mL) that continues to ooze for 24 to 48 hours after the leech has detached. This local bleeding is related to pharmacologically active anticoagulants and vasodilator substances introduced by the leech bite. Each bite can be encouraged to bleed further by gently removing clots that form. Research has demonstrated that new vessels begin to grow around the flap margins after approximately 72 to 120 hours.

Thus the leeches can demonstrate both pathogenic and beneficial effects on humans and wild and domesticated animals.

> **TECHNICIAN'S NOTE** The benefit of the medicinal leech is not in the blood it ingests but in the bleeding that occurs after it releases. This blood seems to help mimic the venous flow of blood to impaired tissues.

CHAPTER FIFTEEN TEST

MATCHING—Match the term with the correct phrase or term.

A. Class Hirudinea

B. *Haemopis sanguisuga*

C. Swimming

D. Stepping

E. Leech bite

F. Hirudin

G. Hirudiniasis

H. *Hirudo medicinalis*

I. Beneficial use of leeches

J. Incentive for leech to release

1. 64–amino acid peptide with a function similar to that of antithrombokinase; the most powerful anticoagulant known

2. Method of locomotion when a leech is in the water

3. The European medicinal leech

4. Reconstructive and microvascular surgery in both humans and animals

5. Y-shaped skin incision

6. Leeches

7. Method of locomotion when a leech is on land

8. The horse leech

9. Concentrated salt solution, strong vinegar, or touching with a lighted match or cigarette

10. Invasion of the nose, mouth, pharynx, or larynx by leeches or attachment of leeches to the skin

QUESTIONS FOR THOUGHT AND DISCUSSION

1. Compare pediculosis, siphonapterosis, acariasis, and linguatulosis with hirudiniasis. Why do you think these terms are important?

2. What was once old-fashioned is now back in style! What were leeches used for during the eighteenth and nineteenth centuries? Discuss the potential for their use in the twenty-first century.

Parasites of Public Health Importance in Veterinary Parasitology

LEARNING OBJECTIVES

After studying this chapter, the reader should be able to do the following:

- Detail the types of zoonotic diseases that might be encountered in a veterinary clinical practice.
- Communicate the symptoms, diagnostic procedures, and prevention of major zoonotic diseases that might be encountered in a veterinary clinical practice.

- Understand that veterinarians and veterinary technicians should never provide direct treatment for a human patient infected with a zoonotic disease.
- Understand that veterinarians and veterinary technicians should act only in an advisory capacity regarding zoonotic diseases.

KEY TERMS

Acquired toxoplasmosis	Ground itch	Ocular larva migrans (OLM)	Swimmer's itch
Bradyzoites	Hydatid disease	Oncosphere	Tachyzoites
Canine scabies	Hymenolepiasis	Papules	Toxocaral larva
Coccidiostats	Incidental nymphal	Paratenic host	migrans
Congenital	pentastomiasis	Pernicious anemia	Toxoplasmosis
toxoplasmosis	Measly beef/beef	Plumber's itch	Trichinosis/
Creeping eruption	measles	Pulmonary	trichinellosis
Cryptosporidiosis	Measly pork/pork	dirofilariasis	Trichostrongyliasis
Cutaneous larva	measles	Rat tapeworm	Unilocular hydatid
migrans (CLM)	Multilocular hydatid	Sandworms	disease
Dermal larva migrans	disease	Schistosome cercarial	Vesicles
Dipylidiasis	Neural larva	dermatitis	Visceral larva migrans
Dwarf tapeworm	migrans	Sparganum	(VLM)
	Neurocysticercosis		Zoonosis

Chapter 1 defines zoonosis as any disease or parasite that is transmissible from animals to humans. In veterinary clinical practice it is important for veterinarians to inform their clients concerning zoonotic diseases or parasites that may be transmitted from their domestic animals. Such zoonotic parasites include *Toxoplasma gondii, Trichinella spiralis, Ancylostoma caninum,* and *Toxocara canis.* This chapter discusses the major parasitic diseases that are of public health importance in veterinary clinical practice.

It is often the veterinarian's role (and also the role of the veterinary diagnostician) to diagnose a parasite in a domestic animal. The veterinary diagnostician must also communicate to the public and often to medical personnel, such as physicians, laboratory personnel, and other public health workers, the significance of many of the zoonotic parasites. It is important for veterinary personnel to understand that in suspected cases of zoonotic parasites or conditions, the client should *always* be referred to a physician, family practitioner, obstetrician, or public health worker as appropriate for diagnosis or treatment. In no instance should a veterinarian or veterinary technician attempt to diagnose or treat any of these zoonotic parasites in humans. The veterinarian's role is to inform, not to

treat. Attempting to diagnose or treat a human is a violation of state veterinary practice acts across the United States. Treatments are included in this chapter for veterinarians strictly for the purpose of advising human health care workers and not for the purpose of treating human patients.

> *TECHNICIAN'S NOTE* It is the role of the veterinarian or technician to educate the client or owner about zoonotic parasites and diseases, *not* to treat the client or owner for zoonoses.

For each zoonotic parasite discussed here the following areas are addressed:
- Symptoms of parasitic infection in humans and the ways in which infection is diagnosed.
- Treatment of the parasitic condition in humans.
- Prevention of the transmission of zoonotic parasites, conditions, or syndromes from animals to humans.

Just as parasites are broken down into major groups in previous chapters, the important zoonotic parasites are divided into zoonotic protozoans, zoonotic trematodes, zoonotic cestodes, zoonotic nematodes, zoonotic arthropods, and zoonotic pentastomes. The acanthocephalans and the leeches have no zoonotic significance.

PROTOZOANS OF PUBLIC HEALTH IMPORTANCE

TOXOPLASMA GONDII (TOXOPLASMOSIS)

Toxoplasmosis in humans is an extremely rare protozoan disease with which humans (particularly a pregnant woman and her developing fetus) can become infected. It is an important zoonotic parasite because a very popular domestic pet, the cat, is the only definitive host for this parasite. The cat can serve as a source of infection for the pregnant woman and her unborn child. Toxoplasmosis can infect the fetus in the womb and produce serious birth defects. This parasite can also wreak havoc in individuals with acquired immunodeficiency syndrome (AIDS).

> **TECHNICIAN'S NOTE** The cat is the only definitive host for *Toxoplasma gondii* and can serve as a source of infection in humans, especially pregnant women and their unborn children.

Although this is a very rare parasite, several precautions must be taken to prevent infection. To sell papers the "sensational press" often exploits this parasite in its headlines, alarming the general public. As a result the veterinary clinical practice may receive phone calls regarding this parasite. Also, uninformed clients may request that veterinarians find a new home for (or even euthanize) the family cat. It is important for the veterinarian to alleviate the client's concerns and to work in conjunction with the obstetrician-gynecologist to answer questions, thwart this parasite, and prevent toxoplasmosis. It is important to note that almost every warm-blooded animal can become infected with *T. gondii*.

> **TECHNICIAN'S NOTE** The news media exploits toxoplasmosis to sell papers; it is the job of the veterinary professional in conjunction with physicians to prevent and thwart this disease with proper client education.

Human Infection With Toxoplasmosis

Humans become infected with toxoplasmosis in one of two ways: congenitally (in the case of unborn babies) or through acquisition. Congenital toxoplasmosis occurs when a woman becomes infected during her pregnancy; the woman ingests sporulated oocysts of *T. gondii* found in the feces of the cat. The domestic house cat with access to the outdoors (and predation) serves as the definitive host for *T. gondii* and will shed unsporulated oocysts in its feces. These unsporulated oocysts sporulate (or become infective) in 1 to 5 days. If a pregnant woman accidentally ingests the sporulated oocyst, the parasite's tachyzoites (rapidly multiplying stages) can infect the developing fetus.

Acquired toxoplasmosis occurs when a human ingests the sporulated oocyst containing tachyzoites or ingests infected meat or tissue stages containing bradyzoites. Many domesticated animals (e.g., cattle, pigs, sheep) serve as intermediate hosts for *T. gondii*. Within their muscle, these intermediate hosts harbor bradyzoites (slowly multiplying stages) that can infect various tissue sites, including the lymph nodes, meninges, eyes, and heart, of humans. The infected human ingests the bradyzoites, which then infect a variety of tissue sites.

> **TECHNICIAN'S NOTE** Unborn babies can be infected with toxoplasmosis if their mothers become infected by ingesting tachyzoites and the infection spreads to the fetus (congenital toxoplasmosis). Acquired toxoplasmosis occurs when humans ingest tachyzoites (in cat feces) or bradyzoites (in meat or muscle).

Symptoms and Diagnosis

If congenital infection occurs early in the pregnancy, abortion is common. If this infection occurs late in the pregnancy, the central nervous system (CNS) may become infected and a variety of neurologic abnormalities may result. These include cerebral calcification, chorioretinitis, hydrocephaly, microcephaly, and psychomotor irregularities. The child may be born dead or alive. If alive, the child may be mentally retarded.

Infected humans with acquired toxoplasmosis exhibit lymphadenopathy, malaise, fever, lymphocytosis, and myocarditis. Most cases, however, are characterized by mild fever and slight enlargement of the lymph nodes.

Diagnosis of clinical toxoplasmosis in humans is quite difficult. Diagnosis relies on the demonstration of organisms or antibodies against it. The best diagnostic test is the inoculation of suspected material into mice and demonstration of the organism multiplying in the mice. Serologic tests are also available. The veterinary diagnostician must remember that these tests need to be delegated to a more sophisticated diagnostic laboratory.

> **TECHNICIAN'S NOTE** The diagnosis of toxoplasmosis in humans is difficult and involves testing for the presence of multiplying organisms or antibodies against the organisms in inoculated mice. Serologic tests are also used.

Treatment

There is no completely satisfactory treatment for toxoplasmosis in humans, although pyrimethamine has been found effective. This drug in conjunction with triple sulfa drugs has shown good results in ocular toxoplasmosis. Remember that suspected cases of toxoplasmosis in humans should *always* be referred to a neonatologist, pediatrician, gynecologist, obstetrician, or family practitioner. The Centers for Disease Control and Prevention (CDC) has many specialists who are qualified to answer questions about the most complex issues of toxoplasmosis in humans.

Prevention of Transmission to Humans

Transmission of *T. gondii* to pregnant women is prevented by having someone else empty the cat's litter box for the duration of her pregnancy. This step eliminates the woman's potential exposure to the sporulated oocysts of *T. gondii*. A person should always wash his or her hands after handling a cat and before eating. Litter boxes should never be placed in the kitchen or dining area. Gloves should be worn while gardening because feral cats often defecate in flower beds. If a child's sandbox is present in the backyard, it should remain covered

when not in use. After gardening, hands should be thoroughly washed. Cats should never be allowed to roam freely and hunt. Likewise, uncooked meat should never be fed to cats. Rodent prey or uncooked meat may contain the tissue stages of *T. gondii,* which will set the life cycle in motion in the cat. Likewise, to avoid acquired infection with *T. gondii* (and a variety of pathogenic bacteria), humans should be wary of undercooked infected meat.

> **TECHNICIAN'S NOTE** Prevention of toxoplasmosis involves reducing exposure in pregnant women by having someone else clean the litter box, washing hands after cleaning the litter box or handling raw meat, covering sandboxes, wearing gloves when gardening, and not eating undercooked meat.

CRYPTOSPORIDIUM PARVUM (CRYPTOSPORIDIOSIS)

Cryptosporidiosis is a rare protozoan disease that produces a prolific, painful, watery diarrhea in humans. This protozoan parasite has been reported in the news because it has contaminated the drinking water supplies of several major metropolitan areas throughout North America and the world. As with toxoplasmosis, cryptosporidiosis is especially harmful in individuals with AIDS. For this reason, it is also an important parasite. Cryptosporidiosis was first reported in farmworkers and individuals who worked around very young calves. This organism is spread by ingestion of infective oocysts in calf feces.

Human Infection With Cryptosporidiosis

Humans become infected with cryptosporidiosis by ingestion of oocysts from feces of young calves or from contaminated supplies of drinking water.

Symptoms and Diagnosis

Cryptosporidiosis produces a transient, painful, watery diarrhea in humans, and all ages are susceptible. The duration of clinical signs in affected individuals varies considerably. Acute cases last from 3 to 7 days, and chronic wasting syndromes can persist for weeks to a few months. The development of natural immunity against the parasite determines the duration of the clinical signs. Most humans infected with *Cryptosporidium* species develop immunity and recover from the infection.

Infections with *Cryptosporidium* species may persist indefinitely in people with immunodeficiencies, particularly AIDS. The prognosis for immunologically compromised individuals with cryptosporidiosis is poor.

Fecal flotation and concentrating solutions such as zinc sulfate and Sheather sugar solution may be used to identify oocysts of *Cryptosporidium* species. These parasites are extremely tiny, less than 5 μm in diameter, and thus may be easily overlooked. Acid-fast stains such as Ziehl-Neelsen or Kinyoun can be used, as well as auramine-rhodamine, Giemsa, and methylene blue. All these stains may be used to improve the identification of the parasite in fecal flotation.

> **TECHNICIAN'S NOTE** Cryptosporidiosis is diagnosed in humans with fecal flotation techniques using zinc sulfate or Sheather solution to identify oocysts.

There are several commercially available enzyme-linked immunosorbent assay (ELISA) tests. These tests have a higher degree of sensitivity and specificity in diagnosing infections with *Cryptosporidium* species than can be obtained from stained fecal flotation smears. A commercially available indirect fluorescent antibody test has been shown to be quite effective in diagnosing infection with *Cryptosporidium* species.

Treatment

Although cryptosporidiosis is caused by a protozoan parasite with a life cycle similar to that of coccidia, coccidiostats have shown minimal to no efficacy when used to treat infected cattle. An effective chemotherapeutic means of eliminating the parasite is not available.

Human cryptosporidiosis is treated symptomatically. Individuals who become dehydrated should be given appropriate fluids either intravenously or orally. Clinical improvement has been demonstrated in patients treated with dialyzable leukocyte extract from calves immunized with *Cryptosporidium* species.

> **TECHNICIAN'S NOTE** Cryptosporidiosis in humans is treated symptomatically.

Prevention of Transmission to Humans

Infection with *Cryptosporidium* species can be prevented by good sanitation and hygiene practices when handling young animals, particularly calves. Infants, young children, or immunologically compromised individuals should not handle animals with diarrhea. Immunocompromised individuals should be advised to wash their hands after handling pets, especially before eating, and should avoid contact with their pet's feces. Many of the agents and processes used to sanitize public drinking water have little effect on *Cryptosporidium* species.

> **TECHNICIAN'S NOTE** Prevention of cryptosporidiosis is best accomplished with good hygiene habits and sanitation.

TREMATODES OF PUBLIC HEALTH IMPORTANCE

SCHISTOSOMES OF WILD MIGRATORY BIRDS (SCHISTOSOME CERCARIAL DERMATITIS, SWIMMER'S ITCH)

Swimmer's itch is a highly pruritic skin condition in humans caused by repeated penetration of the cercariae of the schistosomes (blood flukes) of wild migratory aquatic birds and small mammals native to the water's edge. On first exposure of the cercariae, there is mild redness and edema in the skin; with repeated exposure, however, there is severe pruritus (itching) and a papular or pustular dermatitis (a pus-filled pimple). This dermatitis may persist for several days or even weeks and can become secondarily infected.

Human Infection With Swimmer's Itch

Migratory waterfowl frequently harbor schistosomes (blood flukes) in their blood vasculature. These schistosomes produce eggs that pass in the bird's feces to the watery environment. The eggs hatch, producing miracidia, which in turn penetrate aquatic snails. Within the snail the miracidia undergo asexual reproduction and produce thousands of cercariae. These cercariae exit the snail to penetrate the definitive host, the migratory waterfowl.

Humans serve as incidental hosts for these avian schistosomes. During summer people swim or wade in the lakes, ponds, rivers, and even ocean waters frequented by wild birds. These waters are home to aquatic snails. The cercariae produced within the snails penetrate the skin of humans instead of the skin of migratory birds. The cercariae cannot complete the migration in the human host, and the host's immune system kills the cercariae. At the same time the cercariae release allergenic substances that cause severe dermatitis. Repeated exposure produces the highly pruritic, papular or pustular dermatitis, or schistosome cercarial dermatitis (swimmer's itch). This condition may have many other regional or colloquial descriptive names.

> *TECHNICIAN'S NOTE* Schistosomiasis in humans tends to be self-limiting but can cause severe dermatitis when the cercariae that cause the dermatitis release allergenic substances.

Symptoms and Diagnosis

After the cercaria penetrates the skin, a reddened spot appears at the point of entry. The diameter of this spot increases, and the itching commences. If the area becomes raised, it is called a **papule** and will reach its maximum size in about 24 hours. In severe cases the affected individual may develop a fever, become nauseated, and spend several sleepless nights. The papule itches for several days before subsiding, but in a week or so the symptoms disappear.

Swimmer's itch can be diagnosed by the observation of typical lesions in skin that has come in contact with pond, lake, stream, or ocean water containing infective cercariae from the snail intermediate host. A history of swimming in infested waters also aids in diagnosis. Laboratory findings usually have no role in establishing a diagnosis of swimmer's itch.

Treatment

Suspected cases of swimmer's itch in humans should *always* be referred to a dermatologist or family practitioner. Antihistamines are prescribed to relieve the itch and topical steroid creams to reduce the swelling. Remember that these are prescription drugs and must be prescribed by a physician or dermatologist.

Prevention of Transmission to Humans

During the seasonal occurrence of swimmer's itch, many public health agencies post warnings about swimmer's itch on beaches adjacent to ponds, lakes, streams, or the ocean. The public should heed these warnings and comply with the ban on swimming in infested waters. Swimming in water away from the shore will reduce the chance of contact with the cercariae; cercariae tend to congregate close to the shoreline. If contact is suspected, the swimmer should towel off immediately after leaving the water.

For those who must work in such waters, protective waterproof clothing is available. Repellents such as benzyl benzoate and dibutylphthalate are available. Molluscicides (snail-killing compounds) are available; however, they may have adverse effects on plants and other animals in the environment.

> *TECHNICIAN'S NOTE* The best prevention for swimmer's itch is to avoid water contaminated with schistosomes.

CESTODES OF PUBLIC HEALTH IMPORTANCE

TAENIA SAGINATA (BEEF TAPEWORM)

Taenia saginata, the beef tapeworm, parasitizes the small intestine of humans. Its larval or metacestode stage, *Cysticercus bovis,* is found in the musculature of beef cattle, the intermediate host.

Human Infection With Beef Tapeworm

Humans become infected with the beef tapeworm by ingesting the musculature of beef cattle that contains the cysticercus, or bladder worm, the larval (metacestode) stage for this tapeworm. This cysticercus stage has a scientific name, *C. bovis,* and may be found in a variety of sites in the bovine musculature: skeletal and heart muscle, masseters, diaphragm, and tongue. Humans are infected by ingesting raw or undercooked cysticercus-infected beef. This meat is often referred to as measly beef or beef measles. The covering of the cysticercus is digested away, and the young tapeworm is released and attaches to the wall of the small intestine. This young tapeworm begins to grow its proglottids. The gravid proglottids are released to the outside environment. Each gravid proglottid contains about 80,000 eggs. In the outside environment the gravid proglottids rupture, and the released eggs may be ingested by a beef cow. The eggs hatch, and the embryos penetrate the intestinal mucosa and enter into the general circulation; they are then distributed throughout the musculature of the beef cow.

TECHNICIAN'S NOTE Humans become infected with *Taenia saginata* by ingesting undercooked beef muscle that contains the cysticercus stage of the tapeworm.

Symptoms and Diagnosis

Adult *T. saginata* in the small intestine of humans may cause a variety of nonspecific abdominal signs such as diarrhea, constipation, and cramps. About 10 gravid proglottids are passed in the feces each day; this fact is quite evident to the infected individual. These proglottids are quite motile and will migrate a few centimeters over the human host's body, clothes, or bedding.

The gravid proglottids from human feces are unusual in appearance. Each proglottid has a prominent uterus with 14 to 32 lateral branches. The uterus contains approximately 80,000 eggs. Perianal swabs may be used to detect these eggs. Diagnosis of cysticerci in cattle is usually made by meat inspection procedures.

TECHNICIAN'S NOTE A human infection with *Taenia saginata* will be very evident when the gravid proglottids are seen in the stool specimen upon defecation.

Treatment

Suspected cases of the beef tapeworm in humans should *always* be referred to a family practitioner or internist. The treatment of choice is praziquantel or niclosamide.

Prevention of Transmission to Humans

All infected humans should be treated by a physician. Feedlot employees should be educated concerning transmission of bovine cysticercosis and personal hygiene practices. Adequate and accessible toilet facilities must be provided for all workers. Meat inspection should be thorough. Infected carcasses may be condemned for human consumption or treated by freezing for 10 days to 2 weeks at $-10°C$ or by cooking at $50°C$ to $60°C$. Likewise, humans should be wary of undercooked meat to avoid acquired infection with *T. saginata* (and a variety of pathogenic bacteria).

TECHNICIAN'S NOTE Proper sanitation, personal hygiene, and thorough meat inspection help prevent infection with the beef tapeworm.

TAENIA SOLIUM (PORK TAPEWORM)

Taenia solium, the pork tapeworm, parasitizes the small intestine of humans. The larval, or metacestode, stage of this tapeworm, *Cysticercus cellulosae,* is found in the musculature of pigs, the intermediate host. This is an unusual parasite in that humans can also harbor the larval stage, which may occur not only in the musculature but also within the eye and brain. Therefore humans can serve as both the definitive and the intermediate host for this parasite.

Human Infection With Pork Tapeworm

Humans become infected with the pork tapeworm by ingesting the musculature of pigs that contains the cysticercus, or bladder worm, the larval (metacestode) stage. This cysticercus stage has a scientific name, *C. cellulosae,* and may be found in a variety of muscle sites: skeletal and heart muscle, masseters, diaphragm, and tongue. Humans are infected by ingesting raw or undercooked cysticercus-infected pork. This meat is often referred to as measly pork or pork measles. The covering of the cysticercus is digested away, and the young tapeworm is released and attaches to the wall of the small intestine. This young tapeworm begins to grow proglottids. The gravid (terminal) proglottids are released to the outside environment. Each gravid proglottid contains about 40,000 eggs. In the outside environment the gravid proglottid ruptures; the released eggs must be ingested by a pig. The eggs hatch, and the embryos penetrate the intestinal mucosa and reach the general circulation, to be distributed throughout the musculature of the pig.

> **TECHNICIAN'S NOTE** Pork tapeworm can infect humans if humans ingest undercooked pork meat that contains the cysticercus stage of the tapeworm.

If a human ingests one of the eggs, the egg hatches in the intestine. This embryo penetrates the intestinal mucosa and reaches the general circulation, to be distributed not only throughout the musculature of the human but also in subcutaneous sites and within the brain and eye. In such sites, tremendous damage can result.

When the metacestode stage develops in the brain, the condition is known as neurocysticercosis. The parasite usually develops in the ventricles and is proliferative.

> **TECHNICIAN'S NOTE** If humans ingest pork tapeworm eggs, the eggs can hatch in the intestine and the resulting embryo can reach the general circulation, ending up in the brain, eye, and subcutaneous sites, as well as the musculature.

Symptoms and Diagnosis

Adult *T. solium* in the small intestine of humans may cause a variety of nonspecific abdominal signs such as diarrhea, constipation, and cramps. Chains

of gravid proglottids do not leave the host spontaneously but are passed in the feces each day; this fact is quite evident to the infected individual. These proglottids are quite motile and will migrate a few centimeters over the human host's body, clothes, or bedding.

Neurologic symptoms vary with the site of the offending cysticercus in the nervous tissue. Pain, paralysis, and epileptic seizures have been associated with neurocysticercosis. Ocular lesions may result in blindness.

The gravid proglottids from human feces are unusual in appearance. Each proglottid has a prominent uterus with fewer than 16 lateral branches. The uterus contains approximately 40,000 eggs. Diagnosis of cysticerci in pigs is usually made by meat inspection procedures.

Sophisticated radiographic imaging techniques such as computed tomography (CT) and magnetic resonance imaging (MRI) may reveal the presence of cysticerci within the brain and other sites in the CNS.

> **TECHNICIAN'S NOTE** The symptoms of pork tapeworm infection in humans vary by where the cysticercus ends up in the human (in the case of ingestion of the eggs). Intestinal infection can produce nonspecific abdominal symptoms such as diarrhea, cramps, and constipation.

Treatment

Suspected cases of pork tapeworm in humans should *always* be referred to a family practitioner, neurologist, surgeon, or internist. The treatment of choice is praziquantel. Because of the infectivity of the eggs for humans and the resulting CNS involvement, these cases must be handled with great care. Treatment of human cysticercosis is by surgical removal of the offending lesion.

Prevention of Transmission to Humans

All infected humans should be treated by a physician. Feedlot employees should be educated concerning transmission of porcine cysticercosis and personal hygiene practices. Household workers such as maids and cooks should be educated regarding proper hygiene, such as handwashing before preparation of a meal. Adequate and convenient toilet facilities must be provided for all workers. Meat inspection should be thorough. Infected carcasses may be condemned for human consumption or treated by freezing for 10 days to 2 weeks at −10°C or by cooking at 50°C to 60°C. Likewise, humans should be wary of under-cooked meat to avoid acquired infection with *T. solium* (and a variety of pathogenic bacteria).

> **TECHNICIAN'S NOTE** Pork tapeworm infec-tion can be prevented by proper sanitation, per-sonal hygiene, and thorough meat inspection, as well as by not eating undercooked pork.

ECHINOCOCCUS GRANULOSUS AND ECHINOCOCCUS MULTILOCULARIS (UNILOCULAR AND MULTILOCULAR HYDATID DISEASE)

Hydatid disease is a syndrome characterized by the development of the larval, or metacestode, stage of *Echinococcus* species, a genus of tapeworm found in the small intestine of dogs and cats, the definitive hosts. Hydatid disease is characterized by the forma-tion of large fluid-filled cysts in the internal organs of the intermediate host. There are two species of importance in veterinary parasitology: *Echinococcus granulosus*, a tapeworm that produces a unilocular (large, singular, thick-walled, fluid-filled) hydatid cyst, and *Echinococcus multilocularis*, a tapeworm that produces a multilocular (multiple, extremely invasive, thin-walled, fluid-filled) hydatid cyst. These hydatid cysts may occur in a variety of internal organs in the human intermediate host: the liver, lungs, kidney, spleen, bone, and brain.

> **TECHNICIAN'S NOTE** The hydatid cysts pro-duced by *Echinococcus* species can develop in a variety of organs in the human intermediate host.

Human Infection With Hydatid Disease

Humans become infected with hydatid disease by ingesting the egg of *Echinococcus* species. Once ingested, the egg hatches in the intestine of the human intermediate host. The released oncosphere ("growth ball") penetrates an intestinal venule or lymphatic lacteal and reaches the liver, lungs, or other internal organs. Once in these extraintestinal

sites, the oncosphere develops into the hydatid cyst. *E. granulosus* produces a unilocular hydatid cyst. This cyst has a thick, multilayered wall that keeps the developing cyst restricted to a single compart-ment. The hydatid cyst may grow up to 50 cm in diameter; however, it will not invade the surround-ing tissues of the parasitized organ. *E. multilocularis* produces a multilocular hydatid cyst. In contrast to the unilocular hydatid cyst of *E. granulosus*, this hydatid cyst lacks the thick, multilayered wall. Without this cyst wall, the developing cyst is capable of "budding off," or producing additional compart-ments, which in turn bud off other compartments. As a result, this type of hydatid cyst readily invades the surrounding tissues. This multilocular hydatid cyst takes on a "malignant" invasive role.

Symptoms and Diagnosis

The symptoms of infection with hydatid disease depend on the site where the organism develops; these sites include the liver, lungs, kidney, spleen, bone, and brain. Neurologic symptoms vary with the site of the offending cysticercus in the nervous tissue. Pain, paralysis, and epileptic seizures have also been associated with echinococcosis.

In humans, examination of histopathologic sec-tions of unilocular hydatid cysts reveals the unique structure of the germinal membrane supported by a thicker, acellular, laminated membrane. Protoscoli-ces are contained in the saclike brood capsules. When viewed macroscopically, these brood capsules look like sand. Humans with *E. multilocularis* develop tumorlike masses, or nodules, in their livers. When sectioned, these masses reveal the alveolar-like microvesicles containing protoscolices.

Sophisticated radiographic imaging techniques such as CT and MRI may reveal the presence of hydatid cysts within the brain and other organ sites throughout the body.

> **TECHNICIAN'S NOTE** Diagnosis of echino-coccosis in humans can be made by histopatho-logic sectioning or a CT or MRI scan.

Treatment

Suspected cases of echinococcosis in humans should always be referred to a surgeon, internist, or neurologist. Surgical intervention is recommended for the disease syndromes caused by *E. granulosus* and *E. multilocularis.* For patients in whom the hydatid cyst cannot be removed or for whom surgery is not an option, there may be new therapeutic alternatives. Treatment with mebendazole has shown varied success, although albendazole has been more promising.

State public health officials should be notified when canine or feline echinococcosis is diagnosed. Additionally, the CDC should be notified. The CDC has many specialists who are qualified to answer the most complex questions regarding both unilocular and multilocular hydatid disease in humans.

> **TECHNICIAN'S NOTE** State public health officials and the CDC should be notified if canine or feline echinococcosis is diagnosed.

Prevention of Transmission to Humans
Handwashing, particularly for children, should be emphasized. It is important to prevent exposure to the eggs of *Echinococcus* species. Dogs should never be fed raw livestock viscera or allowed to roam freely to feed on wild rodents.

DIPYLIDIUM CANINUM (HUMAN DIPYLIDIASIS)
Human Infection With *Dipylidium*
Children become infected with the common tapeworm of dogs and cats, *Dipylidium caninum,* by ingesting dog or cat fleas containing cysticercoids of this common canine and feline tapeworm.

Symptoms and Diagnosis
As in the canine or feline host, proglottids are passed in the feces or are found around the anus (if the child is an infant and is still wearing diapers). Most infections occur in children under 8 years of age. Most patients are asymptomatic, but diarrhea, abdominal pain, and anal pruritus may occur. The child may have moderate eosinophilia.

> **TECHNICIAN'S NOTE** Humans, especially children, can be infected with *Dipylidium caninum* by ingesting an infective flea.

Treatment
Suspected cases of *D. caninum* in humans should *always* be referred to a family practitioner or internist. This human disease occurs rarely; humans appear to be highly resistant to the infection given the high frequency of flea infestation on dogs and cats. Suspected cases of dipylidiasis in children should always be referred to a pediatrician or general practitioner. The drugs of choice for human dipylidiasis are praziquantel and niclosamide. For treating *D. caninum* the adult dose of praziquantel is 10 to 20 mg/kg given once; the pediatric dose is the same. The adult dose of niclosamide is 2 g given once. For children weighing 11 to 34 kg, the dose is 1 g given once; for children weighing more than 34 kg, the one-time dose is 1.5 g. Because the method of transmission is by ingestion of dog or cat fleas containing the infected cysticercoids, the child probably is the only family member infected with this canine parasite. It would not be necessary to treat other family members for infection with this canine and feline cestode. All household pets should be treated with anthelmintics; a rigorous flea control program should be instituted for all dogs and cats.

Prevention of Transmission to Humans
Infection in humans or animals by *D. caninum* requires ingestion of the intermediate host, the dog or cat flea containing the larva (cysticercoid) of the tapeworm. Many cases in humans are asymptomatic. Dipylidiasis affects mainly infants and young children who may swallow a flea that hops up while they are crawling on the floor or cuddling the family pet. Again, humans appear to be highly resistant to the infection given the high frequency of flea infestation on dogs and cats and the relative rarity of human disease.

SPIROMETRA MANSONOIDES (BENIGN PLEROCERCOIDOSIS/ MALIGNANT SPARGANOSIS)
Human Infection With *Spirometra* Species
Although human infection with *Diphyllobothrium latum* is an intestinal infection, human infection with *Spirometra* species is usually associated with a

variety of extraintestinal tissue sites. Humans may become infected with the plerocercoid stage, or sparganum, of *Spirometra* species within the tissues. The human is actually serving as the second intermediate host. Infection with the plerocercoid stage of the pseudotapeworm is referred to as *sparganosis.*

There are two forms of infection with *Spirometra* species that may occur in the second intermediate host: the nonproliferative form and the proliferative form. Most infections are of the nonproliferative form (benign plerocercoidosis) and are associated with the presence of a single larva of *Spirometra mansonoides.* Proliferative sparganosis (malignant sparganosis) is caused by the presence of an asexual replication of larvae within host tissues and the subsequent migration of these larvae to new tissue sites, where they grow and repeat the process ad infinitum.

Symptoms and Diagnosis

For benign plerocercoidosis the human ultimately acts as a dead-end host. Symptoms depend on the site(s) of infection.

Proliferative sparganosis in humans may occur in sites from subcutaneous tissue sites to deep visceral forms, involving a variety of internal organs: ocular, CNS, auricular, pulmonary, intraosseous, and intraperitoneal sites. Again, symptoms depend on the severity and site of infection. Once infected with the malignant form, the human may ultimately die. Infections of both benign plerocercoidosis and proliferative sparganosis have been reported primarily in Asia and South America; however, two cases were reported in the United States in the early twentieth century.

Treatment

It would be prudent for a physician to report any occurrence of human sparganosis, especially the malignant form, to the CDC in Atlanta, Georgia.

Depending on the tissue sites where benign plerocercoidosis is occurring in the infected human, surgical intervention may be possible.

In humans infected with proliferative sparganosis, treatment with praziquantel and mebendazole has proven ineffective. Adverse side effects to these anthelmintics include severe nausea, vomiting,

gastritis, sinus tachycardia, muscle tenderness, and a burning sensation at the injection site. Nitazoxanide is an antiprotozoal drug approved for use in humans that has been shown in preclinical trials to be effective against cestodes.

Prevention of Transmission to Humans

Because sparganosis is zoonotic, precautions must be undertaken to prevent infection through consumption of infected water containing the first intermediate host: a *Cyclops* species, an aquatic crustacean containing the procercoid stage. Humans may also become infected by ingesting poorly cooked fish containing the plerocercoid (sparganum) stage. Finally, humans may become infected during the application of medicinal poultices to open wounds; such poultices could contain the plerocercoid stage, which could infiltrate and ultimately infect the open wound.

Although this parasite is not a reportable parasite, it would be wise to report the occurrence of human sparganosis to local public health authorities owing to the severity of infection, particularly with malignant sparganosis, which may develop in humans.

HYMENOLEPIS NANA (HYMENOLEPIASIS)

Human Infection With *Hymenolepis*

Hymenolepis nana, the dwarf tapeworm, is usually found in rodents, primates, and humans. It is common in children under 3 years of age throughout the world and can be passed from human to human. The tapeworms are usually regarded as hand-to-mouth parasites. *Hymenolepis diminuta*, the rat tapeworm, is primarily a parasite of rodents and humans. Children become infected with *Hymenolepis* species by ingesting insects (e.g., rat fleas, mealworms, cockroaches) containing cysticercoids of these tapeworms.

TECHNICIAN'S NOTE The dwarf tapeworm and rat tapeworm are regarded as hand-to-mouth parasites.

Symptoms and Diagnosis

Large numbers of tapeworms can cause necrosis and desquamation of the intestinal epithelial cells.

Light infections cause no significant damage to the mucosa and are either asymptomatic or cause vague abdominal complaints. Young children frequently have loose bowel movements or frank diarrhea with mucus. Bloody diarrhea is rare; diffuse, persistent abdominal pain is the more common complaint. A pruritic anus is another common complaint among infected individuals. Many children also have headaches, dizziness, and sleep and behavioral disturbances, which resolve after therapy. Serious neurologic disturbances have been reported. A moderate eosinophilia (5%-10%) may be associated with hymenolepiasis.

Diagnosis is by finding the characteristic eggs in fecal flotation. Proglottids are usually not found because they degenerate before passage in the stool.

Treatment

In suspected cases of *H. diminuta,* humans should *always* be referred to a family practitioner or internist. Praziquantel is the drug of choice. For treating *H. diminuta* the dose of praziquantel (for both adults and children) is 25 mg/kg given once.

Prevention of Transmission to Humans

Control depends on improved personal and environmental hygiene. Within institutions, all children should be treated.

> *TECHNICIAN'S NOTE* Prevention of the dwarf and rat tapeworm depends on improved personal and environmental hygiene.

DIPHYLLOBOTHRIUM LATUM (DIPHYLLOBOTHRIASIS)

Human Infection With *Diphyllobothrium*

The broad fish tapeworm, or *D. latum,* is often found in many areas of the world where raw, insufficiently cooked, or lightly pickled freshwater fish are consumed. Infected fish contain the plerocercoid, or sparganum, stage; this is the stage eaten by the human. These parasites are often found in northern temperate and subarctic regions. The adult tapeworms are found within the small intestine of the host; humans may also become infected

with the plerocercoid (sparganum) stage. When a homeopathic doctor uses an infected piece of fish as a poultice, the sparganum moves into the wound and sets up an infection in the subcutis, the connective tissue of the muscles, or in other sites within the body.

Symptoms and Diagnosis

Intestinal infections in humans are often asymptomatic. Often the diagnosis is made during routine fecal examination when eggs or chains of proglottids are observed in the feces. Infection in humans may also cause nonspecific abdominal symptoms. Some individuals may complain of abdominal pain, bloating, allergic reactions, hunger pains, loss of appetite, or increased appetite. On rare occasions, mechanical intestinal obstruction may result from tapeworms becoming entangled; intussusception may result. Diarrhea may occur, and infected individuals may pass long sections of spent proglottids in the stool.

> *TECHNICIAN'S NOTE* Intestinal infections in humans with the broad fish tapeworm are often asymptomatic or exhibit nonspecific abdominal symptoms.

Adult tapeworms in the small intestine may successfully absorb vitamin B_{12} from the gut; this loss of vitamin B_{12} produces megaloblastic anemia or pernicious anemia. This condition manifests itself as a macrocytic, hypochromic anemia.

Infection with the sparganum, or sparganosis, produces a severe inflammatory reaction and fibrosis of the infected tissues. Clinical signs include urticaria, painful edema, and irregular nodules containing the plerocercoids. If spargana infect the eye, the infection may lead to exophthalmos, swelling of the eyelids, lagophthalmos, and corneal ulcers.

Treatment

Suspected cases of the intestinal form of the broad fish tapeworm in humans should *always* be referred to a family practitioner or internist. Praziquantel and niclosamide are the drugs of choice. For treating *D. latum* the adult dose of praziquantel is 10 to

20 mg/kg given once; the pediatric dose is the same. The adult dose of niclosamide is 2 g given once. For children weighing 11 to 34 kg, the dose is 1 g given once; for children weighing more than 34 kg, the one-time dose is 1.5 g.

Suspected cases of the sparganum (plerocercoid) form of the broad fish tapeworm in humans should *always* be referred to a surgeon. Spargana within tissue sites in humans must be surgically removed.

> **TECHNICIAN'S NOTE** As with all human zoonotic parasite infections, a physician should be seen for treatment. The broad fish tapeworm can be treated with praziquantel or niclosamide; however, sparganum infection should be referred to a surgeon.

Prevention of Transmission to Humans

Proper cooking of freshwater fish eliminates all possibility of human infection. Likewise, domestic animals such as dogs, cats, and pigs should not be fed raw fish. Freezing at $-10°C$ will kill the infective plerocercoid (sparganum) stage. In the United States smoked salmon is brined before hot smoking; this process eliminates salmon as a source of infection. Food handlers should never taste raw fish while preparing it for cooking. Practitioners of natural medicine should be discouraged from applying poultices made of fish to openings in the skin or to the eye.

NEMATODES OF PUBLIC HEALTH IMPORTANCE

TOXOCARA CANIS AND TOXOCARA CATI (TOXOCARAL LARVA MIGRANS, VISCERAL LARVA MIGRANS, OCULAR LARVA MIGRANS)

Toxocaral larva migrans is a disease of humans caused by the migration of certain parasitic larvae in the organs and tissues. The most incriminated nematodes are the common ascarids of dogs and cats, *T. canis* and *Toxocara cati*, respectively. *Baylisascaris procyonis,* an ascarid of raccoons, causes a similar syndrome.

Human Infection With Toxocaral Larva Migrans

Humans become infected with toxocaral larva migrans when they ingest eggs of *Toxocara* species from the soil or on contaminated hands or other objects. *Toxocara* species require 2 or more weeks before infective larvae develop within the eggs. Persons should also take precautions when handling young puppies still being nursed by their dams. The entire litter area (and their hair coats) may often become extremely contaminated with their aged feces, which may contain infective eggs.

> **TECHNICIAN'S NOTE** Humans become infected with toxocaral larva migrans by ingesting eggs of *Toxocara* species of canine and feline roundworms.

Symptoms and Diagnosis

Infection by a few larvae is usually asymptomatic. Two distinct syndromes are produced by *Toxocara* species: visceral larva migrans (VLM) and ocular larva migrans (OLM). VLM results from the migration of larvae though the human's somatic tissues and organs, including the liver, lungs, heart, and brain. The human is actually serving as a paratenic host for *Toxocara* species. VLM is characterized by fever, leukocytosis, persistent eosinophilia, hypergammaglobulinemia, and hepatomegaly. Pulmonary involvement, with symptoms that include bronchiolitis, asthma, or pneumonitis, may be common. Fatalities may result when the myocardium or CNS becomes involved.

OLM results when larval *Toxocara* species invade the eye. Ocular disease may be seen in the absence of VLM and is often seen in young children. Faulty vision may result; blindness may also occur.

VLM may be diagnosed on the basis of demonstration of lesions and the larvae in biopsy material. Serum samples may be sent to the CDC for serodiagnostic confirmation of toxocariasis. With OLM, the larvae may be observed during an ophthalmic examination.

> **TECHNICIAN'S NOTE** Visceral larva migrans or ocular larva migrans can be seen in humans infected with toxocariasis.

Treatment

Suspected cases of toxocaral larva migrans in humans, particularly young children, should always be referred to a family practitioner, pediatrician, internist, or ophthalmologist. No proven treatment is available. Suggested drugs of choice include mebendazole and diethylcarbamazine. Prednisone helps to control symptoms.

Prevention of Transmission to Humans

Three major methods are used to prevent transmission of *Toxocara* species from dogs and cats to humans. First, it is important to prevent the fouling of backyards and public places, especially playgrounds, with dog and cat feces. All fecal material should be disposed of properly. Second, pet owners should be educated regarding the potential health hazards of roundworms in cats and dogs. Pet owners should be informed of the methods of transmission and of the special risks associated with puppies and their nursing mothers. After handling any young puppy, hands should be thoroughly washed in soap and warm water. Third, it is important that all cats and dogs be routinely tested for intestinal parasites such as ascarids. If infected, pets should be treated with an appropriate anthelmintic.

> **TECHNICIAN'S NOTE** Prevention of toxocariasis uses three methods: prevent fouling of the backyard and public places with dog and cat feces (use proper disposal of fecal material), client education, and routine examination of feces in dogs and cats.

BAYLISASCARIS PROCYONIS (NEURAL LARVA MIGRANS, CEREBROSPINAL NEMATODIASIS)

Neural larva migrans, a variation of VLM, is the prolonged migration and persistence of parasite larvae of *B. procyonis* (an ascarid that normally resides in the small intestine of the raccoon) in the brain and spinal cord of humans and animals. In this case the human or other animal is serving as a **paratenic host**. This syndrome is similar to that of VLM and OLM of *Toxocara* species of both dogs and cats.

Human Infection With Larvae of *Baylisascaris procyonis*

Humans become infected with the larvae of *B. procyonis* by accidentally ingesting eggs that contain its infective second-stage larvae. The eggs are ingested from the environment, from raccoon feces, or from contaminated soil, water, fomites, or hands. The source of these ascarid eggs is the raccoon, a feral animal that should *never* be maintained in any interior or exterior household environment. These eggs are extremely resistant and can remain viable in the environment for several months to years. This resistance increases the likelihood of transmission from animals to humans.

> **TECHNICIAN'S NOTE** Humans contract neural larva migrans by accidental ingestion of infective second-stage larvae from raccoon feces in the environment.

Symptoms and Diagnosis

As mentioned *B. procyonis* can produce VLM and OLM in humans, similar to that produced by *Toxocara* species of both dogs and cats. However, these larvae tend to be more pathogenic because they can migrate through the CNS. Typically, the extent of the infection depends on the number of infective larvae ingested and their locations and behavior in the body. When only a few larvae are ingested, individuals probably are asymptomatic; visceral damage is minor, and most larvae become encapsulated (walled off) in noncritical sites such as skeletal muscle or connective tissue. If larger numbers of larvae are ingested, however, the host may exhibit nonspecific clinical signs or more classic signs attributable to those of classic VLM: fever, leukocytosis, persistent eosinophilia, hepatomegaly, and pneumonitis. These larvae also have an affinity for migration in neurologic tissues, and depending on the location and extent of migration, neurologic signs vary. If enough larvae are ingested, progressive CNS disease can develop rapidly, producing signs such as sudden lethargy, loss of muscle coordination, decreased head control, torticollis, ataxia, and nystagmus. These signs progress to stupor, extensor rigidity or hypotonia, coma, and finally death. Clinical signs of OLM include unilateral loss of vision and photophobia.

Because neither eggs nor larvae of *B. procyonis* are found on fecal flotation or in blood samples from humans, diagnosis of *B. procyonis* in humans must be made on the basis of history, clinical findings, and serologic testing. A history of exposure to raccoons or their feces is important. Clinical findings of VLM include leukocytosis, persistent eosinophilia, hypergammaglobulinemia, hepatomegaly, and pneumonitis. CNS disease may present suddenly and develop progressively. Eosinophilia may be present in both the peripheral blood and the cerebrospinal fluid. OLM may be diagnosed by ophthalmologic examination that reveals inflammatory tracks in the retina and inflammation of the vitreum and choroid. A specific diagnosis may be made by identification of characteristic morphologic features of larval *B. procyonis* in histopathologic section. Serologic tests, such as indirect immunofluorescence, protein immunoblotting, and ELISA, are being evaluated.

> **TECHNICIAN'S NOTE** Diagnosis of neural larva migrans in humans is based on history, clinical findings, and serologic tests.

Treatment

Any person who has contact with raccoons or raccoon feces and develops visual or CNS disturbances should be examined by a physician, who should be alerted to the possibility of infection with *B. procyonis.* Suspected cases of cerebrospinal nematodiasis in humans should *always* be referred to a neurologist, ophthalmologist, internist, or family practitioner. It is unfortunate that effective anthelmintic treatments do not exist for VLM or OLM or for cerebrospinal nematodiasis. Patients with the ocular form of this syndrome can be treated with a laser if the larvae can be localized and visualized with the eye.

Prevention of Transmission to Humans

B. procyonis is more prevalent in raccoons from northern states than in raccoons from southern states, especially those states in the Deep South.

Nevertheless, precautions should be taken around raccoons in all areas of the United States.

First in regard to prevention, raccoons are *not* suitable pets. Wild raccoons should not be encouraged to visit or frequent urban, suburban, or rural dwellings or environments.

For those who rehabilitate raccoons and return them to nature, it is important to prevent shedding of the eggs and to limit exposure of humans and other animals to contaminated areas. Raccoons should be quarantined away from other animals in cages or enclosures that could be decontaminated if needed. All raccoons should be on a strict anthelmintic program to eliminate adult *B. procyonis* from the small intestine.

> **TECHNICIAN'S NOTE** Raccoons should never be kept as pets and should not be encouraged to visit or frequent human environments.

Access by humans, especially children, to known or potentially contaminated areas should be restricted. Raccoon feces should be removed and disposed of daily, in a manner that prevents contact with humans and animals. The feces should be destroyed. Contaminated areas, cages, or traps that have held infected raccoons should be decontaminated. Gloves and rubber boots should be worn by individuals who clean these cages, and hot, soapy water should be used. Protective coveralls should be worn, and these should be washed in near-boiling water and bleach.

ANCYLOSTOMA CANINUM, ANCYLOSTOMA BRAZILIENSE, ANCYLOSTOMA TUBAEFORME, AND *UNCINARIA STENOCEPHALA* (CUTANEOUS LARVA MIGRANS, CREEPING ERUPTION, PLUMBER'S ITCH)

Cutaneous larva migrans (CLM) is a skin condition caused by the migration of hookworm larvae in the skin of humans (Figure 16-1). It is also known as creeping eruption, dermal larva migrans, ground itch, plumber's itch, sandworms, and many other regional or colloquial

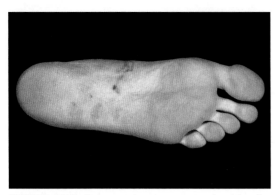

FIGURE 16-1 Cutaneous larva migrans in the sole of a man's foot. This skin condition is caused by migration of hookworm larvae in the skin of humans. It is also known as *creeping eruption, dermal larva migrans, ground itch, plumber's itch,* and *sandworms.*

names. It is a serpentine, reddened, elevated pruritic skin lesion usually caused by the larvae of *Ancylostoma braziliense,* a hookworm of both dogs and cats. Other nematode parasites of domestic and wild animals have been implicated in causing similar lesions in humans. These nematodes include *A. caninum,* the canine hookworm; *Uncinaria stenocephala,* the northern hookworm of dogs; *Bunostomum phlebotomum,* the cattle hookworm; *Gnathostoma spinigerum* (a genus of nematode); *Dirofilaria* species (such as aberrant *Dirofilaria immitis,* the heartworm); *Strongyloides procyonis,* a parasite of raccoons; and *Strongyloides westeri,* an equine parasite. Even the larvae of some of the myiasis-inducing flies (*Gasterophilus* and *Hypoderma* spp.) have been associated with the condition. However, hookworm larvae (*Ancylostoma* spp., particularly *A. braziliense*) are the pathogens most often incriminated.

> *TECHNICIAN'S NOTE*   Cutaneous larva migrans is caused by skin penetration of larvae of *Ancylostoma* species and *Uncinaria stenocephala.*

Human Infection With Cutaneous Larva Migrans

Humans become infected with larvae of canine and feline hookworms when these larvae penetrate unprotected skin. This usually happens when human skin (usually of the bare feet) contacts moist, sandy

soil contaminated with larval hookworms. Larval hookworms penetrate and migrate within the skin; in most cases they do not complete their life cycle or mature to adults in the small intestine.

Three scenarios have been developed regarding cutaneous hookworm infections in humans. The first scenario involves young children and adults who go barefoot in areas frequented by hookworm-infected pets. Children may also become exposed to contaminated sand or soil for extended periods (e.g., by playing in sandboxes or dirt containing larvae).

> *TECHNICIAN'S NOTE*   No matter which scenario of contact is involved, cutaneous larva migrans results from the hookworm larvae penetrating the skin of the affected individual.

The second scenario involves travelers returning from exotic vacation sites around the world who may have walked barefoot or been nude in the sand for an extended time. Third-stage hookworm larvae developing from eggs passed from parasitized dogs and cats can penetrate the naked skin and cause CLM. This dermatitis usually occurs in individuals who frequent beaches; therefore the persons infected are said to be parasitized with sandworms.

The third scenario concerns plumbers, electricians, masons, and technicians working in the crawl space beneath houses and horticulturists tending flower beds and vegetable gardens. If hookworm-infected dogs or cats have been allowed access to these moist sites and have defecated there, infective larvae may penetrate the laborer's skin. These workers are most often infected on their knees, elbows, buttocks, and shoulders. CLM acquired in this manner is also known as *plumber's itch.*

Symptoms and Diagnosis

The skin-penetrating larval hookworms migrate in the dermis of humans and cause distinct symptoms. The human is an abnormal, or incidental, host. The severity of skin lesions is directly related to the degree of exposure to infective larvae. Symptoms are characterized by red, tunnel-like migration tracks with severe pruritus; therefore the common name for the condition is *creeping eruption.* After skin penetration, the larvae reside in the superficial layers of the skin, actively producing and secreting hyaluronidase, an enzyme that aids their tunneling activity. Hookworm dermatitis is characterized by blisters, red bumps, and red tracts within a few days of initial penetration. The reddened site is usually 3 to 4 cm away from the penetration site, with the larva itself 1 to 2 cm ahead of the lesion. Within weeks to months after the initial infection the larva dies and is resorbed by the host.

The skin condition is diagnosed by the observation of typical lesions in skin that has come in contact with moist soil containing infective hookworm larvae. A history of contact with the soil also aids in diagnosis. Laboratory findings usually have no role in the establishment of a diagnosis of CLM.

> **TECHNICIAN'S NOTE** Cutaneous larva migrans is a self-limiting disease because the larvae cannot survive in the human incidental host for more than a few weeks to months.

Treatment

Suspected cases of CLM in humans should *always* be referred to a dermatologist or family practitioner. Patients often receive both oral and topical treatment with thiabendazole. Pruritus often ceases rapidly for all patients after treatment with this anthelmintic. Surgical treatment to extract migrating larvae is often unsuccessful. Because the larva is situated 1 to 2 cm ahead of the visible track, it cannot be localized and removed surgically. The application of liquid nitrogen has been advocated; however, the larvae may continue to migrate. Hookworm larvae are capable of surviving temperatures as low as −21° C for more than 5 minutes.

> **TECHNICIAN'S NOTE** Cutaneous larva migrans has been successfully treated with topical and oral thiabendazole.

Prevention of Transmission to Humans

Pets should be routinely examined for the presence of parasites and treated appropriately with anthelmintics. Pet owners should not allow their pet's feces to accumulate in the lawn or garden environment. Children's sandboxes should remain covered when not in use.

The seaside resort, with its moist, sandy environment, is an excellent locale for propagating larval hookworms. Pet owners should not allow dogs or cats infected with intestinal parasites to frequent beaches either at home or abroad. Infected pets residing in seaside communities are most likely to transmit CLM to humans. Seaside communities should also have leash laws, and well-trained animal control officers should regularly patrol beaches and remove free-roaming dogs and cats.

If an infected pet on a leash defecates in a public area, the feces should be promptly removed from the area, preferably by use of a disposable plastic bag. Burial of feces on the beach is not sufficient because tides and shifting sands are capable of exposing feces at a later time.

Travelers to exotic (or even local) beaches without enforced leash laws are at increased risk of contracting infective hookworm larvae if sandals or appropriate attire are not worn. Likewise, a person should never sit directly in the sand on beaches where infected animals have been allowed to roam and defecate freely.

> **TECHNICIAN'S NOTE** Prevention of cutaneous larva migrans can be accomplished by cleaning the yard of feces on a daily basis before infective larvae are hatched, covering sandboxes when not in use, not allowing infected cats or dogs to walk on beaches, and wearing footwear when traveling, especially in suspected areas of infection.

ANCYLOSTOMA CANINUM (ENTERIC HOOKWORM DISEASE)

Infective larvae of the canine and feline hookworms that penetrate the skin usually produce a cutaneous manifestation. Recently *A. caninum* has been found to grow to the adult stage within the intestine of humans. Human enteric infections with *A. caninum* have been reported in Australia and more recently in the United States. Pulmonary involvement and corneal opacities also have been reported in humans infected with *A. caninum*, and an *Ancylostoma* larva has been recovered from the muscle fiber of a patient with CLM.

TECHNICIAN'S NOTE Although hookworms produce cutaneous larva migrans in humans, *A. caninum* has been able to grow to the adult stage in the human intestines.

Human Infection With Enteric Hookworm Disease

Humans become infected with hookworm when the larval hookworms penetrate unprotected skin. This usually happens when skin (usually of the bare feet) contacts moist, sandy soil contaminated with larval hookworms. Larval hookworms penetrate and migrate within the skin; in most cases they do not complete their life cycle or mature to adults in the small intestine. In the case of enteric hookworm disease, however, they do complete the life cycle and mature to adults in the small intestine.

Symptoms and Diagnosis

It is interesting that *A. caninum* has caused enteric infections in humans residing in developed, urban communities in northeastern Australia. Although the infections may be subclinical, the chief symptom is abdominal pain, which is frequently severe with sudden onset. After biopsy the chief pathologic finding is focal or diffuse eosinophilic inflammation resulting from a type 1 hypersensitivity response to secreted antigens. Additionally two cases of eosinophilic enterocolitis attributable to canine hookworms have been reported in the United States. Canine hookworms adapt poorly in the human host; the infection is scant, and the worms do not produce eggs. Therefore fecal flotation will not reveal the presence of hookworm eggs.

TECHNICIAN'S NOTE The common symptom of human hookworm infection is abdominal pain.

A. caninum also has been reported to occur sporadically in the human intestine in several locales throughout the world, such as the Philippines, South America, and Israel. In these instances *A. caninum* did not produce clinically evident disease, was not fully developed, or was not capable of producing eggs. Three cases of infection with a single adult *A. caninum* were reported in eastern Australia, with results confirmed by ELISA and Western blot testing. Not all recent cases of canine

hookworm infection in humans have been restricted to Australia, however. Cases of eosinophilic enterocolitis in two female children were reported in the United States in Louisiana.

TECHNICIAN'S NOTE Enteric hookworm infection has been reported in two female children in the United States.

Treatment

Suspected cases of enteric hookworm infection in humans should *always* be referred to a family practitioner or gastroenterologist. In the Australian study, canine hookworms were extracted using biopsy forceps during either laparotomy or colonoscopy. After removal of the worms, all patients recovered and remained well. Both patients in the United States were treated with mebendazole (100 mg twice a day for 3 days), with repeated treatment in 2 to 6 weeks.

Prevention of Transmission to Humans

Human exposure to the infective third-stage larvae of hookworms is directly related to the prevalence of the parasite in the local canine population. The same precautions as listed for CLM should be observed. Because most of the world's population shares the environment with dogs infected with *A. caninum,* hookworms could be encountered widely as a human enteric pathogen. As more physicians and human pathologists become aware of this condition, enteric infections with hookworms acquired from pets will become recognized as a major zoonosis. This zoonosis also stresses the need for awareness among public health workers, veterinarians, and pet owners.*

TECHNICIAN'S NOTE Prevention of enteric hookworm infection can be accomplished by cleaning the yard of feces on a daily basis before infective larvae are hatched, covering sandboxes when not in use, not allowing infected cats or dogs to walk on beaches, and wearing footwear when traveling, especially in suspected areas of infection.

*www.emedicine.com, www.peteducation.com, www.diagnosis-me.com

STRONGYLOIDES STERCORALIS (STRONGYLOIDIASIS)

Strongyloidiasis is a disease in humans caused by *Strongyloides stercoralis,* the threadworm. Humans can be infected with this parasitic nematode by dogs, cats, and other carnivores that have the parasite.

Human Infection With *Strongyloides stercoralis*

The female parasite lays eggs in the intestines of the host where the eggs hatch into larvae. The larvae are typically passed in the feces. The larvae develop into third-stage infective larvae, which can then penetrate the skin of a human host and migrate to the intestines. There will often be inflammation at the site of skin penetration. The larvae can migrate through the lungs on their way to the intestine. Once in the intestine, the larvae mature to an adult worm. The adult worms then produce eggs that hatch in the human intestinal tract. In immune-compromised patients, the larvae can remain in the patient, repenetrate the intestinal mucosa, and develop into adult worms (autoinfection). This autoinfection increases the number of adult worms in the intestines, thus making the disease and symptoms worse.

Symptoms and Diagnosis

The larvae can migrate through the lungs on their way to the intestines, causing respiratory symptoms such as coughing and other symptoms associated with respiratory disease. These symptoms can include mild to severe pneumonia. Once in the intestines, the larvae can cause inflammation of the intestinal mucosa and diarrhea. The diarrhea can lead to exhaustion and emaciation in the human host. The human patient can be asymptomatic, or the worms can cause a mild to severe infection, even causing death. Most fatal infections have been linked to autoinfection increasing the worm burden and causing the symptoms to become more severe.

> **TECHNICIAN'S NOTE** Symptoms of strongyloidiasis can include death to the host, most often occurring from autoinfection causing a significant increase in the worm burden on the host.

Diagnosis in humans is essentially the same as seen in animals. A direct fecal smear can be used to identify the larvae in the feces. Fecal flotation or the Baermann technique can also be used for identification of the larval stage of the parasite.

Treatment

All suspected infections of *S. stercoralis* in humans should be referred to the individual's family physician or gastroenterologist. Ivermectin at 200 mcg/kg per day given orally for 1 to 2 days has been successful in many human patients. Thiabendazole at 50 mg/kg per day given every 12 hours for 2 days has also been successful in human patients. However, thiabendazole may need to be given for 7 to 10 days with hyperinfection caused by autoinfection.

> **TECHNICIAN'S NOTE** Humans can be given ivermectin subcutaneously if oral administration does not build up enough serum levels.

Prevention of Transmission to Humans

Human exposure to the infective third-stage larvae of threadworms is directly related to the prevalence of the parasite in the local canine or feline population. The same precautions as listed for CLM should be observed. Because most of the world's population shares the environment with dogs infected with *S. stercoralis,* threadworms could be encountered widely as a human enteric pathogen. This zoonosis also stresses the need for awareness among public health workers, veterinarians, and pet owners.*

TRICHOSTRONGYLUS AXEI

(Trichostrongyliasis)

Human Infection With *Trichostrongylus axei*

The stomach worm of horses or *Trichostrongylus axei* is commonly seen in large animals around the world. According to the Centers for Disease

---

*www.emedicine.com, www.peteducation.com, www.diagnosis-me.com

Control (CDC) and Stanford University resources, trichostrongyliasis has been reported in humans. Humans in the livestock industries are more at risk than other human hosts. Livestock animals, such as horses, cows, sheep and goats, pass the eggs in the feces. The eggs hatch into the larval stage, which molts through two more larval stages to reach the infective stage. When a human ingests the infective larvae, the larvae attach to the small intestinal mucosa and mature to adults. Humans are an incidental host for *Trichostrongylus axei*.

Symptoms and Diagnosis

Human infections are diagnosed with fecal flotation techniques. Since human infections tend to be light infections, concentration techniques such as centrifugal flotation are recommended by the CDC. Since the eggs of *Trichostronglyus axei* closely resemble the eggs of *Ancylostoma caninum* and other hookworm species, care needs to be taken to positively identify the genus and species of the parasite egg.

Human infections with *Trichostrongylus axei* are often light and asymptomatic. However, heavy infections can produce anemia, anorexia, diarrhea, and abdominal pain.

Treatment

Suspected cases of human infection with *Trichostrongylus axei* **should be** referred to the family physician or internist. According to the CDC, the drugs of choice for human infection are albendazole and pyrantal pamoate. In addition, ivermectin has been used successfully.

Prevention of Transmission to Humans

Proper pasture management and good deworming programs will reduce the spread of *Trichostrongylus axei* to other animals and humans. Good hygiene practices in conjunction with the pasture management and deworming programs will further reduce risk to humans. In endemic areas, humans should refrain from eating raw vegetables.

TRICHINELLA SPIRALIS (TRICHINOSIS OR TRICHINELLOSIS)

Trichinosis (also known as trichinellosis) is a disease caused by parasitic nematodes of the genus *Trichinella*. The most common cause of clinical trichinosis in humans is *T. spiralis*, a parasite acquired from domestic pigs.

Human Infection With Trichinosis

Humans become infected with trichinosis by eating pork products containing infective larvae of *T. spiralis*. Pork products have been found to be the cause of approximately two thirds of the reported cases and disease episodes of trichinosis. These products usually are obtained through commercial outlets. Humans become infected by eating lightly processed, partially cooked, or raw pork sausage or spiced pork. Home-raised or locally purchased swine also serve as an important source for human infection. Another important source of infection in humans is the consumption of wild game, particularly bear and boar.

> **TECHNICIAN'S NOTE**   Human trichinosis infection is caused primarily by eating lightly processed, undercooked, or raw pork sausage or spiced pork.

Symptoms and Diagnosis

The severity and clinical outcome of the disease are related to the number of larvae ingested, the species of *Trichinella*, and a variety of host factors such as age, gender, ethnic group, and immune status. Most cases of trichinosis in humans are subclinical, related to the low infection level. Mild, moderate, and severe cases also occur. These clinical manifestations increase in severity and may be life threatening. The clinical manifestation can be classified into two types: early abdominal syndrome and later general trichinosis syndrome. In early abdominal syndrome, clinical signs may commence 2 to 7 days after infection and may last for many weeks. This syndrome is typified by an enteritis caused by the development and maturity of the worms parasitizing the small intestine and by the penetration of the newborn larvae into the intestinal wall. Infected humans may exhibit malaise, nausea, vomiting, anorexia, mild fever, abdominal pain, or diarrhea. Diarrhea may become persistent.

> **TECHNICIAN'S NOTE** The severity of symptoms is directly linked to the number of larvae ingested by the human host, the species of *Trichinella*, and the signalment of the host.

Later general trichinosis syndrome may appear weeks to months after the abdominal syndrome. On penetration of the intestine, the larvae migrate throughout the body via the circulatory system. Although these larvae invade various tissues, encysts are found only in striated skeletal muscle cells. Infected individuals develop an allergic vasculitis. This appears as vascular leakage and hemorrhage and may be observed as periorbital edema and fingernail-bed and conjunctival hemorrhages. Myalgia (muscle pain) and muscle weakness are common signs related to invasion of the skeletal muscle, inflammation, and related damage. In severe cases patients may also develop immune-mediated myocarditis, pneumonitis, encephalitis, and other, even more serious complications.

Human trichinosis is usually diagnosed during the muscle phase of the disease. Cases of trichinosis may be diagnosed by blood hemograms and serum chemistries. Persistent eosinophilia is a characteristic sign of trichinosis in humans. Patients may also exhibit a leukocytosis. Serum chemistries may reveal increased immunoglobulin E (IgE), creatine kinase, and lactate dehydrogenase values.

Treatment
Suspected cases of trichinosis in swine should *always* be reported by the veterinarian to both state and federal authorities. Humans infected with trichinosis should *always* be referred to a physician. The benzimidazole anthelmintics, particularly mebendazole, flubendazole, and cambendazole, are highly effective against the muscle larvae. The CDC has many specialists who are qualified to answer questions about the most complex issues regarding trichinosis in humans.

Prevention of Transmission to Humans
Trichinosis can be contracted only by eating infected meat containing live *Trichinella*. People must assume that pork and wild game may be infected

and should prepare the meat accordingly. Pork should be cooked at a uniform temperature of 140°F (60°C) throughout for at least 1 minute. Consumers at home are encouraged to cook pork at a temperature of 160°F (71°C), which ensures that all larval *Trichinella* are killed. Because microwave cooking often produces "cold spots" in meat, it is considered least effective for killing larvae. People must take care to ensure uniform heating of pork products in microwave ovens.

> **TECHNICIAN'S NOTE** Because trichinosis can be contracted only by eating infected meat, pork and wild game should be fully cooked and hands should be washed after handling raw meat.

Larval *Trichinella* also may be killed by freezing. Meat less than 15.25 cm (6 inches) thick should be frozen to 5°F (−15°C) for 20 days, −10°F (−23°C) for 10 days, and −22°F (−30°C) for 6 days. Gamma irradiation of pork by the packing industry may also safeguard consumers from infection with this parasite.

DIROFILARIA IMMITIS (PULMONARY DIROFILARIASIS)
Only *D. immitis,* the canine heartworm, causes pulmonary dirofilariasis in humans. Pulmonary dirofilariasis has been reported in more than 20 instances outside the United States and more than 90 times within the borders of the United States. Because humans are an incidental host for this parasite, most cases of pulmonary dirofilariasis result in the formation of a single, isolated nodule containing one necrotic (rotting) heartworm at its center.

> **TECHNICIAN'S NOTE** Pulmonary dirofilariasis is caused only by *Dirofilaria immitis* in humans.

Human Infection With Dirofilariasis
Mosquitoes are the intermediate host for *D. immitis,* the canine heartworm. Infected mosquitoes must readily attack both the canine definitive host and

the human incidental host. The infective third-stage larvae emerge from the proboscis of the mosquito and are contained in a small drop of the mosquito's body fluid. These moist larvae must be close to the puncture wound made by the mosquito; the larvae enter this wound. After passage through the puncture wound made by the mosquito, the larva continues to develop in the subcutaneous tissues. It begins its wandering migration. Rather than residing in the right ventricle and pulmonary arteries, the larva finds its way to the lungs. In the lungs the single larval *D. immitis* produces an infarction that results in a solitary pulmonary nodule. This infarction is caused by the occlusion (blockage) of an arteriole when a thrombus (blood clot) forms around an impacted worm. The nodule assumes a spherical shape from the secondary granuloma and the fibrotic reaction that occurs when the antigen from the degenerating worm diffuses into the surrounding pulmonary tissues. These nodules have been reported to occur in every lobe of the lung.

Symptoms and Diagnosis

Most cases of pulmonary dirofilariasis in humans are asymptomatic. Infected patients usually are found by radiographic detection of a density or an opacity in the lung field after routine radiography of the chest. The patient is scheduled for exploratory thoracic surgery, and the nodule is excised. Histopathology usually reveals the presence of a single, necrotic worm at the center of the fibrotic nodule. Special stains are available for identification of necrotic worm fragments. Tissue samples from suspected cases should be sent to a pathologist who is familiar with the appearance of these parasites in histopathologic section.

TECHNICIAN'S NOTE Radiographs of the thorax will reveal a nodule or density in the lung field. Surgical histopathology will usually reveal the presence of a single, necrotic worm at the center of the nodule.

Eosinophil counts vary considerably among humans with pulmonary dirofilariasis and consequently are of little value. Both immunoglobulin M

and immunoglobulin G ELISA for *D. immitis* antibodies have been used in studies of human populations. An ELISA has also been used to detect *D. immitis*–specific IgE in human sera.

Treatment

Suspected cases of pulmonary dirofilariasis in humans should *always* be referred to a thoracic surgeon or human histopathologist. Additionally, the CDC has many specialists who are qualified to answer questions about the most complex issues of pulmonary dirofilariasis in humans.

Prevention of Transmission to Humans

The transmission cycle of dirofilariasis can be interrupted in several different ways. Veterinarians play an important role in the prevention of dirofilariasis in humans by encouraging pet owners to provide their dogs with preventive medicine. The daily or monthly administration of larvicidal drugs is an effective means of controlling the disease in dogs and preventing "spillover" infection in humans. These drugs are safe and effective. Because the weather in many southern states in the United States is mild, preventive medication should be given throughout the year. Control of stray and feral dogs also is an important consideration in the control of dirofilariasis. These animals represent a major reservoir for this disease.

TECHNICIAN'S NOTE Human infection with canine heartworm can be prevented by the use of heartworm preventative to control the spread of the disease in dogs, mosquito-control methods, and use of mosquito repellent.

Control of mosquitoes can reduce the exposure of humans and dogs and cats to these parasites. The removal of mosquito breeding sites and proper drainage of low-lying areas can be helpful. Mosquito larvicides may be used in some cases; however, resistance to these compounds can occur, and such compounds also disrupt the normal ecologic balance in the area. Recently the biologic control of mosquitoes has been attempted in some areas, and the use of various species of fish to reduce larval populations has been successful.

A final line of defense is the prevention of mosquito bites in both humans and animals. People can prevent mosquito bites by the application of repellents and by wearing protective clothing. All effective mosquito repellents contain **DEET** (diethyltoluamide). Walking dogs in the early evening hours when mosquitoes are most abundant should be avoided to reduce exposure in both humans and animals. Mosquitoes are not attracted to light, so electrocution devices are not helpful for their control; use of these devices may actually be detrimental because they destroy insects that may feed on adult mosquitoes.

> **TECHNICIAN'S NOTE** Avoid walking dogs in the early evening hours when mosquitoes are most abundant.

ARTHROPODS OF PUBLIC HEALTH IMPORTANCE

SARCOPTES SCABEI VARIETY CANIS (CANINE SCABIES)

Canine scabies is a zoonotic skin condition caused by the ectoparasitic, tunneling sarcoptiform mite *Sarcoptes scabei.* Both human and canine varieties of this mite are found; these varieties are classified as *S. scabei* variety *hominis* (**human scabies**) and *S. scabei* variety *canis,* respectively. Although these varieties are morphologically identical, they are different in their primary definitive host and in the characteristic lesions they produce.

Human Infection With Canine Scabies
Humans become infected with canine scabies by coming into direct contact with infested dogs. During most of their life cycle, these mites tunnel in the cornified layer of the epidermis (the outermost layer of the skin). During a short period, however, they reside on the surface of the skin and are capable of transferring from one host to another. Infested dogs can pass mites to uninfested dogs or humans through direct contact. It is important to remember that this mite is transitory and does not establish itself in the skin of humans.

> **TECHNICIAN'S NOTE** *Sarcoptes scabei* variety *canis* can be passed to humans but does not establish itself in the skin of the human incidental host.

Symptoms and Diagnosis
Canine scabies in humans, particularly children, is characterized by the presence of characteristic lesions on the trunk, arms, abdomen, and rarely the face and genitalia. These lesions have been described as papules (red bumps) or vesicles (tiny blisters). Although these mites tunnel in the canine definitive host, they do not tunnel in human skin. The lesions caused by these mites are extremely pruritic; the onset of the pruritus commences with the appearance of the lesions.

Skin scrapings of the infested human's papular or vesicular lesions are rarely positive. The skin condition is diagnosed by the observation of typical lesions in skin that has come in contact with infested dogs. A history of contact with such dogs also aids in the diagnosis. Laboratory findings usually have no role in the establishment of a diagnosis of canine scabies.

> **TECHNICIAN'S NOTE** Typically, laboratory findings do not play a role in diagnosing human scabies infections caused by canine scabies mites.

Treatment
Suspected cases of canine scabies in humans should *always* be referred to a dermatologist or family practitioner. Antihistamines are prescribed to relieve the itch and topical steroid creams to reduce the papules and vesicles. Antibiotics may be administered to prevent secondary bacterial infection. Remember that these are prescription drugs and must be prescribed by a dermatologist or physician.

Prevention of Transmission to Humans
Transmission of this mite to humans can be prevented by avoiding contact with infested dogs harboring *S. scabei* variety *canis.* Naturally, when one dog is diagnosed with this parasitic mite, all dogs

in the household must be treated to kill the offending ectoparasite.

PENTASTOMES OF PUBLIC HEALTH IMPORTANCE

REPTILIAN PENTASTOMIASIS

Reptilian pentastomiasis is the presence of encysted, wormlike nymphal stages of snake pentastomes within the mesenteric lymph nodes, liver, lungs, omentum, and other visceral organs of humans. One mammalian pentastome, *Linguatula serrata,* the tongue worm of dogs, behaves similarly and should be handled with precautionary measures as thorough as those for the reptilian pentastomes.

Human Infection With Reptilian Pentastomes

> **TECHNICIAN'S NOTE** Humans can act as intermediate hosts for reptilian pentastomes when the infective larvae are ingested.

Adult reptilian pentastomes occur within the lungs, trachea, and nasal passages of the reptilian definitive host, feeding on tissue fluids and blood cells. Female pentastomes can produce several million fully embryonated eggs, each containing a single larval stage with two or three pairs of rudimentary, jointed legs that are clawed. These eggs are "coughed up" by the host, swallowed, and passed to the outside environment in snake feces. An oval-tailed larva with four (or six) stumpy legs, each of which has two retractable pincerlike claws, hatches from the egg and is infective for the intermediate host. Intermediate hosts include rodents, herbivores, carnivores, nonhuman primates, and in this case humans. The larva bores into the intestinal wall of the intermediate host and passes with the blood to the mesenteric lymph nodes, liver, lungs, omentum, or other visceral organ, where it becomes encysted. The larva becomes quiescent and metamorphoses into a wormlike nymphal stage. The reptilian definitive host is infected by ingesting the intermediate host with its encysted nymphal pentastomes. The infective nymphs penetrate the snake's intestine, bore to the lungs, and become sexually mature

adult parasites. It is important to note that humans serve as incidental intermediate hosts.

Symptoms and Diagnosis

Most cases of nymphal pentastomiasis in humans are asymptomatic; the patient is unaware of the infection. Incidental nymphal pentastomiasis in humans is diagnosed during exploratory surgery, on radiographic examination, and by histopathologic examination of autopsy specimens. The nymphal pentastome may assume a characteristic C shape during its development in the intermediate host. On histopathologic examination, certain morphologic features of the nymphal pentastome can be used for definitive diagnosis.

Antemortem diagnosis of pentastomiasis in humans can be accomplished by radiographic examination. Nymphal pentastomes often die in the human incidental intermediate host. In response, the human host calcifies the dead parasite. These dead, calcified parasites may be visible on radiographic examination. There are no satisfactory laboratory tests for antemortem diagnosis of nymphal pentastomiasis in humans.

> **TECHNICIAN'S NOTE** Pentastomiasis in humans is diagnosed by radiographic examination finding the calcified, dead nymphal stage.

Treatment

Persons having contact with snakes or snake feces and who suspect that they may be serving as an incidental host for reptilian pentastomes should be examined by an internist, who should be alerted to the possibility of pentastomiasis. In cases of limited infection in humans, free or encysted nymphs can be surgically removed. If tissues are removed for biopsy or autopsy purposes, a histopathologist should be alerted to the suspicion. Additionally, the CDC has many specialists who are qualified to answer questions about the most complex issues of nymphal pentastomiasis in humans.

Prevention of Transmission to Humans

It is now "trendy" or "fashionable" to keep snakes and other reptiles as pets. Many individuals believe erroneously that reptiles are easier to maintain than either cats or dogs; reptiles do not require daily feeding. Many drawbacks await the unsuspecting owner, including the zoonotic potential of reptilian pentastomes.

In the United States snakes and other reptiles can be easily obtained in pet stores in almost any mall or shopping center. The initial sources of these snakes often are unknown to the proprietor and owner. Snakes and other reptiles can originate from across town, from across the continent, or from the other side of the globe. The public is largely unaware of the potential risks involved in caring for snakes. It is the veterinarian's duty to educate the client regarding the severity of incidental nymphal pentastomiasis and to instruct the owner in the proper care and husbandry of captive snakes and other reptiles.

> **TECHNICIAN'S NOTE** The most important part of preventing pentastomiasis infection in humans is proper education of reptile owners.

A newly acquired reptile, whether purchased or collected from the wild, should be presented to the veterinarian for physical examination. This visit should include a routine fecal flotation. If the result of this initial fecal examination is negative, examinations should be performed on at least two successive fecal specimens to reduce the possibility of false-negative results. If pentastome eggs are present in the feces, the client should be warned of the zoonotic potential

of these parasites and advised to select another reptile. Anthelmintic drugs are probably ineffective against pentastomes because of the location of the adult parasites within the lungs of snakes. Clients who insist on maintaining poisonous reptiles as pets should be referred to zoos or herpetaria for instructions regarding proper hygienic procedures and good husbandry techniques. Owners and veterinarians should wash their hands after handling snakes, snake feces, or cage and aquarium items. Water bowls and cages must be cleaned regularly.

Snake owners should be instructed about the intricate life cycle of the pentastomes. Because rodent intermediate hosts cannot be identified antemortem, the one practical preventive measure is to feed only clean, laboratory-reared rodents to captive snakes, lizards, crocodilians, and tuataras. Feeding wild, potentially pentastome-infected rodents to reptiles should be avoided.

CONCLUSION

Because of the public health significance of the parasites discussed in this chapter, it is the veterinarian's responsibility to inform and protect the general public in regard to pathogenic zoonoses.

> **TECHNICIAN'S NOTE** It is up to the veterinary professional to properly educate clients on the zoonotic potential of parasites that their pets may have.

CHAPTER SIXTEEN TEST

MATCHING—Match the term with the correct phrase or term.

A. Diagnosing or treating humans

B. Cat

C. Tachyzoites

D. Bradyzoites

E. Methods of acquiring cryptosporidiosis

F. Swimmer's itch

G. Acquiring *Taenia saginata*

H. Acquiring *Taenia solium*

I. Neurocysticercosis

J. *Echinococcus granulosus*

K. Acquiring *Dipylidium caninum*

L. Acquiring *Diphyllobothrium latum*

M. Pernicious anemia

N. *Baylisascaris procyonis*

O. *Ancylostoma braziliense*

P. *Trichinella spiralis*

Q. Papules

R. Vesicles

S. *Linguatula serrata*

T. Prevention of trichinosis

U. Human

V. Raccoons

W. Paratenic host

X. Diagnosis of ocular larva migrans (OLM) in a child

Y. Diethyltoluamide (DEET)

Z. Advisory capacity

1. Ingesting pork products containing infective larvae in muscle cysts

2. Ingesting fish containing plerocercoid, or sparganum, within fish muscle

3. Tiny blisters in the skin

4. Schistosome cercarial dermatitis from penetration of cercariae of bird flukes

5. Violation of state practice act

6. Rapidly multiplying stages of *Toxoplasma gondii*

7. Cerebrospinal nematodiasis

8. Definitive host for both *Taenia saginata* and *Taenia solium*

9. Red bumps in the skin

10. Communication with human health care workers

11. Ophthalmic examination

12. *Cysticercus cellulosae* in the brain of a human (serving as an intermediate host)

13. Vitamin B_{12} deficiency due to *Diphyllobothrium latum*

14. Only definitive hosts for *T. gondii*

15. Tongue worm of dogs

16. Cooking pork at a temperature of 160° F (71° C)

17. Ingesting cysticercoids within flea intermediate host

18. Slowly multiplying stages of *T. gondii*

19. Mosquito repellent

20. Ingesting measly pork

21. Cutaneous larva migrans

22. Ingesting oocysts from the feces of young calves or from contaminated drinking water

23. Ingesting measly beef

24. Human infected with visceral larva migrans or OLM

25. Unilocular hydatid cyst in human intermediate host

26. Definitive host for *Baylisascaris procyonis*

QUESTIONS FOR THOUGHT AND DISCUSSION

1. There are 18 zoonotic parasites discussed in this chapter. Of these parasites, which three do you think would be most important in a small animal veterinary practice?

2. Of these parasites, which three do you think would be most important in a large animal veterinary practice?

3. Veterinarians and veterinary technicians should always be concerned about the zoonotic potential of parasites. Who do you think knows more about zoonotic diseases, veterinarians or other health care workers?

17 Common Laboratory Procedures for Diagnosing Parasitism

LEARNING OBJECTIVES

After studying this chapter, the reader should be able to do the following:
- Recognize the various types of diagnostic procedures that are used in a parasitology laboratory.
- Detail the types of parasites the various diagnostic procedures can be used to identify.
- Understand the importance of maintaining a well-managed, well-equipped diagnostic facility.
- Understand the importance of good parasitology practices in a diagnostic laboratory.

KEY TERMS

Accession number	Calcareous bodies/	Central record	Feathered edge thin
Baermann	calcareous	book	blood smear
technique	corpuscles	Correct fecal sample	Fecal flotation
Buffy coat	Cellophane tape	submission	Fecal sedimentation
preparation	preparation	Ear smear procedure	Field

KEY TERMS—cont'd

Magnesium sulfate solution	Ocular micrometer	Quantitative fecal procedures	Sodium nitrate solution
Modified Knott technique	"Pooled fecal samples" from herds	Saturated sodium chloride solution	Specific gravity
Modified Wisconsin technique	Preputial washes	Sheather solution	Sporulation Stage micrometer
Occult blood	Qualitative fecal procedures	Simple flotation Skin scrapings	Urine sedimentation Zinc sulfate solution

The term **parasite** represents many different types of organisms that live within or on animals, feeding on tissues or body fluids or competing directly for the animal's food. These parasites demonstrate amazing variety in size and appearance. Although no bacteria or viruses are visible to the naked eye, parasites range in size from those that must be observed with the most powerful microscopes to organisms that measure more than a meter in length. Parasites also show great variety in the locations in which they live within animals and the ways in which they are transmitted from one animal to another. Because of the wide variations in size and life cycles, there is no one particular diagnostic procedure to identify all parasites.

This chapter describes many of the procedures that a veterinary diagnostician may perform to diagnose both internal and external parasites. Generally these procedures are used to detect the presence of parasites or their offspring—their eggs or larval stages—on the skin or in the animal's excretions or blood. Additionally, serologic tests are being used more frequently in veterinary clinical practice. Many of the diagnostic procedures described in this chapter are not in common use in most veterinary practices; however, they are mentioned because they may be useful to technicians employed in diagnostic or research laboratories.

> **TECHNICIAN'S NOTE** There are many procedures used to diagnose internal and external parasites. Some of these tests will not be seen in the clinic but will be of value to a technician working in a research laboratory or reference laboratory.

It is important to note that these tests by themselves are not totally reliable. Sometimes an animal is infected with parasites, but because the infection is slight, no detectable stages can be observed. If the wrong test is used, no parasite will be detected. For this reason, veterinary practitioners use not only these tests but also the animal's history, clinical signs, and other laboratory tests, such as blood values, to arrive at a specific diagnosis of internal parasites.

> **TECHNICIAN'S NOTE** The tests described may not identify parasites if the parasite burden is low, the female is not actively producing eggs, or there are no detectable stages to be observed. Therefore if the results are negative, these tests should not be the only ones relied on to make a diagnosis of parasites.

DIAGNOSIS OF PARASITES OF THE DIGESTIVE TRACT

The following procedures can be used as aids in the diagnosis of parasitism of the esophagus, stomach, liver, bile ducts, and large and small intestines. They can also be used for the diagnosis of parasitic infections in other parts of the body when the eggs or the larval stages are passed by way of the digestive tract (e.g., the "coughed up and swallowed" eggs of lung parasites).

COLLECTION OF THE FECAL SAMPLE

Veterinary diagnosticians usually do not have the opportunity to collect fecal samples and must rely on samples brought in by clients or samples collected during farm calls. Regardless of how the samples are obtained, it is important to have fresh feces for testing; this fact must be emphasized to clients. Feces collected from the yard, pen, or litter box may be old, and as a result parasite eggs may have embryonated or larvated, oocysts may have sporulated, or pseudoparasites may be present. Some protozoans are recognized by their distinctive movements, and in old feces these parasites may have died. The need for fresh feces stems from the rapid development and changes that occur in some common parasites' eggs or larvae once they are passed from the animal. If fresh feces cannot be promptly submitted, clients should be advised to refrigerate the sample for no more than 24 hours.

> **TECHNICIAN'S NOTE** Fecal samples should be fresh when used for parasite diagnosis. The feces should not be older than 24 hours and should be as fresh as possible when collected; if necessary, the feces should be refrigerated to prevent eggs from larvating, oocysts from sporulating, or larvae from changing.

Feces should be submitted in a sealed glass or plastic container that is clearly marked with the time and date of collection, species of animal, animal's name, owner's name, and any other information relevant to the case. The condition of the stool should be noted for color, consistency, and the presence of parasites. Adult nematodes or tapeworm segments observed by the client may be overlooked by the veterinary practitioner.

Clients are often confused about the amount of feces needed to perform a fecal examination. An excellent rule of thumb is that the amount of feces submitted should be approximately the size of an adult man's thumb.

Small Animal Samples

For small animal samples, it is best that the client actually witness the animal defecating to be sure of the source of the sample and to note any straining, blood in the feces, or other problems. Again, all samples should be properly identified. In laboratories that process a large number of fecal samples, it

is sometimes convenient to assign samples an "accession number" to ensure that they are processed in the order in which they are received and to aid in thorough recordkeeping.

> **TECHNICIAN'S NOTE** The owner should be instructed to collect a fecal sample that he or she actually sees defecated by the animal to be sure of the source of the sample.

Large Animal Samples

Large animal fecal samples should be collected directly from the animal's rectum if possible. While wearing a disposable plastic glove, the veterinarian performing the rectal examination of cattle or horses can grasp a handful of feces and retrieve it from the rectum. These feces can then be placed in a sealed container and the container appropriately marked with the owner's name, animal's name or number, and date and time of collection.

The practice of turning the disposable palpation glove inside out while removing it and tying the open end with a knot, thus containing the feces, should be discouraged. These makeshift containers are difficult to label, and the process of removing collected feces from such a flexible container can be difficult and distasteful.

Samples from pigs, feedlot cattle, or other grouped animals are often "pooled" samples; that is, several fecal samples are collected from a pen without the specific animal of origin being known. Again, these samples should be as fresh as possible, and each sample should represent only one group of animals in direct contact with one another. Disposable, zipper-locking plastic bags make good containers for pooled large animal fecal samples. These samples should be labeled with the owner's name, specific location of the pen, number of animals, and date and time of collection. The basic rule of thumb is to always have clean containers that can be tightly sealed to prevent spillage or loss of samples. Any fecal sample that cannot be examined within an hour after collection should be refrigerated to slow down or stop the parasite's development and reduce unpleasant odors.

TECHNICIAN'S NOTE Large animal samples should be taken fresh when the veterinarian is doing a rectal examination. In the case of group-housed animals, one "pooled" sample per group is used. All samples should be properly labeled to avoid confusing the samples later.

EXAMINATION OF THE FECAL SAMPLE

Several procedures commonly used to examine feces for internal parasites are described in this section. Before these procedures are attempted, the following rules should be remembered:

- *Always handle fecal samples carefully.* Some parasites, bacteria, and viruses in animal feces are a threat to human health. When examining the samples, the diagnostician should always wear appropriate outer clothing (e.g., a clean laboratory coat) and rubber or plastic gloves. If gloves are not available, hands should be washed thoroughly with a disinfectant soap when the diagnostic tests have been completed. Under no circumstances should food or drink be consumed or tobacco products used in the area where these tests are performed. Likewise, makeup or contact lenses should never be applied in the diagnostic laboratory.

TECHNICIAN'S NOTE The technician should always wear latex or plastic gloves and proper outerwear when handling feces because some parasites are zoonotic and can even enter through the skin.

- *Always clean up immediately after the tests have been performed.* Leaving spilled fecal material or dirty glassware or equipment lying about creates a source of contamination and can lead to serious infections in both animals and humans. The surface top of the area should be thoroughly cleaned with Roccal-D™, Nolvasan™ solution, or other parasiticide cleaning solution.
- *Always keep good records.* A central record book should be kept in the laboratory area, and every sample should be listed by date, owner's name, and animal's name or number. Any observations about the appearance of the fecal sample and any parasites found should be written down immediately. If no parasites are recovered, that fact should be reported; otherwise it will appear that a particular diagnostic test has not been performed. In recording negative results the phrase "No Parasites Observed" should be written in the results column. It is always important to transfer the results from the central record book to the animal's permanent veterinary medical record and to the clinic's central computer file.

The record book serves as a backup for veterinary medical records and provides a catalog of parasites that are prevalent in the pet and livestock population of that geographic area. An accurate diagnosis of parasitism is based primarily on the diagnostician's awareness of parasites prevalent within the geographic region. Because twenty-first century humans are extremely mobile, however, the movement of pets and livestock to and from other geographic regions should also be considered when parasitism is suspected.

TECHNICIAN'S NOTE Laboratory results should be recorded in a central laboratory results book and also recorded in the patient's medical record. The central results book is used as a backup to make sure tests were run. If results are not recorded in the central book or in the record, the tests were not performed.

Gross Examination of Feces

The following characteristics of feces should be recorded and relayed to the attending veterinarians:

- *Consistency.* The condition of the feces, that is, soft, watery (diarrheic), or very hard (constipation), should be noted. This description will vary with the animal species. For example, cattle feces are normally softer than those of horses or sheep.
- *Color.* Unusual fecal colors should always be reported. For example, light-gray feces may indicate excessive fat in the feces, a sign of poor intestinal absorption.
- *Blood.* In fresh feces, blood may appear dark brown to black and tarlike or may demonstrate

the red color associated with fresh blood. Blood may indicate severe parasitism, as well as other intestinal disease. It is important to record the presence of blood because this assists the veterinary practitioner in identifying certain diseases.

- *Mucus.* Mucus on the surface of fresh feces may be associated with intestinal parasitism or some other metabolic disease.
- *Age of the feces.* If the feces appear old and dry, this should be noted. In aged samples, as noted earlier, parasite eggs may have embryonated or larvated, oocysts may have sporulated, or pseudoparasites may be present. Some protozoan parasites are recognized by their distinctive movements. In old feces, these parasites may have died.
- *Gross parasites.* Some parasites, portions of parasites, or larvae are large enough to observe with the naked eye. Probably the most common are the proglottids of tapeworms, entire roundworms, or even larval arthropods (horse bot fly larvae).

TECHNICIAN'S NOTE The physical appearance of the feces should be recorded in the central laboratory record book as well as on the animal's medical record (i.e., color, consistency, presence of blood, gross parasites seen, and presence of mucus).

Figure 17-1 shows tapeworm segments (**proglottids**) in fresh feces. These should be gently removed from the feces with thumb forceps and examined with a handheld lens or dissecting microscope. Figure 17-2 shows segments of two common tapeworms (*Dipylidium caninum* and *Taenia pisiformis*) found in the feces of dogs and cats; their morphology, shape, size, and movement may aid in identification. Short segments of ruminant and equine tapeworms may also be recovered from feces (Figure 17-3). Of interest, swine in the United States do not demonstrate adult tapeworm segments in their feces.

Occasionally clients will bring in dried tapeworm segments that they have found in their pet's bedding or hair coat. For identification these segments must be rehydrated by soaking for 1 to 4 hours in a Petri dish or small container of water or

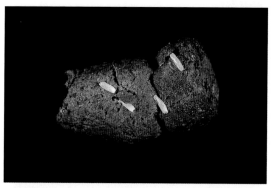

FIGURE 17-1 Fresh dog feces containing tapeworm proglottids (segments). Proglottids may be motile and exit from the feces into the surrounding environment.

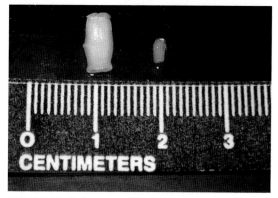

FIGURE 17-2 Segments of two common tapeworms (*Dipylidium caninum* and *Taenia pisiformis*) found in the feces of dogs and cats. Morphology, shape, size, and movement of these common small animal tapeworms may aid in their identification.

physiologic saline. These segments will resume their natural state and can then be identified by their morphologic features. Alternatively they may be "teased" open in a small amount of water on a glass microscope slide. If they are **gravid** (egg-containing) proglottids, they may release their eggs and be easily identified.

The diagnostician should always attempt to identify the parasite in terms of genus and species so that the veterinarian can use this information in the control and treatment of the tapeworm infection. The morphology of the segment can assist in the identification of the tapeworms. For example, with *D. caninum*, the tapeworm of dogs and cats

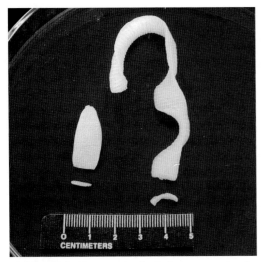

FIGURE **17-3** Chains and individual mature proglottids of tapeworms of ruminants, *Moniezia* species *(left)*, and horses, *Anoplocephala* species *(right)*.

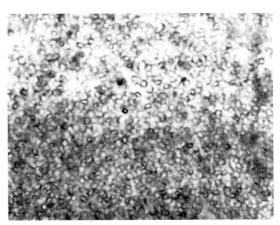

FIGURE **17-4** Microscopic calcium deposits (calcareous bodies, or calcareous corpuscles) are unique to tapeworm tissue (140× magnification).

that is transmitted by fleas, the diagnostician can observe with a handheld magnifying lens the "double-pored effect," the presence of a genital pore on both sides of every segment. Segments of tapeworms of the genus *Taenia*, which use rodents and mammals as intermediate hosts, have a single pore on each segment. These pores are irregularly alternating. Again, tapeworm segments can also be definitively identified by teasing them open and demonstrating the characteristic eggs they contain.

> **TECHNICIAN'S NOTE** Parasites should be identified by genus and species when possible so the veterinarian can use proper control and treatment measures (i.e., some medications work for some types of parasites and not others, some types of parasites [tapeworms] have different intermediate hosts).

Segments of some uncommon tapeworm species may be "spent" proglottids; that is, the proglottids have dispelled their eggs and the uteri are empty. If the diagnostician is confused about whether these are tapeworms, the suspect material can be macerated between two microscope slides and examined microscopically to determine whether the tissue has small mineral deposits (called **calcareous bodies**,

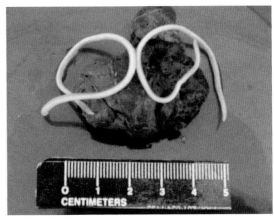

FIGURE **17-5** Two roundworms (*Toxocara canis*) in canine feces after treatment with a nematocide.

or **calcareous corpuscles**) that are unique to tapeworms (Figure 17-4).

Other types of parasites are large enough to be observed in animal feces. These include adult worms expelled from their host by drug treatments or overcrowding by fellow parasites (Figure 17-5). Horse feces may contain **bots**, which are the larvae of a certain type of fly (i.e., *Gasterophilus* species). The larval flies are parasitic in the stomach of horses and are passed in the feces to complete their life cycle outside the body of the equine host (Figure 17-6).

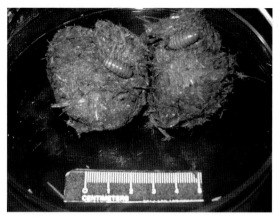

FIGURE 17-6 Two larvae (bots) of bot flies (*Gasterophilus* spp.) in equine feces.

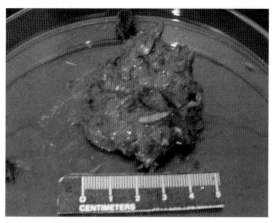

FIGURE 17-7 Free-living fly larvae (maggots) in 2-day-old bovine feces.

TECHNICIAN'S NOTE Aged feces may contain pseudoparasites picked up from the environment or nonparasitic larvae from flies that have grown after defecation occurred.

Aged feces may also contain nonparasitic fly larvae called **maggots** (Figure 17-7). The maggots do not live within the animal's intestines but instead develop from eggs laid by free-living adult flies after the feces have been passed. Flesh flies of the genus *Sarcophaga* deposit larvae (rather than eggs) on the feces of many domestic animals. Usually fly maggots seen in feces voided more than 12 hours previously should not be mistaken for internal parasites; they should be considered **pseudoparasites**. There is one exception to this rule: *Gasterophilus* species, or horse bot fly larvae, may be found in fresh horse feces.

In general, when the veterinary diagnostician cannot identify parasite-like material (whether parasite or pseudoparasite) found within feces, the unidentified specimen should be sent to a diagnostic facility (a university or state diagnostic laboratory) for proper identification. These specimens should be preserved in 70% alcohol or 10% formalin and shipped as described later in this chapter. An up-to-date history should accompany each specimen.

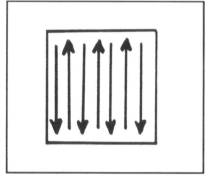

FIGURE 17-8 Pattern of movement of microscopic field for thorough examination of the area under the coverslip.

Microscopic Examination of Feces

Compound microscopes used in a veterinary diagnostic setting vary widely in features and in the magnifications they provide. For parasitologic diagnostic examinations, objective lenses with magnification powers of 4×, 10×, and 40× are most often used. Oil-immersion objectives (e.g., 100× magnification) are occasionally used in veterinary practice, particularly in blood smear preparations. A mechanical stage is preferable and convenient for parasitologic work because it allows for smooth, uniform movement in a thorough search of the microscope slide. Regardless of how the slide is moved, the area under the coverslip must be thoroughly and uniformly searched (Figure 17-8).

To search the slide thoroughly, the diagnostician must begin using an objective lens that magnifies at least 10× and, with experience, should be able to scan the slides more rapidly at 4×. The edge of the coverslip can be used for adjusting the coarse focus, and any debris under the coverslip can be used for fine focus adjustment. Each circular area of the slide seen through the coverslip is called a field. The slide should be moved so that the field follows either of the patterns of arrows shown in Figure 17-8. Each time the edge of the coverslip is reached, a piece of debris or other object at the edge of the field (in the direction of the search) should be identified. The slide is then moved until the piece of debris or other object is at the edge of the field. In this manner, every field scanned slightly overlaps the previous field, and every area beneath the coverslip is examined. When the slide is being scanned in this manner, it is important to move the fine focus knob continually back and forth slightly to aid in visualization of parasite eggs or cysts not in a single plane of focus. When a parasite egg or cyst is observed at low magnification, higher-power objectives (10× or 40×) may be used to more closely examine it.

Calibrating the Microscope

The size of various stages of many parasites is often important for correct identification. Some examples are eggs of *Trichuris vulpis* versus eggs of *Capillaria* species and microfilariae of *Acanthocheilonema reconditum* versus microfilariae of *Dirofilaria immitis*. Accurate measurements are easily obtained by using a calibrated eyepiece on the microscope. Calibration must be performed on every microscope used in the laboratory. Each objective lens (4×, 10×, 40×) of the microscope must be individually calibrated.

Instruments

The stage micrometer is a microscope slide etched with a 2-mm line marked in 0.01-mm (10-μm)

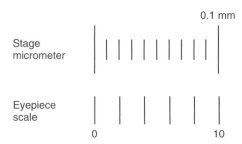

FIGURE 17-9 Stage micrometer *(upper scale)* and eyepiece scale *(lower scale)* used to calibrate a microscope.

divisions (Figure 17-9). Note that 1 micron (micrometer, μm) equals 0.001 mm. Also note that the stage micrometer is used only once to calibrate the objectives of the microscope. Once the ocular micrometer within the compound microscope has been calibrated at 4×, 10×, and 40×, it is calibrated for the service life of the microscope; the stage micrometer will never be used again. Therefore it is a good idea not to purchase a stage micrometer but instead to borrow one from a university or some other diagnostic laboratory and return it after calibration.[1]

The eyepiece scale (or ocular micrometer) is a glass disk that fits into and remains in one of the microscope eyepieces. The disk is etched with 30 hatch marks spaced at equal intervals (see Figure 17-9). The number of hatch marks on the disc may vary, but the calibration procedure does not change.[2]

The stage micrometer is used to determine the distance in microns between the hatch marks on the ocular micrometer for each objective lens of the microscope being calibrated. This information is recorded and firmly affixed to the base of the microscope for future reference.

[1]Item numbers 59 to 1430; Carolina Biological Supply Company, Burlington, NC.
[2]Item numbers 59 to 1423 or 59 to 1425; Carolina Biological Supply Company, Burlington, NC.

Procedure

Start at low power (10×) and focus on the 2-mm line of the stage micrometer. Note that 2 mm equals 2000 μm. Rotate the ocular micrometer within the eyepiece so that its hatch-mark scale is horizontal and parallel to that of the stage micrometer (see Figure 17-9). Align the *0* points on both scales.

Determine the point on the stage micrometer aligned with the *10* hatch mark on the ocular micrometer. In Figure 17-9, this point is at 0.1 mm on the stage micrometer.

Multiply this number by 100. In this example 0.1 mm × 100 = 10 μm. This means that at this power (10×) the distance between each hatch mark on the ocular micrometer is 10 μm. Any object may be measured with the ocular micrometer scale, and that distance is measured by multiplying the number of ocular units by a factor of 10. For example, if an object is 10 ocular units long, its true length is 100 μm (10 ocular units × 10 μm = 100 μm).

This procedure should be repeated at each magnification (4× and 40×). For each magnification this information is recorded and labeled on the base of the microscope for future reference.

Objective Distance between Hatch Marks (Microns)
4×–25 μm
10×–10 μm
40×–2.5 μm

Direct Smear

The simplest method of microscopic fecal examination for parasites is the direct smear, which consists of a small amount of feces placed directly on the microscope slide (Box 17-1). The advantages of the direct smear are the short procedure time and minimal equipment needed. Some veterinary

---

BOX 17-1 | Direct Fecal Smear Procedure

1. Place several drops of saline or fecal flotation solution on a slide with an equal amount of feces.
2. Mix the solution and feces together with a wooden applicator until the solution is homogeneous.
3. Smear the solution over the slide into a thin film. The film should be thin enough to read print through.
4. Remove any large pieces of feces.
5. Place a coverslip over the smear.
6. Examine the area of the slide under the coverslip with the compound microscope (see text), and record any protozoan cysts, eggs, larvae, or gross parasites seen.

---

practitioners make direct smears with only the amount of feces that clings to a rectal thermometer after the animal's temperature has been recorded. The direct smear allows the diagnostician to observe eggs and larvae undistorted by the procedures discussed later.

A disadvantage to the direct smear technique is that the small amount of fecal material required for this procedure is not a good representative sample size; this procedure can be inaccurate. Such a small quantity of feces may not contain the larvae or eggs of the adult parasite the animal is harboring. The animal may be incorrectly assumed to be free of parasites. This procedure also leaves much fecal debris on the slide, which may be confusing to the veterinary diagnostician.

CONCENTRATION METHODS FOR FECAL EXAMINATION

The greatest disadvantage of the direct smear procedure is the small amount of feces used, which greatly reduces the chance of finding parasite eggs or larvae or protozoan cysts. To overcome this problem, methods have been developed to concentrate parasitic material from a larger fecal sample into a smaller volume that can be examined microscopically. Two primary types of concentration methods are used in veterinary practice: fecal flotation and fecal sedimentation.

> **TECHNICIAN'S NOTE** Fecal concentration methods are preferred for identifying parasite ova, larvae, and oocysts in the feces because larger volumes of feces are used, making it more likely the developmental stages will be seen if present in the feces.

Fecal Flotation

Fecal flotation procedures are based on differences in the specific gravity of parasite eggs, cysts, and larvae and that of fecal debris. Specific gravity refers to the weight of an object (e.g., the parasite egg) compared with the weight of an equal volume of pure water. Most parasite eggs have a specific gravity between 1.1 and 1.2 (g/mL), whereas tap water is only slightly higher than 1 g/mL. Therefore parasite eggs are too heavy to float in tap water. To make the eggs float, a liquid with a higher specific gravity than that of the eggs must be used. Such liquids are called **flotation solutions** and consist of concentrated sugar or various salts added to water to increase its specific gravity. Flotation solutions usually have specific gravities between 1.2 and 1.25. In this range, fecal material, much of which has a specific gravity of 1.3 or greater, does not float (Figure 17-10). The result of using flotation solutions is that parasite eggs float to the surface of the liquid and large particles of fecal material sink to the bottom, making eggs easier to observe (Box 17-2).

> **TECHNICIAN'S NOTE** Fecal flotation solutions with a specific gravity of 1.2 to 1.25 are used to "float" parasite ova, cysts, and larvae while the fecal material sinks to the bottom of the container.

If the specific gravity is below the desired range (1.2 to 1.25), add more reagent until the hydrometer

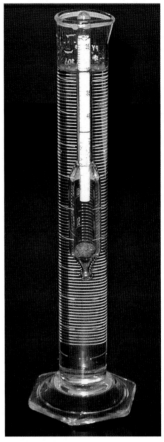

FIGURE 17-10 Measuring the specific gravity of a flotation solution with a hydrometer.

indicates this range. If the specific gravity is above 1.25, add water until the proper reading is obtained.

Sugar (Sheather solution), saturated sodium chloride (table salt), magnesium sulfate (Epsom salt), zinc sulfate, and sodium nitrate solutions are the flotation solutions most often used in veterinary practices. Veterinarians may select from among these solutions according to personal preference, availability of reagents, and target parasites. Sheather solution is less efficient than sodium nitrate solution because it floats fewer eggs and is messy to work with (it is quite sticky). Sugar, however, is readily available and inexpensive, does not distort roundworm eggs, and floats an adequate percentage of the eggs. Sodium nitrate solution is the most efficient flotation solution, but it forms crystals and

| BOX 17-2 | Preparation of Flotation Solutions |

Sugar Flotation Solution (Sheather Solution)

Determine the amount of sugar solution required, and use about half that amount of water. Use an appropriately sized pot (e.g., cooking pot). Heat the water, but be careful not to let it boil. Add granulated pure cane sugar (table sugar) to the water while stirring. About 454 g (1 lb) is required for every 355 mL (12 oz) of water. Add 6 mL of 40% formaldehyde solution or 1 g of crystalline phenol for every 100 mL of solution; these chemicals serve as preservatives and prevent mold from growing in the sugar solution. The solution's specific gravity should always be checked with a hydrometer (see Figure 17-10), an instrument available from scientific supply houses.

Sodium Nitrate Flotation Solution

While stirring, add about 315 g of sodium nitrate for every liter of water. Heating is not necessary but hastens the dissolution process. Adjust the solution to a specific gravity of 1.2 to 1.25, as discussed for the sugar solution.

Zinc Sulfate Flotation Solution

While stirring, add 386 g of zinc sulfate for every liter of water. Heating the water is not necessary but hastens the dissolution process. Using a hydrometer, adjust the solution to a specific gravity of 1.2 to 1.25, as discussed for the sugar solution.

Magnesium Sulfate Flotation Solution

While stirring, add about 350 g of magnesium sulfate (Epsom salt) for every liter of water. Heating the water hastens the dissolution process. Using a hydrometer, adjust the solution to a specific gravity of 1.3, as discussed for the sugar solution.

Saturated Sodium Chloride Flotation Solution

Add sodium chloride (table salt) to boiling water until the salt no longer dissolves and settles to the bottom of the pot. There is no need to adjust the specific gravity because it cannot go above 1.2 with this solution.

---

distorts the eggs after a time. Sodium nitrate may be difficult to acquire, but it can be purchased through chemical supply houses. Sodium nitrate solution is used in commercial fecal diagnostic kits and may be purchased already prepared in the form of refill bottles for these kits. Sodium nitrate solution is more expensive than sugar solution.

Saturated sodium chloride solution is the least desirable flotation solution. Its main disadvantages are that it corrodes expensive laboratory equipment, such as compound microscopes and centrifuges; forms crystals on the microscope slide; and severely distorts the eggs. Because it reaches a specific gravity of 1.2, some heavier eggs may not float in this solution. However, sodium chloride is inexpensive, easily prepared, and readily available.

> **TECHNICIAN'S NOTE** The fecal solutions of choice are Sheather sugar solution, sodium nitrate solution, and zinc sulfate solution; however, the specific gravity of the solution will determine how many different types of eggs, larvae, and cysts are able to be floated.

Zinc sulfate solution is similar in efficiency to sugar solution and can be purchased through chemical supply houses or from veterinary suppliers in ready-to-mix gallon containers. Cystic stages of intestinal protozoans such as *Giardia* are best concentrated with zinc sulfate solution. Magnesium sulfate solution (Epsom salt) also forms crystals on the microscope slide. It is an inexpensive solution and is easily prepared and readily available.

Simple Flotation

The simple flotation method is probably the second–most common parasitologic test performed in veterinary practices after the direct smear (Box 17-3). A specimen of 2 to 5 g of feces is placed in a suitable container, such as a paper cup. Flotation solution is added directly to the feces, mixed thoroughly with a tongue depressor, and strained through a metal tea strainer (or cheesecloth) into a second paper cup. The contents of the second paper cup are poured into a test tube, and the flotation medium is added until a meniscus is formed (Figure 17-11). A glass coverslip is placed over the

BOX 17-3 | Simple Flotation Procedure

1. Place about 2 g (tsp) of the fecal sample in a 90- to 150-mL waxed paper cup. Add approximately 30 mL of flotation medium. Using a tongue depressor, make an emulsion by thoroughly mixing the solution with the feces until a fecal slurry has been made.

2. Bend the side of the waxed paper cup into a spout, and cover the spout with a piece of cheesecloth. Pour the emulsion through the cheesecloth into a straight-sided shell vial. A tea strainer may be used instead of cheesecloth: Pour the contents of the cup through the strainer into a second waxed paper cup and the contents of that cup into the shell vial. Wash the tea strainer thoroughly in hot, soapy water before using it again.

3. Fill the shell vial to the top, then slightly overfill it so that a meniscus forms above the lip of the vial (see Figure 17-11). If there is not enough fluid in the cup to fill the shell vial, a small amount of fresh flotation medium may be added.

Place a glass coverslip gently on top of the fluid, and allow it to settle on the meniscus.

4. Allow the coverslip to remain undisturbed on top of the vial for 10 to 20 minutes (sugar solution requires longer than sodium nitrate). If the coverslip is removed before this time, all the eggs may not have had time to float to the top. If left for more than 1 hour, some eggs may become waterlogged and begin to sink or become distorted.

5. Remove the coverslip carefully, picking it straight up, and immediately place it on the microscope slide. When placing the coverslip on the slide, be sure to hold the coverslip with one edge tilted slightly up, and allow it to gradually settle levelly on the slide. This reduces the number of air bubbles beneath the coverslip.

6. Examine the area of the slide under the coverslip with the compound microscope (see text), and record any protozoan cysts, eggs, larvae, or gross parasites seen.

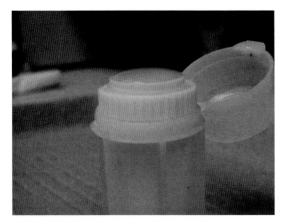

FIGURE 17-11 Fecalyzer vial filled with flotation medium, showing meniscus.

meniscus and allowed to remain for 10 to 15 minutes (depending on the flotation medium used), after which the coverslip is removed and placed on a glass microscope slide. The parasite eggs are lighter than the solution and float to the top of the tube (or vial) of flotation solution. The coverslip is removed from the liquid and examined with a microscope. This method is less efficient than the centrifugal flotations described next, but it does not require a centrifuge.

Some veterinary diagnostics companies have packaged simple flotation kits consisting of a prepared flotation solution, disposable plastic vials, and strainers; examples include the Ovassay, Fecalyzer, and Ovatector (Figure 17-12).[3] Instructions for use are included with these kits. The main disadvantages to these kits are the expense and the environmental contamination created by the disposal of plastics.

Centrifugal Flotation

The centrifugal flotation procedure more efficiently recovers parasite eggs and cysts and requires less time than the simple flotation procedure (Box 17-4 and Figure 17-13). However, it does require a

---

[3]Ovassay manufactured by Synbiotics Corp., San Diego, CA; Fecalyzer manufactured by EVSCO Pharmaceuticals, Buena, NJ; Ovatector manufactured by BGS Medical Products, Inc., Venice, FL.

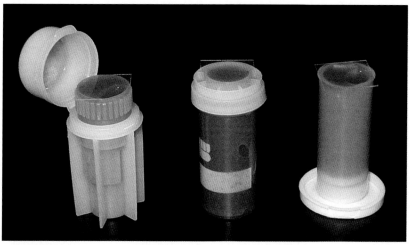

FIGURE 17-12 Three commercially available fecal flotation kits: Fecalyzer *(left)*, Ovassay *(center)*, and Ovatector *(right)*. These kits are based on the principles of the simple flotation procedure.

BOX 17-4 | Centrifugal Flotation Procedure

1. Using a paper cup and tongue depressor, mix approximately 1 tsp of feces with enough water to make a semisolid suspension.
2. Place a wire tea strainer (or piece of cheesecloth) over a second paper cup and empty the fecal suspension into it. Use the tongue depressor to press out most of the liquid; return the solid waste to the first cup and discard. Wash the strainer in hot running water; soak it in water containing dishwashing solution.
3. Pinch the rim of the second paper cup to form a pouring spout, and transfer the contents into a 15-mL centrifuge tube (a test tube). Place the tube into the centrifuge, remembering to counterbalance the tube with an identical tube filled to the same level with water. Be sure that all tubes are marked so they can be identified after centrifugation.
4. Centrifuge for 3 minutes at 400x to 650x *g*. For many centrifuges, this is about 1500 rpm. Decant the supernatant, which contains fats and dissolved pigments that interfere with the identification of parasite eggs, larvae, or cysts.
5. Add concentrated flotation solution to within 1/2 to 3/4 inch of the top of the tube, and resuspend the sediment using a stirring action with a wooden applicator stick. Insert a rubber stopper, and mix by four or more inversions so

that the solution is thoroughly mixed with the sediment.

Variation A
Return the tube to the centrifuge, remembering to counterbalance the tube with an identical tube filled to the same level with the same flotation solution. Centrifuge for 5 minutes. Without removing the tube from the centrifuge, pick up the surface film containing eggs, larvae, or cysts by touching the surface gently with a wire loop (bent at a 90-degree angle) (see Figure 17-13) or a glass rod. Transfer the surface film to a glass microscope slide and add a coverslip. Examine the slide under the compound microscope using the 10x objective (see text).

Variation B
Return the tube to the centrifuge, and fill the centrifuge tube with the flotation solution until a meniscus is formed. Apply a coverslip to the top of the tube. Remember to counterbalance the tube with an identical tube filled to the same level with the same flotation solution and covered with a coverslip. Centrifuge for 5 minutes. After centrifugation lift the coverslip straight up and place it on the glass slide. This modification works only if a variable-angle (not a fixed-angle) centrifuge is used. Examine the slide under the compound microscope, using the 10x objective (see text).

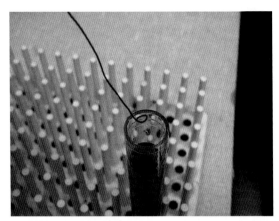

FIGURE 17-13 Use of a bacteriologic loop to transfer a drop from the top of a fecal flotation emulsion after a centrifugation procedure. Note that the loop is bent at a 90-degree angle to the wire handle.

centrifuge capable of holding 15-mL test tubes and producing a centrifugal force of 400× to 650× *g*. Most tabletop centrifuges are capable of producing this force. Centrifuges with a fixed-angle headpiece are not suitable for such centrifugal flotation procedures.

> *TECHNICIAN'S NOTE* Fecal centrifugation is the method of choice for fecal flotation testing because it has been shown in multiple studies to float a higher concentration of ova, cysts, and larvae than simple fecal flotation.

Fecal Sedimentation

Sedimentation procedures concentrate both feces and eggs at the bottom of a liquid medium, usually water (Box 17-5). Sedimentation detects most parasite eggs but is not as good as flotation for providing a clear sample for microscopic examination. Sedimentation is primarily used to detect eggs or cysts that have too high a specific gravity to float or that would be severely distorted by flotation solution.

Sedimentation can be used for roundworm and tapeworm eggs, but there is usually too much fecal debris hiding the eggs to make it worthwhile. Therefore this procedure is not used routinely and has its greatest use in suspected trematode (fluke)

BOX 17-5 | Sedimentation Procedure

1. Using a tongue depressor, mix about 2 g of feces with tap water in a cup or beaker. Strain the mixture through cheesecloth or a tea strainer into a centrifuge tube, as described for centrifugal flotation.
2. Balance the centrifuge tubes and centrifuge the sample at about 400× *g* (about 1500 rpm). If a centrifuge is unavailable, allow the mixture to sit undisturbed for 20 to 30 minutes.
3. Pour off the liquid in the top of the tube without disturbing the sediment at the bottom.
4. Using the pipette and bulb, transfer a small amount of the top layer of sediment to a microscope slide. If the drop is too thick, dilute it with a drop of water. Lugol iodine solution (diluted 1 : 5 in water) may be used for dilution instead of water to aid in identification of protozoan cysts. Apply a coverslip to the drop. Repeat the procedure using a drop from the bottom layer of the sediment.
5. Examine both slides microscopically (see text).

---

infections. Fluke eggs are somewhat denser and sometimes larger than roundworm eggs. Some fluke eggs float in flotation solutions, and others do not. Some laboratories increase the specific gravity of their flotation solutions to 1.3 to ensure recovery of fluke eggs by the flotation technique. The problem with the use of flotation methods for recovery of fluke eggs is that the eggs may be damaged by the high concentration of the solution and may become difficult to identify.

> *TECHNICIAN'S NOTE* Fecal sedimentation is rarely used for routine fecal analysis. It is more commonly used to test for trematode eggs, which are heavier than other parasite eggs and thus do not float as well.

QUANTITATIVE FECAL EXAMINATION

All the procedures previously described are qualitative, which means they reveal the presence or absence of parasite ova or cysts. Quantitative procedures indicate the number of eggs or cysts present in each gram of feces. The results of these procedures are a rough, or approximate, indication of the number of adult parasites present within the host (the severity of the infection). These procedures are not completely accurate because different species of parasites produce different numbers of eggs. Also, the most severe signs of disease are produced by parasites that have not yet started to produce eggs or larvae.

> **TECHNICIAN'S NOTE** Qualitative procedures tell you whether parasite ova or cysts are present in a fecal sample, whereas quantitative procedures provide the number of ova or cysts in 1 g of feces.

Several procedures are used to estimate the numbers of parasite eggs or cysts per gram of feces, including the Stoll egg-counting technique, the modified Wisconsin sugar flotation method, and the McMaster technique. These techniques are used most often in research laboratories and are not usually performed in veterinary clinical practice. Of these tests, the modified Wisconsin sugar flotation method is used most often (Box 17-6).

> **TECHNICIAN'S NOTE** Quantitative procedures are used more often in research facilities than in the veterinary clinic.

EXAMINATION OF FECES FOR PROTOZOANS

All the procedures for microscopic fecal examination are useful for detection of cysts of intestinal protozoans. However, some protozoans do not form cysts and are passed in the feces as **trophozoites** (motile forms). Cyst-forming protozoans may also pass trophozoites in the feces in large numbers when the host has diarrhea. Trophozoites lack the rigid wall of cysts, and they collapse and become difficult to recognize in flotation solutions.

To observe live trophozoites, a fecal smear should be prepared as previously described, but physiologic saline must be used to dilute the feces. Trophozoites are recognized by their movement, which varies among the different groups of protozoans. *Balantidium coli*, a parasite of humans, pigs, and

| **BOX 17-6** | Modified Wisconsin Sugar Flotation Method |

1. Fill a 20-mm × 150-mm test tube with Sheather solution 1 inch below the top of the tube.
2. Using scales, weigh exactly 3 g of the fecal sample and place into a paper cup.
3. Pour the Sheather solution from the test tube into the paper cup containing the feces and mix well.
4. Place a tea strainer in a second paper cup, and pour the Sheather solution and feces mixture through the strainer. Using a tongue depressor, press all the liquid out of the fecal pat and through the tea strainer.
5. Return the Sheather solution and strained feces mixture to the test tube originally containing the Sheather solution and place it in a test tube rack.
6. Add Sheather solution to the test tube until a small meniscus forms. Carefully place a glass coverslip on top of the meniscus.
7. Allow the test tube with its coverslip to stand undisturbed for 4 hours.
8. Remove the coverslip, place it on a glass microscope slide, and examine the entire coverslip on low power (10×), counting parasite eggs, cysts, or oocysts. This count represents the number of eggs, cysts, or oocysts per 3 g of feces.

dogs, moves in a slow, tumbling manner. *Giardia* species, which are found in several species of animals, swim in a jerky motion. Trichomonads, also found in several different types of hosts, appear to wobble and have a sail-like, undulating membrane that ripples as they swim. Amoebae, found in humans and dogs, move by extending part of their cell body (the pseudopod) and moving the rest of the body after it.

> **TECHNICIAN'S NOTE** *Giardia* appendages (trophozoites) swim in a jerky motion in a fecal smear.

Many methods have been used to stain and preserve intestinal protozoans. The simplest method to stain cysts is a direct smear stained with an iodine

BOX 17-7	Preparation of Modified D'Antoni's Iodine Solution

1. Before preparing this solution the technician should remove all jewelry because this iodine solution can permanently stain precious metals.
   Distilled water, 100 mL
   Potassium iodide, 1 g
   Powdered iodine crystals, 1.5 g
2. The potassium iodide solution should be saturated with iodine, with some excess remaining in the bottle. It should be stored in brown, glass-stoppered bottles and kept in the dark. The solution is ready for use immediately and should be decanted into a brown glass dropping bottle. When the solution lightens, it should be discarded and replaced with fresh stock. The stock solution is good as long as an excess of iodine remains in the bottom of the bottle.
3. When using this solution in the laboratory around the compound microscope, the technician should take great care not to spill the solution onto the metal parts of the microscope because it is extremely corrosive.

solution (as described under the direct smear procedure). This method does not preserve the sample but highlights any protozoans in the smear, facilitating identification. Several iodine solutions are available for staining. Modified D'Antoni's iodine or Lugol iodine is often used in diagnostic laboratories to stain protozoan cysts (Box 17-7).

> **TECHNICIAN'S NOTE** Modified D'Antoni's iodine or Lugol iodine can be used to stain protozoan cysts on a direct smear.

Fecal smears containing protozoal trophozoites can be allowed to dry and then can be stained with Giemsa, Wright, or Diff-Quik stain.[4] Once stained in this manner, the slides may be sent to a diagnostic laboratory for identification of the organism.

Other procedures for the concentration, staining, and preservation of intestinal protozoans

---

[4]Diff-Quik, product number B4132-1; Baxter Diagnostics, Scientific Products Division, McGaw Park, IL.

include merthiolate-iodine-formaldehyde (MIF) solution, polyvinyl alcohol, and iron hematoxylin. These staining procedures are generally too complex and time-consuming for use in veterinary practice.

FECAL CULTURE

Fecal culture is used in diagnostic parasitology to differentiate parasites whose eggs and cysts cannot be distinguished by examination of a fresh fecal sample. For example, the eggs of large strongyles in horses are very similar to those of small strongyles. To distinguish between them, feces containing strongyle eggs are allowed to incubate at room temperature for several days while the larvae hatch from the eggs. The newly hatched larvae can then be identified.

Nematode (Roundworm) Eggs

The procedure for culture of nematode (roundworm) eggs in feces is simple; however, identifying the larvae once they are recovered is much more tedious (Box 17-8). Diagnosticians who need to culture and identify nematode larvae are referred to state or private diagnostic laboratories.

> **TECHNICIAN'S NOTE** The culturing and identification of nematode larvae are often referred to state or private diagnostic laboratories.

Coccidial Oocysts

Another type of fecal culture that has some use in veterinary practices is sporulation of coccidial oocysts (Box 17-9). Sporulation is a process of development that takes place within the oocyst. In fresh feces, oocysts of various species of coccidia may appear similar to one another; however, once sporulation occurs, coccidia of the genus *Eimeria* can be easily distinguished from those of the genus *Cystoisospora*. A fully sporulated oocyst of the genus *Eimeria* contains four sporocysts, whereas a fully sporulated oocyst of the genus *Cystoisospora* has two sporocysts (Figure 17-14).

> **TECHNICIAN'S NOTE** *Cystoisospora* species have two sporocysts when sporulated, whereas *Eimeria* species have four sporocysts.

BOX 17-8	Fecal Culture of Roundworm Eggs

1. Place 20 to 30 g of fresh fecal sample in a jar. Break up the feces with a tongue depressor and moisten slightly with tap water. The mixture should not be so wet as to appear soupy.
2. Place the jar on a shelf, away from direct sunlight, and allow it to incubate at room temperature for 7 days. There should be enough moisture so that droplets of condensed water can be seen on the sides of the glass jar. If moisture does not form, add a few drops of water.
3. Some species of nematode larvae can migrate up the walls of the jar. These may be recovered by removing condensation drops from the glass with an artist's paintbrush and transferring them to a drop of water on a microscope slide. Other species must be recovered with the Baermann technique (see p. 322).
4. Apply a coverslip to the slide (a drop of modified D'Antoni's iodine may be added), and pass it over the open flame of a Bunsen burner once or twice to kill the larvae while they are in an extended position. Place the slide on the microscope slide stage and identify the larvae.

BOX 17-9	Fecal Culture of Coccidial Oocysts

1. When coccidial oocysts are found in a fresh fecal sample, place 10 to 20 g of the sample in a beaker or a paper cup and cover with about 60 mL of 2.5% potassium dichromate solution. Mix this solution thoroughly with a tongue depressor.
2. Pour the solution into a Petri dish and let incubate at room temperature for 3 to 5 days. Open the plate daily and swirl the contents gently to allow air to reach the developing oocysts.
3. After incubation, centrifuge the plate's contents as described under the sedimentation procedure (see p. 316).
4. Process the fecal sediment by the centrifugal flotation procedure to recover the oocysts; then examine them microscopically.

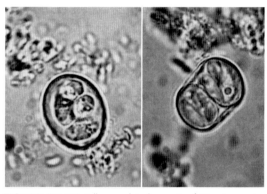

FIGURE 17-14 Fully sporulated oocysts of *Eimeria* species *(left)* and *Cystoisospora* species *(right)* (1400×).

SAMPLE COLLECTION AT NECROPSY

Necropsy, or postmortem examination, is an important method for diagnosing parasitism of the digestive tract. Lesions of internal organs are often fairly indicative of the type of parasites that produce them. The veterinary technician is responsible for assisting during necropsy procedures and in particular helping with the preservation and processing of the samples collected. During necropsy and the processing of samples, all workers should wear gloves.

TECHNICIAN'S NOTE Technicians are usually responsible for assisting with necropsy examinations, and all participants should wear gloves.

The contents of the digestive system may contain many types of parasites, some of which may be nematodes (roundworms). Trematodes (flukes) and cestodes (tapeworms) are easily seen and can be individually isolated. The two preferred methods for recovering roundworms are the decanting method (Box 17-10) and the sieving method (Box 17-11). With either method, the contents of

BOX 17-10 | Decanting Method for Sample Collection at Necropsy

1. Using wrapping twine, tie off each portion of the digestive tract (the stomach, duodenum, small intestine, large intestine, and so on). Open each organ, and pour its contents into a bucket marked with the animal's identification and the organ being examined. Scrape the interior lining of the organ with a spatula or the blunt edge of a pair of scissors, and add the scrapings to the bucket.
2. Add an equal volume of water to the contents in each labeled bucket and mix thoroughly with a stirring spoon or paddle.
3. Allow the heavier part of the contents to settle to the bottom of the bucket. This usually takes about 45 minutes. Carefully pour off the liquid on top, leaving the sediment.
4. Add an equal volume of water to the sediment and stir again. Allow this to resettle. Repeat this process until the water over the sediment becomes clear.
5. Pour off the clear water over the sediment; then transfer the sediment to the dissection pan.
6. Using the dissecting microscope, examine a small amount of the sediment at a time. Any parasite found should be gently removed from the sediment with thumb forceps and should be preserved (see text). Each parasite should be identified using a compound microscope.

BOX 17-11 | Sieving Method for Sample Collection at Necropsy

1. Using wrapping twine, tie off each portion of the digestive tract (the stomach, duodenum, small intestine, large intestine, and so on). Open each organ, and pour its contents into a bucket marked with the animal's identification and the organ being examined. Scrape the interior lining of the organ with a spatula or the blunt edge of a pair of scissors, and add the scrapings to the bucket.
2. Add an equal volume of water to the contents in each labeled bucket and mix thoroughly with a stirring spoon or paddle.
3. Pour the mixture through a 1-mm mesh (No. 18) sieve and then through a 0.354-mm mesh (No. 45) sieve. Reverse wash the contents of the sieve with water. Sieves are available from Fisher Scientific, Pittsburgh, PA.
4. Using the dissecting microscope, examine a small amount of the sieve's contents at a time. Any parasite found should be gently removed from the contents with thumb forceps and should be preserved (see text). Each parasite should be identified using a compound microscope.

the different parts of the digestive tract should be separated into individual containers.

It is not always necessary to examine all sediment or sievings. An estimate of the number of worms may be obtained by counting an **aliquot** (a known percentage of the total volume) of the sediment.

When parasites are recovered from the digestive tract or other parts of the body, it may be necessary to preserve them for identification later. **Nematodes** (roundworms) should be briefly washed in water to remove any attached debris and then placed in hot 70% ethyl alcohol (ethanol). Isopropyl alcohol may be used but is not preferred. The alcohol is allowed to cool, after which the worms are examined. The worms may be stored in the alcohol after adding glycerine to make a 5% concentration. **Cestodes**

(tapeworms), including the scolices (heads), should be placed in water at about 37° C (98.6° F) for about 1 hour and then stored in a mixture of 5% glycerine or 70% alcohol or 5% to 10% formalin. **Trematodes** (flukes) may be preserved in the same manner as tapeworms. If tapeworms and flukes are to be stained later, they should be "relaxed" in alternate changes of ice water and tap water for about 3 hours and then lightly pressed between sheets of glass immersed in 10% formalin.

TECHNICIAN'S NOTE Parasites may be preserved and stored for future analysis. The preservation technique depends on the type of parasite. Nematodes are preserved differently than cestodes or trematodes.

Sometimes during necropsy of domestic animals, **cysticerci**, or bladder worms, are seen in the abdomen, muscles, or other internal organs. These

BOX 17-16	Buffy Coat Method

1. Fill a hematocrit tube with the whole-blood sample and seal one end with hematocrit clay.
2. In the hematocrit centrifuge, centrifuge the hematocrit tube for 5 minutes.
3. If desired, read the packed-cell volume to determine whether the animal is anemic. Observe the location of the buffy coat layer between the red cell layer and the plasma (Figure 17-17).
4. Place the hematocrit tube on the stage of the compound microscope. Using the 4× objective, examine the zone between the buffy coat layer and the plasma for the presence of microfilarial activity. Use the iris diaphragm to decrease the light because low light intensity and high contrast increase visualization of the motile microfilariae.
   or
   Using a small file or glass cutter, deeply scratch the hematocrit tube at the level of the buffy coat. Snap the hematocrit tube by applying thumb pressure opposite the scratch. Immediately take the part of the buffy coat and plasma and tap the buffy coat onto the center of a microscope slide, including some plasma with it. Add a drop of physiologic saline and a drop of methylene blue stain and cover with a coverslip. Using the 10× objective, examine the slide for the presence of microfilariae.

BOX 17-17	Modified Knott Technique

1. In a centrifuge tube with a conical end, mix 1 mL of the whole-blood sample and 9 mL of 2% formalin (2 mL of 40% formaldehyde per 98 mL of distilled water). Stopper the tube, and rock it back and forth for 1 to 2 minutes until the mixture becomes a clear, red-wine color.
2. Centrifuge the tube at 1500 rpm for 5 minutes.
3. Pour off the liquid supernatant. It is permissible to let the tube stand with the open end down for 45 minutes to 1 hour if time permits. The purpose of this step is to remove as much fluid as possible, leaving sediment only.
4. Add 1 drop of methylene blue stain to the sediment at the bottom of the tube. Transfer a drop of the mixture to a glass slide and apply a coverslip.
5. Examine the slide for the presence of microfilariae using the 10× objective. When microfilariae are found, use a higher-power objective (40×) to observe the fine differences between them (see Table 17-1).
6. The diagnostician may stop this procedure at one of two stopping points:
   (a) The diagnostician has identified microfilariae as those of *Dilofilaria immitis* or *Acanthocheilonema reconditum,* or
   (b) the diagnostician runs out of the sediment/stain mixture.

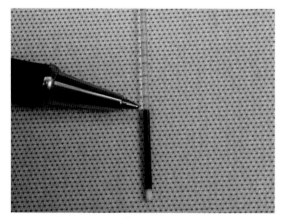

FIGURE 17-17 Buffy coat in a hematocrit tube.

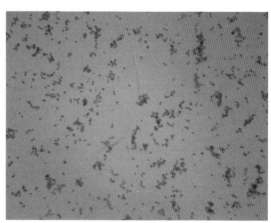

FIGURE 17-18 Microfilariae in a buffy coat smear of canine blood (500×).

the modified Knott procedure and may not be indicative of other tests that depend on observation of morphologic features of the microfilariae. The most accurate features are the total length of the microfilaria, the midbody width, and the shape of the cranial end. Body length and width should be measured using an ocular micrometer (see p. 310). The body length of the microfilaria of *D. immitis* ranges from 295 to 325 µm (average, 310 µm), whereas the body length of the microfilaria of *A. reconditum* ranges from 250 to 288 µm (average, 280 µm). The midbody width of the microfilaria of *D. immitis* ranges from 5 to 7.5 µm, whereas the midbody width of the microfilaria of *A. reconditum*

ranges from 4.5 to 5.5 µm. It is important for the differentiation of the morphologic parameters of the parasites on the modified Knott procedure that veterinary clinics own and calibrate an ocular micrometer within at least one compound microscope. The anterior end of the microfilaria of *D. immitis* tapers gradually from its midbody (Figure 17-19), whereas the microfilaria of *A. reconditum* has a blunt anterior end, much like the end of a wooden broom handle. Likewise, the posterior end of the microfilaria of *D. immitis* is said to be straight, whereas the microfilaria of *A. reconditum* may have a curved or "buttonhook" or "shepherd's crook" tail. It is important to remember that the bending, or hooking, of the tail of the microfilaria of *A. reconditum* is an artifact of 2% formalin fixation and may not be observed as a consistent diagnostic feature. Likewise, other microfilarial tests (e.g., commercial filter tests) will not produce this hooking characteristic. Veterinary diagnosticians should remember to measure several microfilariae to confirm that the microfilaremia is not a concomitant infection (i.e., both parasites may be present). In some areas of North America (those with high indigenous populations of both mosquitoes and fleas), infection with both filarial parasites is quite possible.

TABLE 17-1	Morphologic Characteristics for Differentiation of Microfilariae of *Dirofilaria Immitis* and *Acanthocheilonema Reconditum*	
CHARACTERISTIC	DIROFILARIA IMMITIS	ACANTHOCHEILONEMA RECONDITUM
Body shape	Usually straight	Usually curved
Body length	295-325 µm (average, 310 µm)	250-288 µm (average, 280 µm)
Anterior end	Tapered	Blunt ("broom handle")
Posterior end	Straight	Curved or hooked (artifact of formalin fixation)

> **TECHNICIAN'S NOTE** The morphologic features of *Dirofilaria immitis* and *Acanthocheilonema reconditum* are used for differentiation.

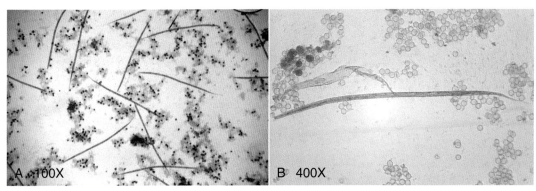

FIGURE 17-19 Microfilariae of *Dirofilaria immitis* using the modified Knott test.

Immunologic Heartworm Tests

About 25% of dogs with adult heartworm infection in the heart and pulmonary vasculature do not have circulating microfilariae in the peripheral blood. These infections may consist of (1) heartworms that are too young to produce microfilariae, (2) a "unisex" or "single-sex" infection, (3) an infection in which circulating microfilariae are produced by the adult female heartworms but for some reason are removed by the host, or (4) an infection in which the circulating microfilariae have been killed by a drug but the adults have not been affected. This type of infection is referred to as an **occult infection**. The hosts are said to be **amicrofilaremic**, without microfilariae. It is important to remember that cats also can be infected with canine heartworms. Because the heartworms are in cats rather than in their natural host (the dog), the adult heartworms produce either low numbers of microfilariae or none at all.

> **TECHNICIAN'S NOTE** With the monthly heartworm preventatives being used, animals are amicrofilaremic because the preventatives kill the microfilariae.

To detect infections, tests have been developed in which antibodies against antigens of adult *D. immitis* react with chemicals to produce a color change when these antigens are in a blood sample. These tests are available commercially and are easy to perform and fairly rapid (15 to 20 minutes) when the directions are carefully followed and samples are correctly labeled. Older styles of kits detected only canine antibodies in response to heartworm and were unsuitable for use in cats.

> **TECHNICIAN'S NOTE** Many heartworm immunologic test kits now are sensitive enough to detect antibodies in cats. However, it is recommended that an antibody test and an antigen test be used for cats because the worm burden is so low.

BOX 17-18 | Serum Collection

1. Using a needle and syringe, dispense 10 mL of blood into a blood collection vacuum tube lacking anticoagulant (tube with a red stopper). Slowly dispense the blood from the syringe into the tube to avoid lysis of the red blood cells. Lysis of red blood cells often interferes with the functions of many tests.
2. Keep the blood at room temperature (25° C) for 2 to 3 hours to allow a solid clot to form.
3. Remove the formed blood clot with a wooden applicator stick by gently "rimming" the clot and then sliding it up the side of the tube with the applicator stick. Discard the clot. (Some laboratories request that the clear serum then be transferred to a new tube.)
4. Correctly label each tube of serum with the client's name, animal's name or number, and practitioner's name. Refrigerate the sample until it can be shipped.
5. Ship samples to the laboratory packed in an insulated container with ice or a cool pack. Use the fastest shipper possible for next-day delivery.

Other tests for parasites such as *Toxoplasma gondii* can be performed by diagnostic laboratories. The laboratory will provide information on the nature and amount of specimens it requires. Box 17-18 provides a method for collecting serum for these immunologic tests.

Miscellaneous Methods for Microfilarial Identification

Other heartworm diagnostic procedures used in the detection and differentiation of microfilariae include staining with brilliant cresyl blue and acid phosphatase. These procedures are often too cumbersome and time-consuming to be used in a veterinary practice. Many of the reagents used in the processing of these specimens are not found in the practice setting. Diagnostic referral laboratories usually are able to perform both procedures.

DIAGNOSIS OF PARASITISM OF THE RESPIRATORY SYSTEM

FECAL EXAMINATION FOR RESPIRATORY PARASITES

> **TECHNICIAN'S NOTE** Because lungworms use the digestive system to pass their eggs or larvae after the animal coughs them up and swallows them, routine fecal flotation techniques and the Baermann technique can be used to find most of these parasite infections.

The life cycles of helminth (nematode and trematode) parasites of the lungs are completed through the passage of their eggs or larvae up the airways to the pharyngeal region, from which they are swallowed and passed to the outside environment in the feces. Because of this dependence on fecal transmission, parasitism of the lungs and airways is often diagnosed by microscopic examination of the feces, as described previously. The Baermann technique can be used to recover the larvae of lungworms from feces. Again, this method takes advantage of the fact that warm water stimulates the larvae in a sample to move about. Once the larvae move out of the sample, they relax in the water and sink to the bottom of the container. The Baermann apparatus should be employed when parasitism with lungworms is suspected (see p. 322).

EXAMINATION OF SPUTUM AND TRACHEAL WASHES

The larvae and eggs of respiratory parasites have the same characteristics as those found in the feces. An exception is *Dictyocaulus* species, lungworms of cattle and sheep, which are usually seen in the sputum as eggs containing larvae rather than as free larvae in the feces.

A drop of sputum or nasal discharge on a microscope slide is easily examined. Several slides should be examined. When the sputum is especially viscous, a drop of the material should be placed between two microscope slides and both slides examined microscopically. Larger quantities of fluid obtained from the respiratory tract should be concentrated by centrifugation at 1500 rpm for 5 minutes. A drop of the sediment can then be placed on a slide and examined microscopically.

> **TECHNICIAN'S NOTE** Some endoparasites do not use the digestive tract to complete their life cycle but instead use sputum. Therefore the sputum can be examined for eggs or larvae by either a direct smear or centrifugation performed like a fecal sample.

Dogs may occasionally become infested with the nasal mite, *Pneumonyssoides caninum,* or the tongue worm, *Linguatula serrata.* A cotton swab dipped in mineral oil may be inserted into the nose of a suspect dog and rubbed against the nasal membranes. *Pneumonyssoides* mites have eight legs and are white, hairless, and 1 to 1.5 mm long. The eggs of *L. serrata* measure 90×70 µm and contain a mitelike larval stage. Tiny hooked feet may be observed in the interior of the egg.

DIAGNOSIS OF PARASITISM OF THE URINARY SYSTEM

Roundworms are common parasites of the kidney and urinary bladder. They complete their life cycle by passing eggs out of the host's body in the urine. These nematodes include *Capillaria* species, which inhabit the walls of portions of the urinary system of both dogs and cats, *Dioctophyma renale,* the giant kidney worm of dogs, and *Stephanurus dentatus,* the swine kidney worm.

> **TECHNICIAN'S NOTE** Some endoparasite eggs can be found in the urine of the animal.

COLLECTION OF THE URINE SAMPLE

Urine for parasitologic examination may be collected during normal urination. Catheterization and cystocentesis are usually not necessary unless part of the sample will be used for bacteriologic or cytologic examination. A waxed paper cup (3-5 mL) with a lid or other clean container may be used for collection. The cup is held in the urine stream and filled. Unless the sample is to be used for other tests, it is not necessary to collect the sample at a certain time during urination. Clients can be instructed to collect a sample at home. Urine samples should be properly labeled with the client's name and the animal's identification and refrigerated until the examination can be conducted.

URINE EXAMINATION FOR PARASITES

The primary method of examining urine for parasites is by microscopic examination of the sediment (Box 17-19). Just as with microscopic examination of feces using the compound microscope, uniform movement and a thorough search of the microscope slide must be performed. Regardless of how the slide is moved, the area under the coverslip must be thoroughly and uniformly searched (see Figure 17-8). When a parasite egg is observed at low magnification, higher-power objectives may be used to examine it more closely.

> *TECHNICIAN'S NOTE* **Urine sedimentation** is used to find parasite eggs in the urine of an animal.

DIAGNOSIS OF PARASITISM OF THE SKIN

SKIN SCRAPINGS

Skin scraping is one of the most common diagnostic tools used in evaluating animals with

dermatologic problems. Equipment required includes an electric clipper with a No. 40 blade, a scalpel or spatula, mineral oil in a small dropper bottle, a microscope slide, a coverslip, and a compound microscope. Typical lesions or sites likely to harbor the particular parasite should be scraped (e.g., margins of the ear for *Sarcoptes scabiei*).

The scraping is performed with a No. 10 scalpel blade used with or without a handle. A stainless steel spatula is preferred by some clinicians. The scalpel blade should be held between the thumb and the second finger, with the first finger used to help prevent cutting the animal (Figure 17-20). Before the skin is scraped, the blade is dipped in a drop of mineral oil on the slide or a drop of mineral oil may be placed on the skin.

During the scraping process, the blade must be held perpendicular to the skin. Holding it at another angle may result in the animal being incised. The average area scraped should be 6 to 8 cm^2.

> *TECHNICIAN'S NOTE* Skin scraping is performed with a No. 10 scalpel blade held perpendicular to the skin so the blade does not incise the animal.

The depth of the scraping varies with the typical location of the parasite in question. When scraping for mites that live in tunnels (e.g., *Sarcoptes* spp.) or

BOX 17-19	Urine Sedimentation

1. Thoroughly mix the urine sample, and put 5 to 10 mL into a centrifuge tube with a conical tip.
2. Centrifuge the sample for 5 minutes at 1500 rpm.
3. Pipette all but about 0.5 mL of the fluid from the centrifuge tube, leaving the sediment at the bottom undisturbed.
4. Mix the remaining fluid and sediment together with the pipette; transfer a drop of the mixture to a microscope slide and apply a coverslip.
5. Thoroughly examine the drop of sediment microscopically using the 10× objective.

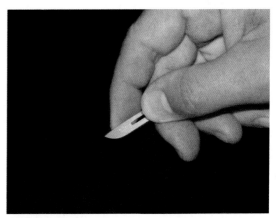

FIGURE 17-20 Safe method of holding a scalpel blade with the thumb and second finger for skin scrapings.

hair follicles and sebaceous glands (e.g., *Demodex* spp.), the skin should be scraped until a small amount of capillary blood oozes from the area. Clipping the area with a No. 40 blade before scraping enables better visualization of the lesion and removes excess hair that could impede proper scraping and interfere with collection of epidermal debris. For surface-dwelling mites (e.g., *Chorioptes* spp., *Cheyletiella* spp.), the skin is scraped superficially to collect loose scales and crusts. Clipping before scraping is not always necessary when infestation with surface-dwelling mites is suspected.

> **TECHNICIAN'S NOTE** The depth of the skin scrape depends on the type of ectoparasite suspected of causing the skin problem.

All the scraped debris on the forward surface of the blade is then spread in a drop of mineral oil on a glass microscope slide. A glass coverslip is placed on the material, and the slide is ready for microscopic examination using the 4× (scanning) objective. The slide should be examined systematically in rows so that the entire area under the coverslip is evaluated (see Figure 17-8). Low light intensity and high contrast increase visualization of mites and eggs. If necessary the slide may be evaluated using the 10× (low-power) objective.

Demonstration of a characteristic mite or egg is frequently diagnostic for most diseases. In certain circumstances, however, more than identification of the parasite is necessary. For example, determining live/dead ratios and observing immature stages of demodectic mites are important in evaluating a patient with demodicosis. A decrease in the number of live mites and eggs during therapy is a good prognostic sign.

CELLOPHANE TAPE PREPARATION

When attempting to demonstrate the presence of lice or mites that live primarily on the surface of the skin (e.g., *Cheyletiella* spp.), use a cellophane tape preparation instead of a skin scraping. Clear cellophane tape is applied to the skin to pick up epidermal debris. A ribbon of mineral oil is placed on a glass slide, and the adhesive surface of the tape is placed on a glass slide and then placed on the mineral oil. Additional mineral oil and a coverslip may be placed on the tape to prevent it from wrinkling, but this is not necessary. The slide is then examined systematically in rows.

GROSS SPECIMENS

Unknown large **ectoparasites** such as fleas, ticks, chigger mites, biting flies, and myiasis-producing maggots are often collected from the surface of the animal's skin. It is important that these arthropods be placed in a sealed container in either 10% formalin or 95% ethyl alcohol for shipment to a diagnostic laboratory. As many intact specimens as possible should be collected and shipped to a diagnostic laboratory capable of **speciating** these important ectoparasites. Again, containers should be properly labeled with the client's name and the animal's identification.

> **TECHNICIAN'S NOTE** Unknown large ectoparasites being sent to a diagnostic laboratory should be preserved in either 10% formalin or 95% ethyl alcohol for shipment.

DIAGNOSIS OF PARASITISM OF MISCELLANEOUS BODY SYSTEMS

PARASITES OF THE EYE

Thelazia species are nematodes that live within the conjunctival sac and on the surface of the eye of several species of domestic animals including cattle, sheep, goats, horses, dogs, and cats. The adult parasites are milky white and 7 to 17 mm long and reside in the conjunctival sac, just under the eyelids, particularly the third eyelid. Diagnosis is made by anesthetizing the eye with a local ophthalmologic anesthetic and directly examining the eye for parasites. If observed, these nematodes should be removed while the eye is anesthetized.

> **TECHNICIAN'S NOTE** Parasites found in the eye should be removed by the veterinarian while the eye is anesthetized for examination.

Another nematode parasite often associated with the eye is *D. immitis,* the canine heartworm. This parasite is often associated with aberrant locations throughout the body of both dogs and cats. A site that may become infected is the anterior chamber of the eye; this is usually noted with alarm by the pet owner. Treatment is by surgical extraction of the wandering ("lost") parasite by a veterinary ophthalmologist.

PARASITES OF THE EAR

Otodectes cynotis, the ear mite, is a common cause of external ear irritation in both dogs and cats. These white mites are frequently observed during otoscopic examination. *O. cynotis* are approximately the size of a grain of salt; they may be seen on a cotton swab after it has been moistened with mineral oil and used to clean the dark, waxy debris from the ears of infested animals. This material may be transferred to a drop of mineral oil on a microscope slide and spread out with the swab. A coverslip is applied to the debris, and the slide is examined microscopically in a systematic manner (Box 17-20). This mite has suckers on short stalks at the tips of some of its legs (Box 17-20).

> *TECHNICIAN'S NOTE* The ear smear is used to diagnose parasites of the ear.

PARASITES OF THE GENITAL TRACT

Tritrichomonas foetus is a protozoan parasite of the reproductive tract of cattle. These parasites reside in the prepuce of infected bulls and in the vagina, cervix, and uterus of infected cows. They may also be found within the stomach contents of aborted fetuses. *T. foetus* is pear-shaped and 10 to 25 μm

---

BOX 17-20 | Ear Smear Procedure

1. Obtain a sample of debris from the affected ear.
2. Place 2 or 3 drops of mineral oil on the slide and an equal amount of ear debris.
3. Mix the ear debris and mineral oil with a wooden applicator to form a homogeneous solution.
4. Remove large pieces of debris.
5. Place a coverslip over the smear.
6. Examine the slide under the compound microscope and record any parasites or parasite eggs found.

---

long, with a sail-like, undulating membrane and three rapidly moving, whiplike anterior flagella. In fresh specimens, these protozoans move actively with a jerky motion. Diagnosis is by finding the organisms in washings from the predilection sites or from the stomach of the aborted fetus. Fluid material should be centrifuged at 2000 rpm for 5 minutes. The supernatant is then removed and a drop of sediment transferred to a slide for microscopic examination for the organisms. Several slides should be examined. For more accurate diagnosis, fluid material from the predilection sites can be cultured in a special medium. Laboratories specializing in diagnostic parasitology should be consulted for information on these techniques.

> *TECHNICIAN'S NOTE* Fluid samples from the genital parasite's predilection site should be centrifuged to concentrate the parasites, and the sediment should be examined for organisms.

CHAPTER SEVENTEEN TEST

MATCHING—Match the term with the correct phrase or term.

A. Mineral deposits unique to tapeworms

B. Stage micrometer

C. Ocular micrometer

D. Specific gravity

E. Flotation solutions

F. Sheather solution

G. Sodium nitrate solution

H. Saturated sodium chloride

I. Zinc sulfate solution

J. Simple flotation technique

K. Fecal sedimentation technique

L. Quantitative procedures

M. Modified D'Antoni's iodine

N. Sporulation

O. Sporulated oocyst of *Eimeria*

P. Sporulated oocyst of *Cystoisospora*

Q. Cellophane tape preparation

R. Baermann apparatus

S. Modified Knott procedure

T. Immunologic heartworm tests

U. Occult heartworm infection

V. Amicrofilaremic

W. Microscopic examination of urine sediment

X. Skin scraping

Y. *Tritrichomonas foetus*

Z. *Otodectes cynotis*

1. Eyepiece scale

2. Does not require the use of a centrifuge

3. Process of development that takes place within a coccidian oocyst

4. Flotation medium that best concentrates cystic stages of *Giardia*

5. Used primarily in suspected trematode (fluke) infections

6. Calcareous bodies or calcareous corpuscles

7. Concentrated sugar or various salts added to water to increase its specific gravity and thus make parasite eggs float because they are lighter than the solution

8. Weight of an object compared with the weight of an equal volume of pure water

9. Two sporocysts, each with four sporozoites

10. Apparatus used to collect larval nematodes from fresh feces; a funnel is an essential part of this apparatus

11. Used to stain protozoan cysts such as *Giardia*

12. Four sporocysts, each with two sporozoites

13. Messy to work with because it is quite sticky; it is a sugar solution

14. Instrument used to calibrate a compound microscope

15. "Color change" test kits, many of which use antibodies against adult *Dirofilaria immitis* antigen

16. Term meaning "without microfilariae"

17. Collection of eggs of pinworms such as *Oxyuris equi*

18. Most efficient flotation solution, but it forms crystals and distorts eggs

19. Indicate the number of eggs or cysts present in each gram of feces

20. Least desirable flotation solution; can corrode the microscope

21. Diagnosed using the ear smear procedure

22. Used to differentiate microfilariae of *D. immitis* from those of *Acanthocheilonema reconditum*

23. Finding organisms in preputial washings of infected bulls

24. Dog with adult heartworms but no demonstration of circulating microfilariae

25. Performed using a No. 10 scalpel blade

26. Detection of ova of *Dioctophyma renale* or *Stephanurus dentatus*

QUESTIONS FOR THOUGHT AND DISCUSSION

1. For the following parasites, what is the best procedure for identifying each of the following parasites?
   - *Giardia* assemblages
   - *Aelurostrongylus abstrusus* larvae (feline lungworms)
   - *Fasciola hepatica*
   - *Dirofilaria immitis*
   - *Stephanurus dentatus*
   - *Sarcoptes scabiei* variety *canis*
   - *Acanthocheilonema reconditum*
   - *Tritrichomonas foetus*
   - *Dipylidium caninum*

2. Discuss the importance of accurate identification of the following parasites in a veterinary clinical situation.
   - *Giardia* assemblages
   - *Aelurostrongylus abstrussus* larvae (feline lungworms)
   - *Fasciola hepatica*
   - *Dirofilaria immitis*
   - *Stephanurus dentatus*
   - *Sarcoptes scabiei* variety *canis*
   - *Acanthocheilonema reconditum*
   - *Tritrichomonas foetus*
   - *Dipylidium caninum*

18 Reference to Common Parasite Ova and Forms Seen in Veterinary Medicine

OUTLINE

A major part of the veterinary technician's job is identifying parasites in feces, blood, skin scrapings, and cellophane tape techniques. This chapter is a quick reference guide for identifying those parasites often seen in feces, in blood, and on the skin of dogs, cats, horses, ruminants, swine, and exotic animals.

COMMON PARASITES OF DOGS AND CATS

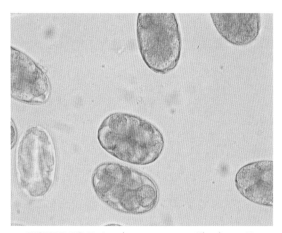

FIGURE 18-1 *Ancylostoma caninum* ("hookworm").

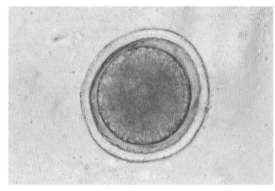

FIGURE 18-2 *Toxocara canis* ("roundworm").

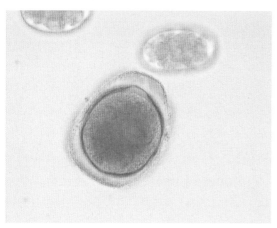

FIGURE 18-3 *Toxocara cati* ("roundworm").

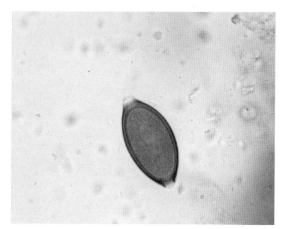

FIGURE 18-4 *Trichuris vulpis* ("whipworm").

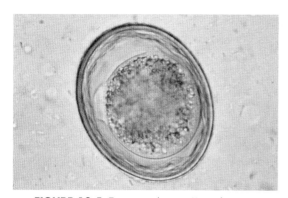

FIGURE 18-5 *Toxascaris leonina* ("roundworm").

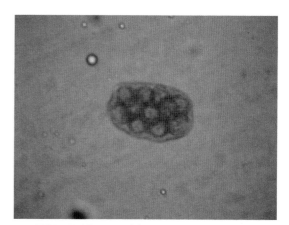

FIGURE 18-6 *Dipylidium caninum* ("tapeworm").

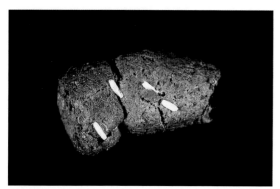

FIGURE 18-7 *Dipylidium caninum* segments in stool ("cucumber seed tapeworm").

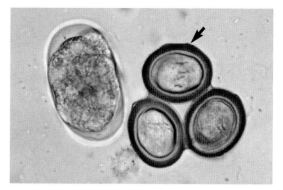

FIGURE 18-8 *Taenia pisiformis* ("tapeworm").

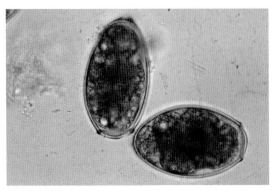

FIGURE 18-9 *Paragonimus kellicotti* ("lung fluke").

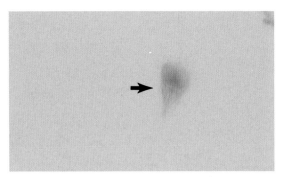

FIGURE 18-10 *Giardia* species trophozoite.

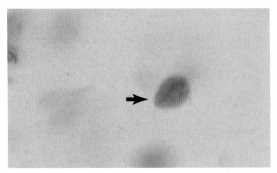

FIGURE 18-11 *Giardia* species oocyst.

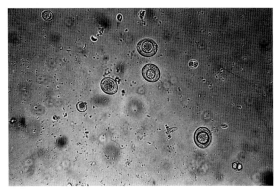

FIGURE 18-12 *Cystoisospora canis*, large oocysts ("coccidia").

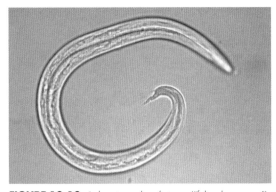

FIGURE 18-13 *Aelurostrongylus abstrusus* ("feline lungworm").

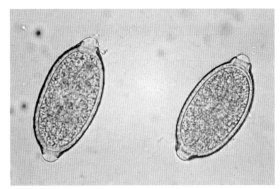

FIGURE 18-14 *Left*, *Trichuris vulpis* (whipworm). *Right*, *Eucoleus aerophilus* (lungworm).

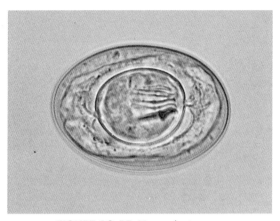

FIGURE 18-15 *Hymenolepis nana.*

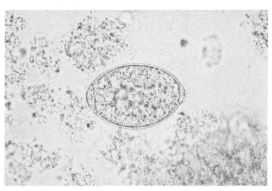

FIGURE 18-16 *Spirometra mansonoides* ("zipper tape-worm").

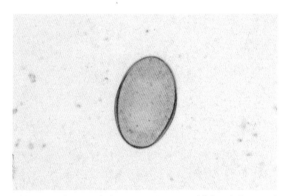

FIGURE 18-17 *Alaria* species ("intestinal fluke of dogs and cats").

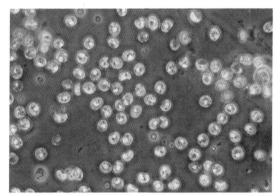

FIGURE 18-18 *Cryptosporidium* species ("cryptosporidium" or "cryptosporidiosis").

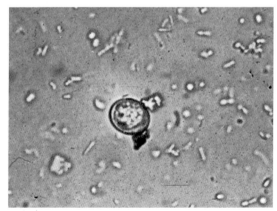

FIGURE 18-19 *Toxoplasma gondii* ("toxoplasma or toxo-plasmosis").

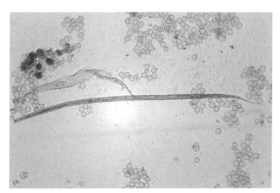

FIGURE 18-20 *Dirofilaria immitis* microfilariae ("heart-worm").

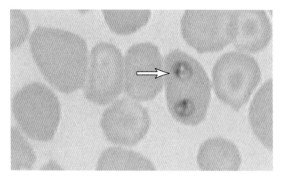

FIGURE 18-21 *Babesia canis* ("babesia").

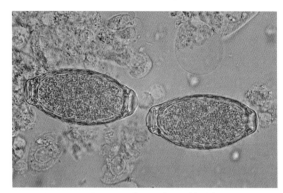

FIGURE 18-22 *Capillaria plica* ("bladder worm").

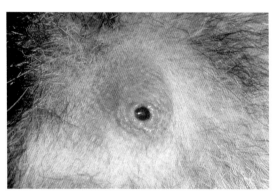

FIGURE 18-23 *Cuterebra* species ("warbles or wolves").

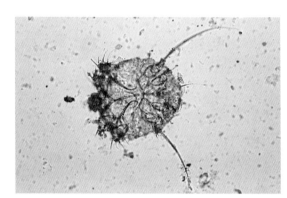

FIGURE 18-24 *Sarcoptes scabei* variety *canis* ("scabies").

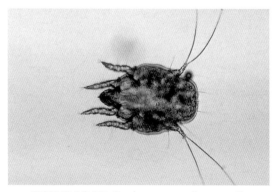

FIGURE 18-25 *Otodectes cynotis* ("ear mites").

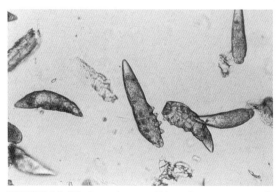

FIGURE 18-26 *Demodex canis* ("demodectic mange mite").

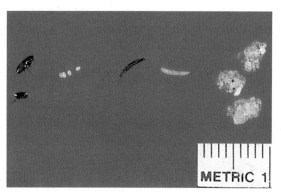

FIGURE 18-27 Flea life cycle stages (adults, eggs, larvae, and pupae).

COMMON PARASITES OF HORSES

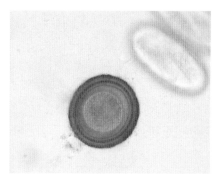

FIGURE 18-30 *Parascaris equorum* ("equine roundworm").

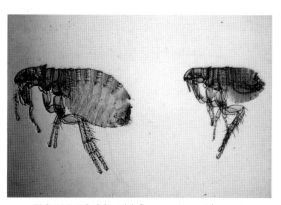

FIGURE 18-28 Adult fleas (male and female).

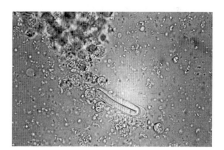

FIGURE 18-31 *Habronema* species ("equine stomach worm").

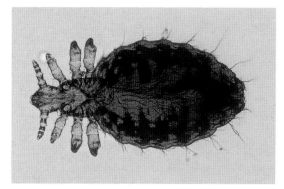

FIGURE 18-29 *Linognathus setosus* ("sucking louse of dogs").

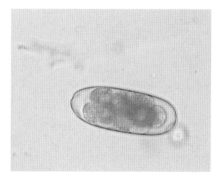

FIGURE 18-32 *Strongylus vulgaris* ("equine hookworm").

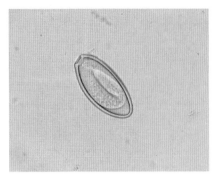

FIGURE 18-33 *Oxyuris equi* ("equine pinworm").

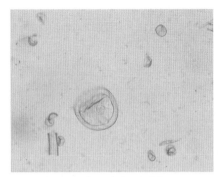

FIGURE 18-34 *Anoplocephala perfoliata* ("equine tapeworm").

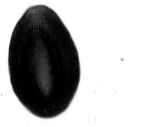

FIGURE 18-35 *Eimeria leuckarti* ("equine coccidia").

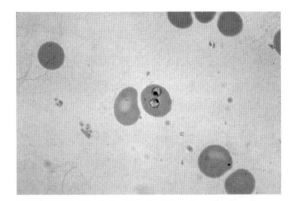

FIGURE 18-36 *Babesia caballi* ("equine piroplasm").

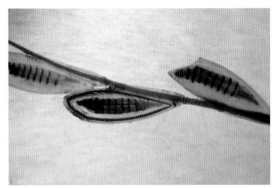

FIGURE 18-37 *Gastrophilus* species eggs ("horse bot fly eggs").

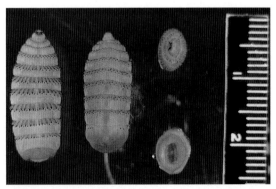

FIGURE 18-38 *Gastrophilus* species larvae ("horse bot fly larvae").

COMMON PARASITES OF RUMINANTS

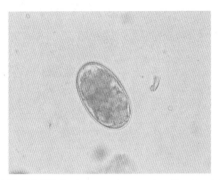

FIGURE 18-39 *Trichostrongylus* species ("ruminant hookworm").

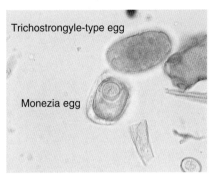

Trichostrongyle-type egg

Monezia egg

FIGURE 18-42 *Moniezia* species, square ("ruminant tapeworm").

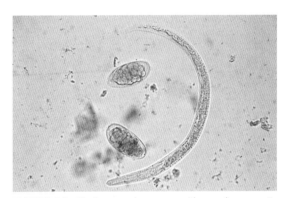

FIGURE 18-40 *Dictyocaulus viviparus* ("bovine lungworm").

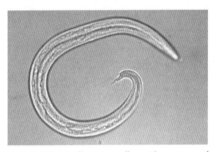

FIGURE 18-43 *Muellerius capillaris* ("lungworm of sheep and goats").

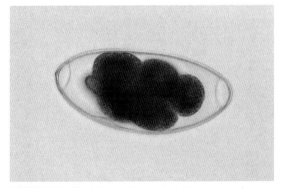

FIGURE 18-41 *Nematodirus* species ("ruminant trichostrongyle").

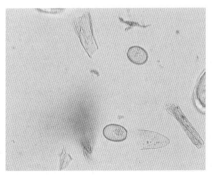

FIGURE 18-44 *Eimeria species* ("ruminant coccidia").

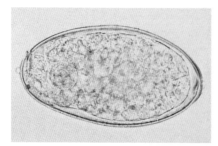

FIGURE 18-45 *Fasciola hepatica* ("ruminant liver fluke").

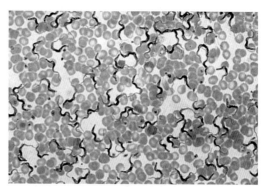

FIGURE 18-46 *Trypanosoma* species in bovine blood ("trypanosome").

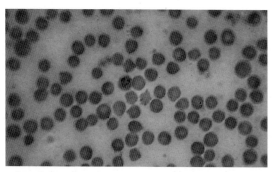

FIGURE 18-47 *Babesia bigemina* in bovine red blood cells ("babesia").

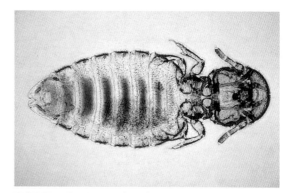

FIGURE 18-48 *Damalinia bovis* ("biting/chewing lice of cattle").

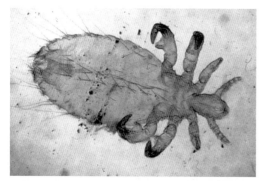

FIGURE 18-49 *Solenopotes capillatus* ("sucking louse of sheep").

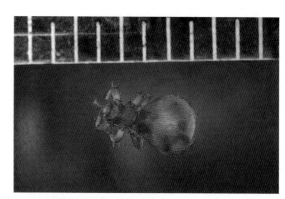

FIGURE 18-50 *Melophagus ovinus* ("sheep ked").

COMMON PARASITES OF SWINE

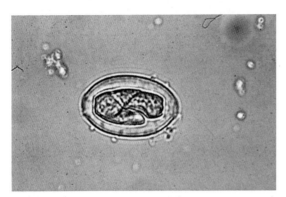

FIGURE 18-51 *Ascarops strongylina* ("swine stomach worm").

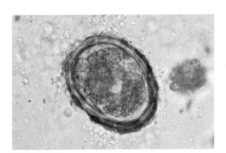

FIGURE 18-52 *Ascaris suum* ("swine roundworm").

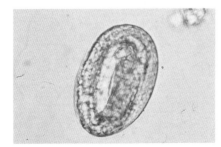

FIGURE 18-53 *Metastrongylus apri* ("swine lungworm").

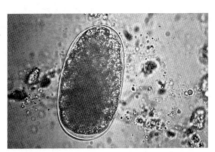

FIGURE 18-54 *Stephanurus dentatus* ("swine kidney worm").

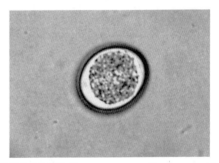

FIGURE 18-55 *Cystoisospora suis* ("swine coccidia").

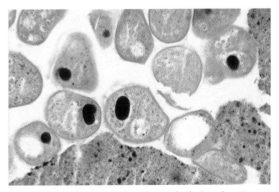

FIGURE 18-56 *Balantidium coli* ("balantidium").

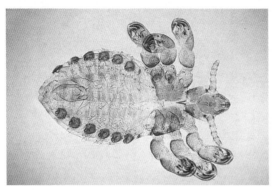

FIGURE 18-57 *Haematopinus suis*, adult ("sucking lice of pigs").

COMMON PARASITES OF EXOTIC PETS AND BIRDS

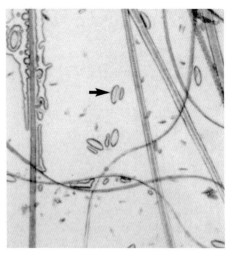

FIGURE 18-59 *Syphacia muris* ("pinworm of mice and rats"—cellophane tape technique).

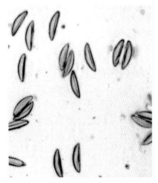

FIGURE 18-58 *Syphacia obvelata* ("pinworm of mice").

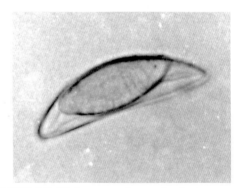

FIGURE 18-60 *Dentostomella translucida* ("pinworm of gerbils").

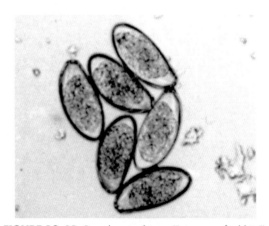

FIGURE 18-61 *Passalurus ambiguus* ("pinworm of rabbits").

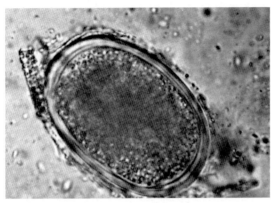

FIGURE 18-62 *Ascaridia* species ("roundworm of birds").

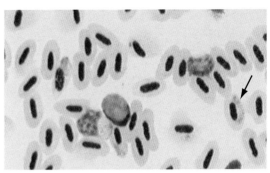

FIGURE 18-63 *Trichomonas gallinae* ("trichomona of birds").

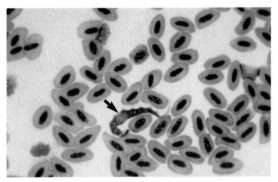

FIGURE 18-64 *Trypanosoma* species ("trypanosomes of birds").

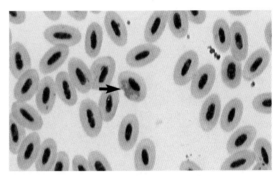

FIGURE 18-65 *Haemoproteus* species ("*Haemoproteus* of birds").

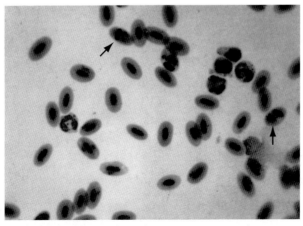

FIGURE 18-66 *Plasmodium* species ("avian malaria").

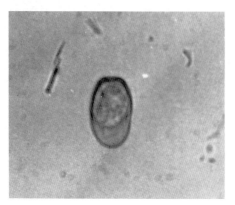

FIGURE 18-67 Unsporulated *Eimeria magna* ("coccidia of rabbits").

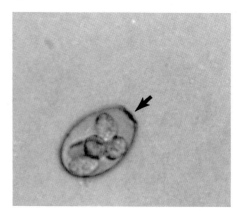

FIGURE 18-68 Sporulated *Eimeria magna* ("coccidia of rabbits").

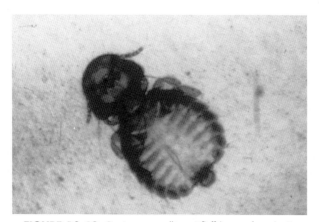

FIGURE 18-69 *Goniocotes gallinae* ("fluff louse of poultry").

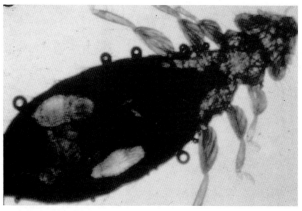

FIGURE 18-70 *Menacanthus stramineus* ("avian body louse").

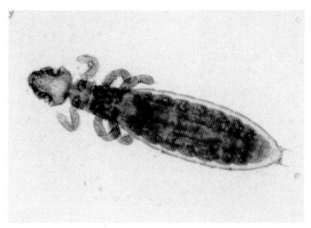

FIGURE 18-71 *Gliricola porcelli* ("guinea pig chewing louse").

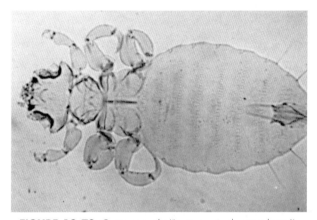

FIGURE 18-72 *Gyropus ovalis* ("guinea pig chewing louse").

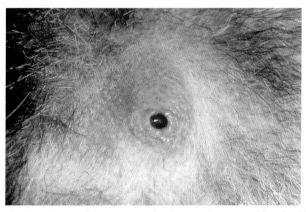

FIGURE 18-73 *Cuterebra* species under skin ("wolves or warbles of rabbits").

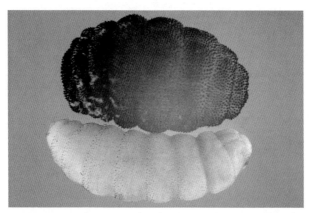

FIGURE 18-74 *Cuterebra* species larval stages ("wolves or warbles of rabbits").

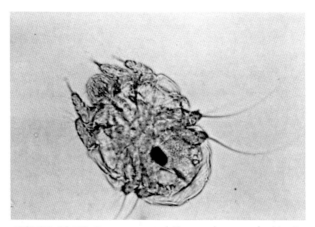

FIGURE 18-75 *Psoroptes cuniculi* ("ear canker mite of rabbits").

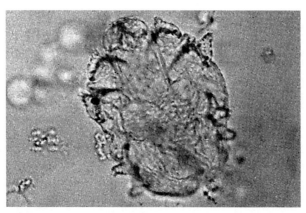

FIGURE 18-76 *Trixacarus caviae* ("sarcoptic mite of guinea pigs").

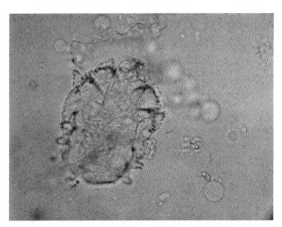

FIGURE 18-77 *Cnemidocoptes pilae* ("sarcoptic mite of birds").

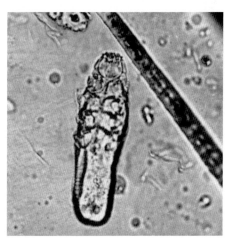

FIGURE 18-78 *Demodex criceti* ("demodectic mite of hamsters").

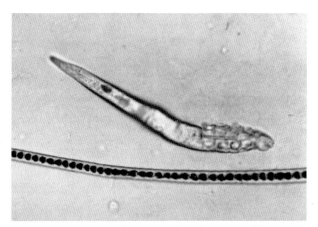

FIGURE 18-79 *Demodex aurati* ("demodectic mite of hamsters").

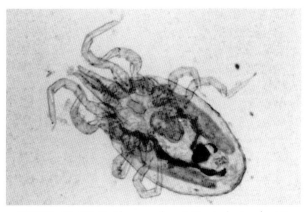

FIGURE 18-80 *Ornithonyssus bacoti* ("tropical mite of rats").

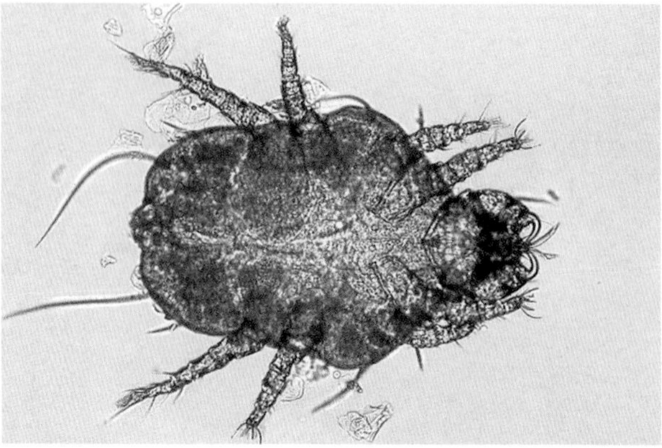

FIGURE 18-81 *Cheyletiella parasitivorax* ("fur mite of rabbits, dogs, and cats").

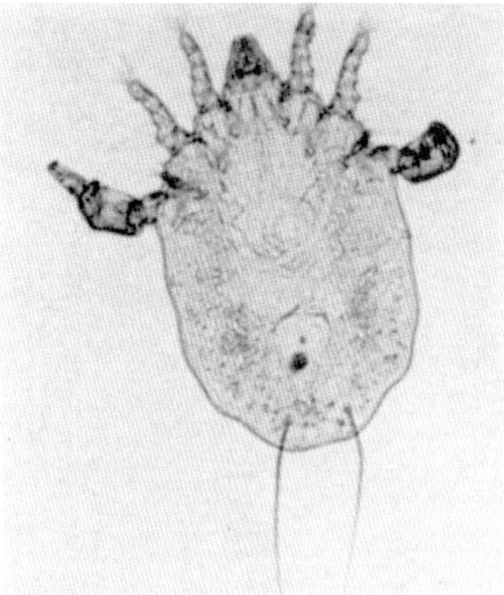

FIGURE 18-82 *Myocoptes musculinus* ("fur mite of mice").

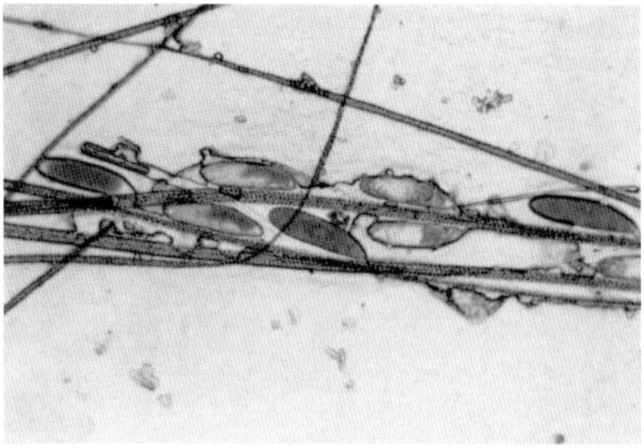

FIGURE 18-83 *Myocoptes musculinus* nits ("fur mite of mice"; nits).

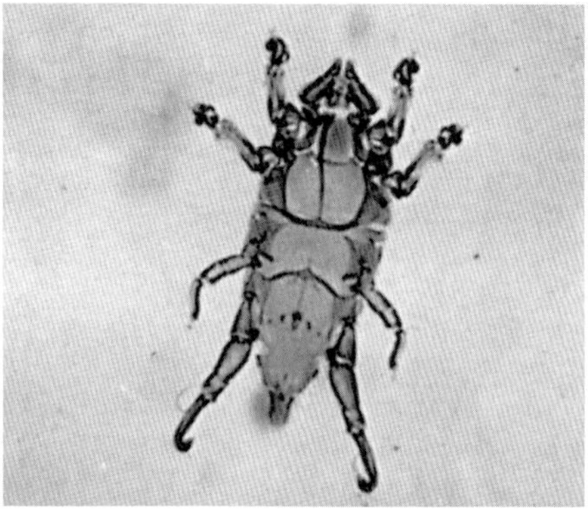

FIGURE 18-84 *Chirodiscoides caviae* ("fur mite of guinea pigs").

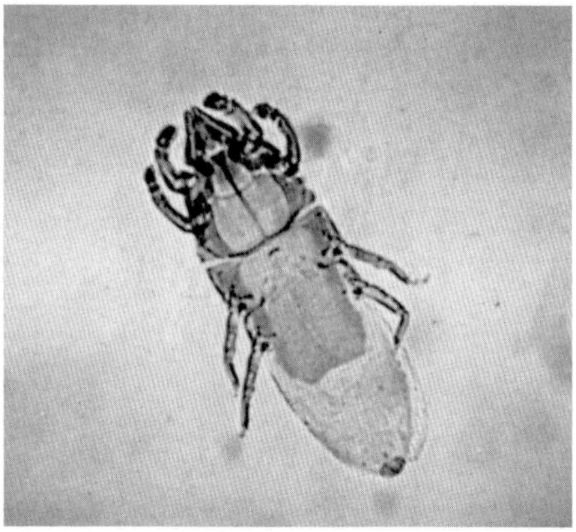

FIGURE 18-85 *Chirodiscoides caviae* (female "fur mite of guinea pigs").

PSEUDOPARASITES

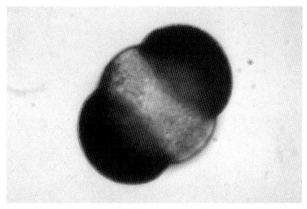

FIGURE 18-86 Pine pollen.

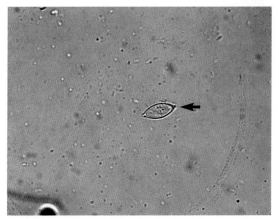

FIGURE 18-87 *Monocystis* (sporulated) parasite of the earthworm.

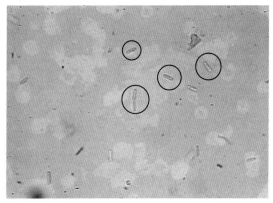

FIGURE 18-89 *Saccharomycopsis guttulatus,* a yeast of the rabbit alimentary tract.

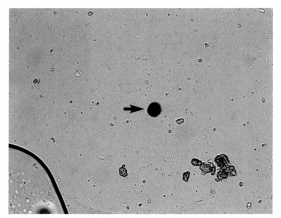

FIGURE 18-88 Pollen.

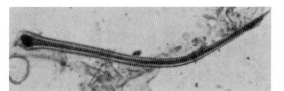

FIGURE 18-90 Plant hair. (From Bowman: *Georgis' parasitology for veterinarians,* ed 9, 2008, Elsevier.)

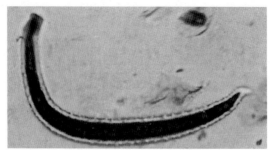

FIGURE 18-91 Plant hair. (From Bowman: *Georgis' parasitology for veterinarians*, ed 9, 2008, Elsevier.)

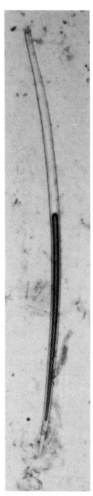

FIGURE 18-92 Plant hair. (From Bowman: *Georgis' parasitology for veterinarians*, ed 9, 2008, Elsevier.)

Parasite Reference List by Species and Parasite Type

PARASITES OF DOGS AND CATS

NEMATODES

Acanthocheilonema reconditum, pp. 39-41, 44, 48-49, 230, 310, 325-328

Aelurostrongylus abstrusus, pp. 31-34

Ancylostoma braziliense, pp. 31-34, 291-292

Ancylostoma caninum, pp. 31-34, 291-293, 296, 336

Ancylostoma tubaeforme, p. 27

Aonchotheca putorii or *Capillaria putorii*, p. 47

Pearsonema (Capillaria) feliscati, p. 47

Pearsonema (Capillaria) plica, p. 47

Dioctophyma renale, pp. 16, 46, 330

Dirofilaria immitis, pp. 38-42, 48, 324, 328, 339

Dracunculus insignis, pp. 48-50

Enterobius vermicularis, p. 37

Eucoleus aerophilus or *Capillaria aerophila*, pp. 45, 338

Eucoleus böehmi, p. 45

Filaroides hirthi, p. 44

Filaroides milksi, p. 44

Filaroides osleri, p. 44

Ollulanus tricuspis, pp. 27-28, 323

Pelodera strongyloides, pp. 47-48

Physaloptera species, pp. 26-27, 323

Spirocerca lupi, pp. 25-26

Strongyloides stercoralis, pp. 34-35, 292-295, 318, 323

Strongyloides tumiefaciens, pp. 34-35

Thelazia californiensis, p. 50

Toxocara canis, pp. 28-29

Toxocara cati, pp. 28-29

Toxascaris leonina, pp. 28-29, 323, 337

Trichuris campanula, pp. 31, 35-37

Trichuris serrata, pp. 31, 35-37

Trichuris vulpis, pp. 31, 35-37

Uncinaria stenocephala, pp. 31-34, 291-292

CESTODES

Diphyllobothrium species, pp. 120-121

Dipylidium caninum, pp. 103-107, 286, 307, 337

Echinococcus granulosus, pp. 103, 113-115

Echinococcus multilocularis, pp. 103, 113-115

Mesocestoides species, pp. 103, 115-116

Multiceps serialis, pp. 112-113

Spirometra species, pp. 119-120, 286-287

Taenia hydatigena, pp. 101, 103, 106-110

Taenia multiceps, pp. 101, 103, 106-110

Taenia ovis, pp. 101, 103, 106-110

Taenia pisiformis, pp. 101, 103, 106-110, 307, 337

Taenia taeniaeformis or *Hydatigera taeniaeformis*, pp. 110-111

TREMATODES

Alaria species, pp. 135-136, 339

Heterobilharzia americanum, pp. 136-139

Nanophyetus salmincola, pp. 134-135

Paragonimus kellicotti, pp. 136-137, 338

Platynosomum fastosum, pp. 134-135

ACANTHOCEPHALANS

Oncicola canis, pp. 142, 146

PROTOZOANS

Babesia canis, pp. 65-66, 340

Balantidium coli, pp. 157, 172-173, 317, 345

Cryptosporidium species, pp. 160-161, 164, 220-222, 339

Cytauxzoon felis, p. 166

Entamoeba histolytica, pp. 156-157

Giardia species, pp. 154-156, 180, 313, 317, 338

Hepatozoon americanum, pp. 166-167

Hepatozoon canis, pp. 166-167

Cystoisospora canis, pp. 158-159

Cystoisospora felis, pp. 158-159

Cystoisospora ohioensis, pp. 158-159

Cystoisospora rivolta, pp. 158-159

Cystoisospora wallacei, pp. 158-159

Leishmania species, p. 165

Sarcocystis species, p. 164

Eimeria zuernii, p. 167
Tritrichomonas foetus, pp. 169-170, 333
Trypanosoma species, pp. 164-165, 168, 344

ARTHOPODS

Aedes species, p. 211
Amblyomma americanum, p. 260
Amblyomma maculatum, p. 260
Anopheles species, pp. 210-211
Calliphora species, pp. 216, 218, 220
Chorioptes bovis, pp. 239-240
Chorioptes caprae, pp. 239-240
Chorioptes ovis, pp. 239-240
Chrysops species, pp. 207-211
Cochliomyia hominivorax, pp. 220-222
Culex species, pp. 210-211
Culicoides species, pp. 210-211
Damalinia bovis, p. 201
Demodex species, pp. 242-244
Dermacentor andersoni, pp. 253-259
Dermacentor occidentalis, pp. 259-260
Glossina species, p. 212
Haematobia irritans, pp. 207, 214
Hippelates species, p. 219
Hypoderma lineatum, pp. 223-224
Lucilia species, pp. 216, 218, 220
Lutzomyia species, pp. 207-209
Melophagus ovinus, pp. 207, 215, 344
Musca autumnalis, pp. 3, 50, 57, 67, 207, 213, 217
Musca domestica, pp. 216-217
Oestrus ovis, pp. 225-226
Otobius megnini, pp. 253, 255-256
Phaenicia species, pp. 216, 218, 220
Phormia species, pp. 216, 228, 220
Psoroptes bovis, pp. 238-239
Psoroptes ovis, pp. 238-239
Rhipicephalus annulatus, pp. 253-254, 257-258
Sarcophaga species, pp. 216, 218, 220
Sarcoptes scabei, pp. 232-236, 299, 331, 340
Simulium species, pp. 207-208, 219
Solenopotes capillatus, pp. 13, 18, 207-208, 219, 344
Stomoxys calcitrans, pp. 212-214, 217
Tabanus species, pp. 207, 211
Trombicula species, pp. 244-245

ANNELIDS

Haemopis terrestris, p. 274

PARASITES OF HORSES
NEMATODES

Dictyocaulus arnfieldi, p. 65
Draschia megastoma, pp. 58-59
Habronema microstoma, pp. 58-59
Habronema muscae, pp. 58-59
Onchocerca cervicalis, pp. 66-67
Oxyuris equi, pp. 63-65, 342
Parascaris equorum, pp. 59-61, 341
Setaria equina, p. 67
Strongyloides westeri, pp. 62-63, 292, 294
Strongylus edentatus, pp. 61-62
Strongylus equinus, pp. 61-62
Strongylus vulgaris, pp. 61-62, 341
Thelazia lacrymalis, p. 67
Trichostrongylus axei, pp. 59, 68

CESTODES

Anoplocephala magna, pp. 102-103
Anoplocephala perfoliata, pp. 102-103
Paranoplocephala mamillana, pp. 102-103

PROTOZOANS

Babesia caballi, pp. 171, 342
Eimeria leuckarti, pp. 170, 342
Giardia equi, pp. 154-156, 170
Klossiella equi, p. 171
Sarcocystis neurona, p. 172
Theileria equi, p. 171

ARTHROPODS

Aedes species, p. 211
Amblyomma americanum, p. 260
Amblyomma maculatum, p. 260
Anopheles species, pp. 210-211
Calliphora species, pp. 216, 218, 220
Chorioptes equi, pp. 239-240
Chrysops species, pp. 207-211
Cochliomyia hominivorax, pp. 220-222
Culex species, pp. 210-211
Culicoides species, pp. 208-210
Demodex equi, p. 242
Dermacentor andersoni, pp. 253-259
Dermacentor occidentalis, pp. 259-260
Gastrophilus species, p. 250
Glossina species, p. 212

Echidnophaga gallinacea, pp. 226-229
Glossina species, p. 212
Goniocotes gallinae, p. 201
Haemaphysalis leporispalustris, pp. 261-262
Lynchia species, p. 216
Menacanthus stramineus, p. 201
Ornithonyssus sylviarum, p. 246
Pseudolynchia species, p. 216

ANNELIDS

Theromyzon tessulatum, p. 274

PARASITES OF RABBITS
NEMATODES

Obeliscoides cuniculi, p. 79
Passalurus ambiguus, pp. 78-79
Trichostrongylus calcaratus, p. 79

PROTOZOANS

Eimeria irresidua, pp. 178-179
Eimeria magna, pp. 178-179
Eimeria media, pp. 178-179
Eimeria perforans, pp. 178-179
Eimeria stiedae, pp. 179-180

ARTHROPODS

Cediopsylla simplex, pp. 226-227
Cheyletiella parasitivorax, pp. 247-248
Cuterebra species, pp. 221-223
Dermacentor occidentalis, pp. 259-260
Dermacentor variabilis, pp. 253-254, 258
Haemaphysalis leporispalustris, pp. 261-262
Hemodipsus ventricosus, pp. 206-207
Listrophorus gibbus, pp. 252-253
Odontopsylla multispinosus, pp. 226-227
Psoroptes cuniculi, pp. 235-238
Sarcoptes scabei, pp. 232-236, 299, 331, 340

PARASITES OF GUINEA PIGS
NEMATODES

Paraspidodera uncinata, pp. 77-78

PROTOZOANS

Cryptosporidium wrairi, pp. 184-185
Eimeria caviae, p. 184

Entamoeba caviae, pp. 183-184
Giardia caviae, p. 183
Giardia muris, p. 180
Tritrichomonas caviae, p. 180

ARTHROPODS

Chirodiscoides caviae, pp. 251-252
Dermacentor andersoni, pp. 253, 259
Dermacentor occidentalis, pp. 259-260
Dermacentor variabilis, pp. 253-254, 258
Gliricola porcelli, p. 206
Gyropus ovalis, p. 206
Notoedres muris, pp. 234-236
Ornithonyssus bacoti, pp. 246-247
Panstrongylus species, p. 200
Rhodnius species, p. 200
Sarcoptes scabei, pp. 232-236, 299, 331, 340
Triatoma species, p. 200
Trixacarus caviae, pp. 232, 235, 237

PARASITES OF RATS
NEMATODES

Aspiculuris tetraptera, pp. 73-75
Syphacia muris, pp. 73-75
Syphacia obvelata, pp. 73-75
Trichosomoides crassicauda, p. 79

CESTODES

Hymenolepis diminuta, pp. 95-96, 287-288
Hymenolepis nana, pp. 95-96, 339

PROTOZOANS

Eimeria nieschultzi, p. 182
Giardia muris, p. 180
Spironucleus muris, pp. 180-181
Tetratrichomonas microti, p. 180
Tritrichomonas muris, p. 180

ARTHROPODS

Cuterebra species, pp. 221-223
Dermacentor andersoni, pp. 253, 259
Dermacentor occidentalis, pp. 259-260
Dermacentor variabilis, pp. 253-25, 258
Notoedres muris, pp. 234-236
Ornithonyssus bacoti, pp. 246-247
Panstrongylus species, p. 200
Polyplax spinulosa, pp. 203-205

Radfordia ensifera, pp. 249-250
Rhodnius species, p. 200
Triatoma species, p. 200

PARASITES OF MICE

NEMATODES

Aspiculuris tetraptera, pp. 73-75
Syphacia muris, pp. 73-75
Syphacia obvelata, pp. 73-75

CESTODES

Hymenolepis diminuta, pp. 95-96, 287-288
Hymenolepis nana, pp. 95-96, 339

PROTOZOANS

Eimeria falciformis, p. 181
Eimeria ferrisi, p. 181
Eimeria hansonorum, p. 181
Eimeria hansorium, p. 181
Giardia muris, p. 180
Klossiella muris, p. 171
Spironucleus muris, pp. 180-181
Tetratrichomonas microti, p. 180
Tritrichomonas muris, p. 180

ARTHROPODS

Cuterebra species, pp. 221-223
Dermacentor andersoni, pp. 253, 259
Dermacentor occidentalis, pp. 259-260
Dermacentor variabilis, pp. 253-254, 258
Ixodes scapularis, pp. 253-254, 257
Myobia musculi, pp. 249-251
Myocoptes musculinus, pp. 249-250
Polyplax serrata, pp. 203-205
Ornithonyssus bacoti, pp. 246-247
Radfordia affinis, pp. 249-251
Radfordia ensifera, pp. 249-251

PARASITES OF HAMSTERS

NEMATODES

Syphacia muris, pp. 73-75
Syphacia obvelata, pp. 73-75

CESTODES

Hymenolepis diminuta, pp. 95-96, 287-288
Hymenolepis nana, pp. 95-96, 339

PROTOZOANS

Giardia species, pp. 154-156, 180, 313, 317, 338
Spironucleus muris, pp. 182-183
Tritrichomonas muris (criceti), pp. 182-183

ARTHROPODS

Demodex aurati, pp. 243, 351
Demodex criceti, pp. 243, 351
Ornithonyssus bacoti, pp. 246-247

PARASITES OF GERBILS

NEMATODES

Dentostomella translucida, pp. 76-77, 346

CESTODES

Hymenolepis diminuta, pp. 95-96, 287-288
Hymenolepis nana, pp. 95-96, 339

ARTHROPODS

Demodex aurati, pp. 243, 351
Demodex criceti, pp. 243, 351
Hoplopleura meridionidis, p. 205

PARASITES OF FISH

PROTOZOANS

Cryptocaryon irritans, p. 185
Ichthyophthirius multifiliis, pp. 150, 185

PARASITES OF REPTILES

PENTASTOMES

Armillifer species, p. 267
Porocephalus crotali, pp. 268-269
Porocephalus species, pp. 267-269
Kiricephalus species, p. 267

ARTHROPODS

Glossina species, p. 212

Glossary

A

Aberrant parasite: Parasite that has wandered from its usual site of infection into an organ or location in which it does not ordinarily live; also called *erratic parasite.*

Acanthella: Larval acanthocephalan within the intermediate host, where the acanthella develops into a juvenile acanthocephalan, the *cystacanth.*

Acanthocephalan: A thorny-headed worm.

Acanthor: Larval acanthocephalan parasite within an egg.

Acariasis: Any infestation or infection by either mites or ticks.

Acaricides: Chemical compounds developed to kill mites and ticks.

Acarines: Mites and ticks.

Accession number: A log-in number to identify a submitted biological sample for a patient (either small or large animal). The assigned accession number identifies all parameters related to the case, especially the results of diagnostic procedures.

Acetabulum: One of four suckers on the anterior end of a true tapeworm (*eucestode*).

Acquired toxoplasmosis: Infection with *Toxoplasma gondii* by ingestion of sporulated oocysts or ingestion of bradyzoites from infected meat.

Adult fluke: The sexually mature stage of a trematode. Flukes have a set of completely functioning male and female reproductive organs making them hermaphrodites.

Aliquot: Percentage of a solution or sample.

Alopecia: Hair loss.

Amastigote: Resting cyst stage of some protozoans.

Amicrofilaremic: Referring to the absence of immature filarial parasites.

Amphistome: Type of digenetic fluke with an oral sucker on one end and a ventral sucker on the other end.

Annelids: Earthworms.

Anoplurans: Members of the class Insecta, order Anoplura. This order includes the sucking lice.

Anthelmintics: Chemical compounds developed to kill roundworms, tapeworms, flukes, and thorny-headed worms; also called *anthelminthics.*

Antiprotozoals: Chemical compounds developed to kill protozoan organisms.

Apicomplexan: Banana-, comma-, or boomerang-shaped protozoans found in epithelial cells of the intestine, in blood cells, and in cells of the reticuloendothelial and nervous systems. Apicomplexans have complex life cycles that are intimately integrated into the physiology of the host's body. Their locomotory (movement) organelles are internal and are not grossly visible as with other types of protozoans.

Argasid: A family of ticks with soft bodies.

Armed tapeworm: True tapeworm that possesses a rostellum on its anterior end.

Arthropodology: The study of arthropods.

Arthropods: The creatures possessing a chitinous exoskeleton and jointed legs.

Ascariasis: Infection with ascarids, either larval or adult.

Ascaroid: One of four egg types produced by nematodes (see Figure 3-9 for characteristic look).

Aseptically: Referring to the use of sterile technique.

Axostyle: A filamentous or hyaline rodlike structure passing through the center of some flagellate protozoans that has a skeletal function.

B

Baermann technique: Type of diagnostic technique in which nematode larvae are collected using gravity (sedimentation).

Benzimidazoles: A family of anthelmintics that include fenbendazole, oxfendazole, and albendazole.

Body cavity: Hollow area of the body that contains the major organs of an organism.

Borreliosis: Lyme disease.

Bothria: Two slitlike holdfast organs on the anterior end of a pseudotapeworm.

Bradyzoites: Slowly multiplying stages of toxoplasmosis within the muscle of an intermediate host.

Buccal cavity: Large opening that connects to the mouth of a nematode; connects the mouth to the esophagus.

Bursal rays: Fingerlike projections that make up the copulatory bursa of a male nematode.

C

Calcareous corpuscles: Microscopic calcium deposits unique to the tissues of cestodes (tapeworms); also called *calcareous bodies*.

Cantharidin: Toxic or blistering compound found in a certain group of beetles; often referred to as *Spanish fly* but has no aphrodisiac effect.

Capitulum: Mouthparts of an acarine (mite or tick).

Catarrhal: Characterized by inflammation of the mucous membranes.

Cercaria: Asexual stage within the life cycle of a digenetic trematode. The cercarial stage emerges from the snail, the first intermediate host. Each cercarial stage produces one metacercarial stage, found in the second intermediate host or on vegetation. Sometimes the cercaria can penetrate the definitive host directly.

Cervical alae: Lateral expansion of the cuticle in the anterior end of nematodes.

Cestodes: Tapeworms.

Chelicerae: Two cutting or lacerating organs of the capitulum.

Chelicerata: Subphylum of the arthropods that includes the mites, ticks, spiders, and scorpions that possess chelicerae mouthparts.

Chelicerates: Arthopods with holdfast and lacerating mouth parts designed for sucking fluid, either blood or lymph.

Ciliophorans: Members of the kingdom Protista, phylum Ciliophora. These are the ciliates.

Chitin: Hard but elastic body covering that envelops the entire body of an arthropod.

Cilia: Tiny hairs that cover the body surface of one type of protozoan, the ciliates, which move by beating these hairs.

Ciliates: Protozoans that possess cilia.

Cloaca: Opening of the intestine of the male nematode to the outside.

Coelom: The true body cavity.

Coenurus: Type of metacestode (larval tapeworm) stage characterized by a large, fluid-filled bladder with a number of invaginated (inside-out) scolices attached to the wall of the bladder.

Coleopterans: Members of the phylum Arthropoda, subphylum Mandibulata, class Insecta, order Coleoptera. These are the beetles.

Commensalism: Type of symbiotic relationship in which one symbiont benefits while the other neither benefits nor is harmed.

Common name: Non-scientific name for a living organism in different regions of the world; may refer to different organisms in different places.

Complex metamorphosis: One of two types of metamorphosis by insects; the four developmental stages are egg, larva (maggot), pupa, and adult. Each stage is morphologically and structurally different from the other stages.

Congenital toxoplasmosis: Infection of *Toxoplasma gondii* acquired by the fetus during pregnancy.

Copepod: An aquatic crustacean.

Copulatory bursa: Flattened, lateral expansion of a nematode's cuticle in the posterior region of certain male nematodes; serves to hold on to or grasp the female nematode during the mating process; composed of fingerlike projections called *bursal rays*.

Coracidium: Ciliated hexacanth embryo unique to the pseudotapeworms (cotylodans); when ingested by the first intermediate host (an aquatic crustacean), forms a procercoid within the intermediate host.

Cotylodan: Pseudotapeworm, or false tapeworm.

Crustaceans: Members of the subphylum Mandibulatat, class Crustacea. The members include the aquatic arthropods: crabs, lobsters, crayfish, and copepods.

Cutaneous larva migrans: Migration of larval stages of a nematode through the skin of humans, most often seen with *Ancylostoma braziliense*.

Cyst stage: Nonmotile, resistant stage of a protozoan parasite.

Cystacanth: Juvenile acanthocephalan that possesses an inverted proboscis.

Cysticercoid: Type of metacestode (larval tapeworm) stage characterized by a small, fluid-filled bladder containing a single, noninvaginated scolex; usually microscopic.

Cysticercus: Type of metacestode (larval tapeworm) stage characterized by a large, fluid-filled bladder containing a single invaginated (inside-out) scolex.

D

Definitive host: Host that harbors the adult, sexual, or mature stage of the parasite.

Demodicosis: Infection with the demodectic (*Demodex*) species of mites.

Dermatitis: Inflammation of the skin.

Dictyopterans: Members of the class Insecta, order Dictyoptera (also known as Orthoptera). These include the cockroaches and the grasshoppers.

Digenetic fluke: Within the life cycle of a trematode, there are two intermediate hosts—a first (usually a snail) and a second intermediate host. There will be a few exceptions where the digenetic fluke only has one intermediate host such as the schistosomes.

Dioecious: Having separate sexes, both male and female; the nematodes and the arthropods are dioecious.

Diptera: Two-winged flies.

Dipterans: Referring to two-winged flies.

***Dipylidium* egg:** Tapeworm egg type containing a packet of multiple hexacanths within one egg.

Direct life cycle: Life cycle that does not involve an intermediate host.

E

Ectoparasite: Parasite that lives *on* the body of the host.

Ectoparasitism: Parasitism by an external parasite; an ectoparasite produces an *infestation* on the host.

ELISA test: Enzyme-linked immunosorbent assay, an immunodiagnostic technique that detects the presence of antigen.

Embryophore: Tapeworm hexacanth embryo with striated eggshell.

Empodia: Clawlike features on the end of the second pair of legs of *Myobia musculi* and *Radfordia affinis*.

Encysted: Encapsulated in suspended animation.

Endoparasite: Parasite that lives *within* the body of the host; an endoparasite produces an *infection* within that host.

Endoparasitism: Parasitism by an internal parasite; an endoparasite produces an infection within the host.

Endosome: A tiny pinpoint center within the nucleus of the amoeba.

Entomologist: One who specializes in the study of insects.

Erratic parasite: See Aberrant parasite.

Eucestode: True tapeworm.

Euryxenous parasite: Parasite with a very broad host range.

Excoriation: Self-induced skin trauma.

F

Face fly: A periodic parasite (genus *Musca*, species *autumnalis*) that feeds on mucus, tears and saliva.

Facultative myiasis: Condition resulting from fly larvae, normally free living, that become parasitic and use a host for their development.

Facultative parasite: Organism that is usually free living (nonparasitic) in nature and develops a parasitic existence in certain hosts.

Feathered edge: Thinnest part of a blood smear at the edges.

Festoons: Indentations or folds along the margin of an external body part.

Fistula: Pore or hole within tissue.

Flagellum: Long whiplike or lashlike appendage that is used by a group of protozoans (the flagellates) as a means of moving about in a fluid medium.

Flea dirt: Partially digested blood defecated by fleas; also called *flea feces* and *flea frass*.

Flotation solutions: Liquids used to float parasite ova, cysts, and larvae for identification.

Fly strike: Lesion(s) produced in the tissues of vertebrate hosts by maggots or fly larvae.

Free living: Life cycle stage that does not require a host to survive.

G

Gadding: Action of a vertebrate host marked by running away from irritating flies.

Gastritis: Inflammation of the stomach.

Genus name: The group a particular type of animal, parasite, or plant belongs to.

Gravid proglottids: Oldest segments of a tapeworm or pseudotapeworm farthest from the scolex or bothria that contain spent or degenerated reproductive organs and viable eggs.

H

Hard ticks: Members of the Ixodid type of ticks.

Helminths: Parasitic worms.

Hemipterans: Members of the class Insecta, order Hemiptera. These are the true bugs.

Hemocoel: A body cavity filled with a bloodlike fluid.

Hemolymph: Bloodlike fluid that bathes the internal organs of arthropods.

Hermaphroditic: Having complete sets of both male and female reproductive organs; the tapeworms and the flukes (except for the schistosomes) are hermaphroditic.

Hexacanth embryos: Type of tapeworm egg containing a six-toothed embryo (an embryo that contains six hooklets).

Hippoboscid flies: Winged dipterans that parasitize wild birds.

Hirsute: Very hairy.

Hirudin: Anticoagulant produced in the oral cavity of leeches.

Hirudineans: Members of the phylum Annelida, class Hirudinea. These are the leeches.

Hirudiniasis: Infestation with leeches.

Holdfast organelle: Scolex or head of the pseudotapeworm.

Homoxenous parasite: Parasite that infects only one type of host; also called *monoxenous parasite*.

Host: In a parasitic relationship, the member in which or on which the parasite lives.

Hydatid cyst: Large, fluid-filled bladder that contains brood capsules, which bud from the internal germinal membrane; each brood capsule contains several protoscolices.

Hydrometer: Tool for measuring the specific gravity of solutions.

Hymenopterans: Members of the class Insecta, order Hymenoptera. These are the stinging bees, wasps, and ants.

Hypodermis: Thin layer beneath the cuticle that secretes the cuticle layer of the nematode.

Hypostome: Penetrating, anchorlike sucking organ of the tick.

I

Idiosoma: Abdomen of a mite or a tick.

Immature proglottids: Youngest segments closest to the scolex or bothria of the tapeworm or pseudotapeworm that contain sexually immature reproductive organs.

Incidental parasite: Parasite that is found in a host in which it does not usually live.

Indirect life cycle: Life cycle of a parasite that requires an intermediate host.

Infection: A condition caused by an endoparasite within the host's body.

Infective third-stage larva: Stage in the life cycle that is able to infect the definitive host.

Infestation: A condition caused by an ectoparasite outside or on the host's body.

Inornate: Species of ticks with a reddish or mahogany color.

Insecticides: Chemical compounds developed to kill insects.

Insects: Members of the phylum Arthropoda, subphylum Mandibulata, class Insecta.

Intermediate host: Host that harbors the larval, juvenile, immature, or asexual stages of the parasite. A parasite may have more than one intermediate host.

Invaginated scolices: Tapeworm heads turned inside out within the bladder worm life stage.

Ixodid: Tick family with hard bodies.

L

Lappets: Round protuberances behind the suckers of the scolex in *Anoplocephala perfoliata*.

Larval pentastome: The stage that hatches from a pentastome egg. It is mitelike with 4-6 legs, each of which ends in pincerlike claws.

Larviparous: Type of female nematode that retains her eggs within the uterus and produces live first-stage larvae.

Leaf crown: The collection of papillae of nematodes.

Leeches: Bloodsucking annelids.

Lepidopterans: Members of class Insecta, order Lepidotera. These are the moths and butterflies.

Life cycle: Development of a parasite through its various life stages. Every parasite has its own distinct, individual life cycle with at least one *definitive host* and may have one or more *intermediate hosts.*

Linguatuliasis: See Pentastomiasis.

Linguatulosis: See Pentastomiasis.

Linnaean classification scheme: Classification for all living organisms (animals, plants, fungi, protozoa, and algae) perfected by Carl Linnaeus, an early Swedish biologist. Every living organism can be classified using the following scheme: kingdom, phylum, class, order, family, genus, and species.

M

Maggots: Fly larvae.

Mandibulata: Subphylum of arthropods that possesses mandibulate mouthparts.

Mature proglottids: The segments in the middle of the tapeworm or pseudotapeworm body that contain sexually mature reproductive organs.

Measly meat: Meat that is infected with the cysticerci (larval stages) of certain human and canine tapeworms; includes measly beef (*Cysticercus bovis*), measly pork (*Cysticercus cellulosae*), and measly mutton (*Cysticercus ovis*).

Megaloblastic anemia: Anemia caused by the loss of vitamin B_{12}.

Metacercaria: Asexual stage within the life cycle of a digenetic trematode. The cercarial stage emerges from the snail (first intermediate host) and produces one metacercarial stage. If the cercaria is ingested by the second intermediate host, it will encyst within its tissues. The metacercarial stage may be found encysted on vegetation.

Metacestode: Larval tapeworm found within the intermediate host; types of metacestodes include cysticercoid, cysticercus, coenurus, hydatid, tetrathyridium, procercoid, plerocercoid, and sparganum.

Metamorphosis: To achieve the adult stage, an insect must undergo a series of developmental changes in size, form, or structure called *metamorphosis;* two types are simple metamorphosis and complex metamorphosis.

Metazoan parasites: Multicellular or complex organisms that include trematodes, tapeworms, pseudotapeworms, roundworms, thorny-headed worms, leeches, and arthropods.

Microfilaria: Immature stage of filarial parasites.

Microfilaricide: Dewormer that kills the immature filarial worm.

Micropyle: A small pore at one end of some protozoan oocysts.

Miracidium: Developmental stage in the life cycle of a digenetic trematode. This stage emerges from the operculated egg and penetrates the first intermediate host, usually a snail.

Molt: Shedding of the outside cuticle.

Monoecious: Hermaphroditic; having both sexes in a single organism.

Monogenetic fluke: A rare type of trematode often parasitizing fish, amphibians, or reptiles. Monogenetic flukes do not occur in domesticated animals. They are not of veterinary significance.

Monoxenous parasite: A parasite that infects only one type of host.

Morula: Type of nematode egg that contains an undeveloped grapelike cluster of cells within the eggshell.

Mucocutaneous: Pertaining to the mucous membrane and the skin.

Mutualism: Type of symbiotic relationship in which both organisms derive some benefit.

Myiasis: Infection or infestation of the tissues or organs of humans or domesticated or wild animals by larval members (maggots) of the order Diptera (two-winged flies).

Myositis: Inflammation of the muscle tissue.

Myriopodans: Members of the phylum Arthropoda, subphylum Mandibulata, class Myriopoda. These are the centipedes and millipedes.

N

Neck: Germinal or growth region of a tapeworm that lies just posterior to the scolex.

Necropsy: Postmortem examination or autopsy of an animal.

Nematodes: Roundworms.

Neotenic: A type of parasite in which the small male lives inside the vagina of the immature female or the uterus of the mature female parasite.

Neurocysticercosis: Infection with the pork tapeworm that develops in the brain of a human.

Nit: Egg of a sucking or chewing louse.

Nymphal Pentastome: The worm-like developmental stage found within the tissues of the intermediate host. It is the stage that is infective for the definitive host.

O

Obligatory myiasis: Lesions caused by fly larvae that require a vertebrate host for their development.

Obligatory parasite: Parasite that must lead a parasitic existence; most parasites of domestic animals are obligatory parasites.

Occult blood: Blood present in small amounts so as not to be visible to the unaided eye.

Occult infection: Parasitic filarial infection without the presence of microfilariae.

Ocular micrometer: The eyepiece scale on a microscope.

Oncosphere: Growth ball released by the ingested egg of *Echinococcus* species.

Operculum: Tiny "door" at either end (pole) of an egg.

Oral sucker: The organ of feeding/attachment on the anterior end of a mature digenetic fluke. The oral sucker connects to a muscular pharynx and the pharynx connects to the blind caeca of the adult fluke.

Ornate: Species of ticks with distinctive white patterns on the dark reddish or mahogany background of the scutum.

Oviduct: Female nematode reproductive organ that connects the tubular ovaries to the uterus.

Oviparous: Type of nematode egg that contains either a single cell or a morula, a grapelike cluster of cells.

Ovoviviparous: Type of nematode egg that contains a first-stage larva.

P

Palpi: Mouthparts.

Palps: Appendages found near the mouth in invertebrate organisms that are used for sensation, locomotion, and/or feeding.

Papillae: Fingerlike or bumplike projections on the cuticle of a nematode.

Papules: Red bumps.

Parasite: In a parasitic relationship, the member that lives on or within the host.

Parasitiasis: Type of parasitic relationship in which the parasite is present on or within the host and is potentially pathogenic (harmful); however, the animal does not exhibit outward clinical signs of disease.

Parasiticides: Chemical compounds (either very simple or very complex) used to treat specific internal and external parasites (endoparasites and ectoparasites); different types include anthelmintics, acaricides, insecticides, and antiprotozoals.

Parasitism: Type of symbiotic relationship between two organisms of different species in which one member (the *parasite*) lives on or within the other member (the *host*) and may cause harm; the parasite is metabolically dependent on the host for its survival.

Parasitology: The study of parasitic relationships.

Parasitosis: Type of parasitic relationship in which the parasite is present on or within the host and causes obvious injury or harm to the host animal; the host exhibits obvious outward signs of clinical parasitism.

Paratenic host: A host used for transport of a parasite. The parasite does not go through any developmental stages.

Parthenogenesis: Modified form of sexual reproduction characterized by the development of offspring by a female nematode from eggs that have not been fertilized by a male nematode; genus best known for parthenogenesis is *Strongyloides*.

Pathogenicity: Disease-causing potential.

Pedicels: Stalks at the tip of sarcoptiform mite legs.

Pediculosis: Infestation by either chewing or sucking lice.

Pedipalps: Two leglike accessory appendages attached to the capitulum that act as sensory support.

Pelage: Hair coat.

Pentastome: Tongue worms, or linguatulids. These annelid-like arthropods have a mitelike larval stage; nymphal stages are found in the visceral organs of many mammalian intermediate hosts; adults usually parasitize snakes and other reptiles. The one pentastome found in domestic animals is *Linguatula serrata*.

Pentastomiasis: Infection with pentastomes.

Percutaneous: Through the skin.

Periodic parasite: Parasite that makes frequent short visits to its host to obtain nourishment or other benefits.

Pernicious anemia: See Megaloblastic anemia.

Phoresis: Type of symbiotic relationship in which the smaller member in the relationship is mechanically carried by the larger member.

Pilose antennae: Antennae covered with fine hairs.

Piroplasmosis: Disease caused by *Babesia canis*.

Pleomorphic: Demonstrating a variety of morphologic forms or body forms.

Plerocercoid: Type of metacestode stage unique to the pseudotapeworms (cotylodans); this solid-bodied metacestode stage with slitlike mouthparts is found within the second intermediate host, usually a fish or an amphibian; also called a *sparganum*.

Predator-prey relationship: Extremely short-term symbiotic relationship in which one symbiont benefits at the expense of the other; for example, a lion (the *predator*) kills a zebra (the *prey*). The prey ultimately pays with its life and serves as a food source for the predator.

Prepatent period: Time from the point of infection by a nematode until a specific diagnostic stage can be recovered.

Preputial washes: Flushes of the prepuce of the male bull for analysis for genital tract parasites.

Probenzimidazoles: Family of anthelmintics that includes thiophanate, febantel, and netobimin.

Proboscis: Retractable "nose" on the anterior end of an acanthocephalan that is covered with tiny, backward-facing spines and serves to anchor the acanthocephalan to the mucosa of the intestine.

Procercoid: Type of metacestode stage unique to the pseudotapeworms (cotylodans). This metacestode stage is found within the first intermediate host, usually a tiny aquatic crustacean.

Proglottid: Individual boxlike components of the tapeworm strobila; three types are immature, mature, and gravid proglottids.

Protoscolices: Multiple tapeworm heads in a hydatid cyst that develop into adult tapeworms when ingested by a definitive host.

Protozoan parasites: Unicellular, or single-celled, organisms that may be flagellates, amoebae, sporozoans, apicomplexans, or ciliates.

Pruritus: Itch or itchiness.

Pseudocoelom: Cavity between the middle layer and inner layer of the three body tissue layers of the nematode.

Pseudocoelomic membrane: The tissue that surrounds and lines the pseudocoelom.

Pseudoparasites: Living creatures or inanimate objects that are not parasitic but may be mistaken for, or erroneously identified as, parasites.

Pseudophyllidean egg: Tapeworm egg type with an operculum at one end and an oval shape.

Pseudopodia: False feet.

Pseudosucker: A false sucker surrounding the mouth of a leech.

Psocids: Primitive insects associated with vegetation.

Psoroptidae: Family of sarcoptiform mites that resides on the surface of the skin or within the external ear canal.

Pyriform apparatus: The innermost lining (third lining) of the covering of certain types of tapeworm eggs; pear-shaped.

Q

Qualitative testing: Indicates the presence or absence of parasite ova, cysts, or larvae.

Quantitative testing: Indicates the number of eggs or cysts present in one gram of feces.

R

Rectum: Opening of the intestine of the female nematode to the outside.

Redia: Asexual stage in the life cycle of a digenetic trematode. This stage is preceded by the sporocyst stage, which produces many rediae; each redia will form many cercariae.

Reportable parasites: Parasites that must be reported to both state and federal authorities (e.g., *Cochliomyia hominivorax, Psoroptes* species in large animals, *Boophilus annulatus*).

Repugnatorial glands: Areas beneath the legs of millipedes that produce caustic substances.

Reservoir host: Vertebrate host in which a parasite or disease occurs in nature and is a source of infection for humans or other domesticated animals.

Rhabditiform esophagus: Type of nematode esophagus that has a corpus, isthmus, and posterior bulb.

Rostellum: Holdfast organ on the anterior end of an armed true tapeworm; has backward-facing hooks used to anchor the tapeworm to the wall of the host's gut.

S

Sarcomastigophorans: Members of the kingdom Protista, phylum Sarcomastigophora. These are the flagellates and amoebae.

Sarcoptic acariasis: Infection caused by *Sarcoptes* mites.

Sarcoptidae: Family of sarcoptiform mites that burrow or tunnel within the epidermis.

Sarcoptiform mites: A classification of mites that can cause severe dermatologic problems in the host.

Scabies: See Sarcoptic acariasis.

Schistosome cercarial dermatitis: Swimmer's itch; highly pruritic papular or pustular dermatitis in humans caused by the cercarial stages of bird schistosomes.

Scientific name: Name for a living organism that is composed of two Latin words, usually written in italics. The *genus name* (capitalized; e.g., *Felis*) indicates the group to which a particular type of animal or plant belongs; the *specific epithet* (lowercase; e.g., *catus*) indicates the type of animal itself.

Scolex: The "head" of a tapeworm.

Scutum: Hard, chitinous plate that covers the body of some ticks.

Seed ticks: Six-legged larval stage of the tick life cycle.

Seminal receptacle: A female nematode's reproductive organ used to store sperm.

Setae: Tiny hairlike bristles found on *Musca domestica* and other arthropods.

Simple metamorphosis: One of two types of metamorphosis by insects; three developmental stages are egg, nymph, and adult. The nymphal and adult stages are similar in morphology and structure; the nymphal stage is smaller than the adult and is not sexually mature.

Siphon: A structure used by larvae to breathe oxygen from the air.

Siphonapterosis: Infestation with fleas.

Skin scraping: A procedure used to find mites on the surface or just under the skin.

Somatic muscular layer: The layer of muscle below the hypodermis that is used by nematodes to move.

Sparganosis: Infection with the plerocercoid stage within the tissues of the second intermediate host.

Sparganum: See Plerocercoid.

Specific epithet: The type of animal in a genus.

Specific gravity: The weight of an object compared with the weight of an equal volume of pure water.

Spicule pouch: Pocket that contains the male reproductive organs used to open the female nematode's vulva.

Spicules: Male nematode's intromittent organs ("penis") associated with the copulatory bursa.

Spiracular plate: Opening on the posterior end of some arthropod larvae used for breathing.

Spiruroid: One of four egg types produced by nematodes (see Figure 3-11 for characteristic look).

Sporocyst: Asexual stage in the life cycle of a digenetic trematode. This miracidium penetrates the snail (first intermediate host) and forms the sporocyst stage.

Stenoxenous parasite: Parasite with a narrow host range.

Stepping: Inchwormlike manner of movement used by leeches when moving on land.

Strike: See Fly strike.

Strobila: Body of the tapeworm composed of individual proglottids (immature, mature, and gravid).

Strobilocercus: Type of metacestode stage found in the liver of rats; has a scolex that attaches to a long neck, which connects to a fluid-filled bladder.

Stylostome: Tube that forms in the host at the attachment site of chiggers.

Symbiont: Each living organism in a symbiotic association.

Symbiosis: Any association (temporary or permanent) between at least two living organisms of different species.

Synathropic: Living with humans.

T

***Taenia* egg:** Tapeworm egg type with a wide outer shell and thicker outer covering and with a single six-hooked hexacanth within.

Tachyzoites: Rapidly multiplying stages of toxoplasmosis in sporulated oocysts.

Tegument: Body wall of a helminth.

Tetrathyridium: Solid-bodied metacestode stage with a deeply invaginated acetabular scolex. This stage is capable of asexual reproduction and divides by splitting into two stages; two then become four, four become eight, and so on.

Tick paralysis: Paralysis seen in animals and humans caused by the toxic saliva in some ticks.

Transport host: Special type of intermediate host in which the parasite does not undergo any development but instead remains arrested or encysted ("in suspended animation") within the host's tissues; also called *paratenic host*.

Trematodes: The flukes.

Trichinelloid: One of four egg types produced by nematodes (see Figure 3-12 for the characteristic look).

Trichoroid: See Trichinelloid.

Trichostrongyle type: One of four egg types produced by nematodes (see Figure 3-10 for the characteristic look).

Trophozoite stage: Motile or moving form of a protozoan.

Trypomastigote: Swimming life stage of trypanosomes.

Tubular ovaries: Female nematode's reproductive organs.

Tubular testes: Male nematode's reproductive organs.

U

Unarmed tapeworm: True tapeworm that lacks a rostellum on its anterior end.

Urticating: The act of stinging.

V

Vas deferens: Male nematode's reproductive organ connecting the tubular testes to the cloaca.

Venation: Possessing veins in a part of the body.

Vermicide: Dewormer that kills the parasite so that it can be broken down by the host's body.

Vermifuge: Dewormer that paralyzes (but does not kill) the adult parasite so it passes in the feces.

Vesicles: Tiny blisters.

Veterinary parasitology: The study of parasitic relationships affecting domesticated, wild, exotic, and laboratory animals.

Visceral larva migrans: Migration of the larval stages of a nematode through the organs or tissues of humans (e.g., lungs, liver, eye); most often seen with *Toxocara canis*.

Vitellaria: Accessory genital gland that secretes the yolk and shell for the fertilized ovum.

W

Warbles: Larvae of dipteran flies found in the skin of domestic or wild animals, producing cutaneous myiasis.

Wolves: See Warbles.

Z

Zoonosis: Any disease or parasite that is transmissible from animals to humans.

Index

Page numbers followed by "*f*" indicate figures, "*t*" indicate tables, and "*b*" indicate boxes.